Small Animal Theriogenology

Editor

BRUCE W. CHRISTENSEN

VETERINARY CLINICS OF NORTH AMERICA: SMALL ANIMAL PRACTICE

www.vetsmall.theclinics.com

July 2018 • Volume 48 • Number 4

ELSEVIER

1600 John F. Kennedy Boulevard • Suite 1800 • Philadelphia, Pennsylvania, 19103-2899
http://www.vetsmall.theclinics.com

**VETERINARY CLINICS OF NORTH AMERICA: SMALL ANIMAL PRACTICE Volume 48, Number 4
July 2018 ISSN 0195-5616, ISBN-13: 978-0-323-61084-1**

Editor: Colleen Dietzler
Developmental Editor: Meredith Madeira

Veterinary Clinics of North America: Small Animal Practice (ISSN 0195-5616) is published bimonthly by Elsevier Inc., 360 Park Avenue South, New York, NY 10010-1710. Months of issue are January, March, May, July, September, and November. Business and Editorial Offices: 1600 John F. Kennedy Blvd., Ste. 1800, Philadelphia, PA 19103-2899. Customer Service Office: 3251 Riverport Lane, Maryland Heights, MO 63043. Periodicals postage paid at New York, NY and additional mailing offices. Subscription prices are $325.00 per year (domestic individuals), $622.00 per year (domestic institutions), $100.00 per year (domestic students/residents), $430.00 per year (Canadian individuals), $773.00 per year (Canadian institutions), $469.00 per year (international individuals), $773.00 per year (international institutions), and $220.00 per year (international and Canadian students/residents). To receive student/resident rate, orders must be accompanied by name of affiliated institution, date of term, and the *signature* of program/residency coordinator on institution letterhead. Orders will be billed at individual rate until proof of status is received. Foreign air speed delivery is included in all *Clinics* subscription prices. All prices are subject to change without notice. **POSTMASTER:** Send address changes to *Veterinary Clinics of North America: Small Animal Practice*, Elsevier Health Sciences Division, Subscription Customer Service, 3251 Riverport Lane, Maryland Heights, MO 63043. Customer Service (orders, claims, online, change of address): Elsevier Periodicals Customer Service, Elsevier Health Sciences Division. Subscription **Customer Service 3251 Riverport Lane Maryland Heights, MO 63043. Tel: 1-800-654-2452 (U.S. and Canada); 314-447-8871 (outside U.S. and Canada). Fax: 314-447-8029. E-mail: journalscustomerservice usa@elsevier.com (for print support); journalsonlinesupport-usa@elsevier.com (for online support).**

Reprints. For copies of 100 or more of articles in this publication, please contact the Commercial Reprints Department, Elsevier Inc., 360 Park Avenue South, New York, NY 10010-1710. Tel.: 212-633-3874; Fax: 212-633-3820; E-mail: reprints@elsevier.com.

Veterinary Clinics of North America: Small Animal Practice is also published in Japanese by Inter Zoo Publishing Co., Ltd., Aoyama Crystal-Bldg 5F, 3-5-12 Kitaaoyama, Minato-ku, Tokyo 107-0061, Japan.

Veterinary Clinics of North America: Small Animal Practice is covered in *Current Contents/Agriculture, Biology and Environmental Sciences, Science Citation Index, ASCA, MEDLINE/PubMed (Index Medicus), Excerpta Medica, and BIOSIS.*

Contributors

EDITOR

BRUCE W. CHRISTENSEN, DVM, MS
Diplomate, American College of Theriogenologists; Veterinarian and Owner, Kokopelli
Assisted Reproductive Services, Franklin Ranch Pet Hospital, Elk Grove, California,
USA

AUTHORS

CHERYL S. ASA, BS, MA, PhD
Advisory Board Chair, AZA Reproductive Management Center, Affiliate Scientist, Saint
Louis Zoo, St Louis, Missouri, USA

JANE BARBER, DVM, MS
Diplomate, American College of Theriogenologists; Veterinary Specialties at the lake,
Sherrills Ford, North Carolina, USA

CARLA BARSTOW, DVM
Theriogenology Resident, Department of Clinical Sciences, Auburn University, Auburn,
Alabama, USA

BRUCE W. CHRISTENSEN, DVM, MS
Diplomate, American College of Theriogenologists; Veterinarian and Owner, Kokopelli
Assisted Reproductive Services, Franklin Ranch Pet Hospital, Elk Grove, California,
USA

NATALIE S. FRASER, DVM, MS
Diplomate, American College of Theriogenologists; Senior Lecturer, Theriogenology,
School of Veterinary Science, The University of Queensland, Gatton, Queensland,
Australia

KRISTINE GONZALES, DVM
Diplomate, American College of Theriogenologists; Staff Veterinarian, Veterinary Services,
Guide Dogs for the Blind, San Rafael, California, USA

RAGNVI HAGMAN, DVM, PhD
Associate Professor in Small Animal Surgery, Department of Clinical Sciences, Swedish
University of Agricultural Sciences, Uppsala, Sweden

AIME K. JOHNSON, DVM
Diplomate, American College of Theriogenology; Associate Professor, Department of
Clinical Sciences, Auburn University, Auburn, Alabama, USA

KARA A. KOLSTER, DVM
Diplomate, American College of Theriogenologists; Springfield Veterinary Center,
Glen Allen, Virginia, USA

MICHELLE ANNE KUTZLER, DVM, PhD
Diplomate, American College of Theriogenologists; Associate Professor, Department of Animal and Rangeland Sciences, Oregon State University, Corvallis, Oregon, USA

CHERYL LOPATE, MS, DVM
Diplomate, American College of Theriogenologists; Veterinarian and Owner, Reproductive Revolutions and Wilsonville Veterinary Clinic, Wilsonville, Oregon, USA

STUART J. MASON, BVSc (Hons), MANZCVS
Diplomate, American College of Theriogenologists; Monash Veterinary Clinic, Oakleigh East, Victoria, Australia

MARGARET V. ROOT KUSTRITZ, DVM, PhD, MMedEd
Diplomate, American College of Theriogenologists; Professor and Assistant Dean of Education, Department of Veterinary Clinical Sciences, University of Minnesota College of Veterinary Medicine, St Paul, Minnesota, USA

WILL SCHULTZ, DVM
Schultz Veterinary Clinic, Okemos, Michigan, USA

KATHERINE SETTLE, DVM
Sanford Animal Hospital, Sanford, North Carolina, USA

ROBYN R. WILBORN, DVM, MS
Diplomate, American College of Theriogenologists; Associate Professor, Theriogenology, Department of Clinical Sciences, Bailey Small Animal Teaching Hospital, Auburn University, Auburn, Alabama, USA

Contents

> Broadening your scope of practice to include theriogenology services of-
> fers a myriad of advantages. Theriogenology services are profitable, offer
> new revenue streams, and optimize the use of support staff and hospital.
> Offering reproductive services sets your practice apart from competitor
> practices. Breeder clients are demanding but loyal and return for repeat
> services; they also request and follow recommendations for "high-end"
> services. Your theriogenology clients often refer locally placed puppies
> and kittens to you for primary care, and you gain new general practice cli-
> ents. And it is fun!

> The demand for feline semen collection, evaluation, and subsequent use is
> growing as a way to preserve important genetic materials. This article de-
> scribes semen collection methods using a variety of techniques that can
> be applicable in almost any setting. Also discussed are cryopreservation
> methods that optimize sperm survival.

> Assisted reproduction in the queen can range from simple ovulation induc-
> tion to more advanced techniques such as in vitro fertilization. This article
> describes techniques available and the success associated with each.

> Semen evaluation of the male dog is a critical step in any canine infertility
> workup. Assessment of total sperm count, sperm viability, and sperm
> morphology are the mainstay of breeding soundness evaluation. Adjunct
> tests, such as ultrasonography and serum hormone levels, can aid in diag-
> nosis. Pharmacologic treatments, dietary supplements, and management
> practices may help improve breeding success in subfertile dogs. This
> article discusses a clinically practical approach to assessing sperm abnor-
> malities and fertility in male dogs.

> A breeding soundness examination is a vital part of any breeding program. These examinations are not performed as frequently in the bitch as they are in the male dog. They allow clinicians to identify any problems at an early stage in a bitch's breeding career and to screen for any genetic abnormalities. A thorough physical examination and accurate history guide the choice of which diagnostics tests are most useful. Ultrasound scan, culture, cytology, and biopsies (surgical and nonsurgical techniques) are discussed. Knowing which stage of the cycle to perform these diagnostics yields the most information and increases the chance of a successful outcome.

> Artificial insemination is the collection of semen from the male and the subsequent insertion of the collected semen into the female. Artificial insemination may be requested for several reasons, including inability to achieve a mating or owing to the use of fresh chilled or frozen semen. A good understanding of the cycle of the bitch is imperative for maximizing pregnancy rates, as poor timing of insemination is the most common cause of subfertility in the bitch. Insemination techniques commonly undertaken in the bitch include vaginal insemination, surgical intrauterine insemination, and transcervical insemination.

> Since 1939, scientists have studied estrous cycle manipulation in dogs resulting in more articles published in this field than any other area of canine reproduction. Estrous cycle manipulation in dogs must be safe and reliable. Dopamine agonists, gonadotropin-releasing hormone agonists, and gonadotropins are hormones that have been used for estrus induction in bitches, but each treatment has advantages and disadvantages. Despite widespread availability of these medications throughout the rest of the world, there are no drugs currently labeled for canine estrus induction in the United States.

> Since 1952, scientists have studied estrus suppression in dogs. Estrus suppression in dogs must be safe and reliable. Medications used for estrus suppression in bitches include gonadotropin-releasing hormone (GnRH) agonists, GnRH antagonists, progestogens, and androgens. Despite widespread availability of these medications throughout the rest of the world, there are no drugs currently labeled for canine estrus induction in the United States.

Natalie S. Fraser

Mismating, or termination of pregnancy, is a commonly requested reproductive procedure for bitches and queens. Surgical treatment via ovariohysterectomy is the preferred choice when bitches or queens are not
desired for future breeding purposes. Animals that are reproductively valuable can be treated with a variety of drugs to terminate the pregnancy. The
choice of specific medical therapy is based on safety, efficacy, availability
of the drug, and gestational age of the pregnancy. Currently, there is no US
Food and Drug Administration–approved treatment of mismating in North
America for dogs or cats.

Cheryl Lopate

This article provides a complete understanding of how radiography and ultrasound imaging can be used to determine gestational age when inadequate breeding data are available. Formulas for calculation of gestational
age using both fetal and extrafetal structures are presented. Ultrasonographic descriptions of organ development and their use in determining
gestational age are discussed. This information may be used to monitor
the health and development of the fetuses and may be useful when the
need to plan an elective or emergency Cesarean section occurs. Ultrasound imaging to assess fetal stress, viability, placental health and to
sex fetuses is also described.

Ragnvi Hagman

 Video content accompanies this article at http://www.vetsmall.
theclinics.com.

Pyometra is a common disease in dogs and cats. Hormones and opportunistic bacteria are fundamental in the development, with progesterone
playing a key role. The disease should be suspected in intact bitches
and queens presenting with illness, and particularly if within 4 months after
estrus. Early diagnosis and treatment are vital to increase chances of survival as endotoxemia and sepsis often are induced. Typical clinical signs
include vaginal discharge, depression, anorexia, polyuria and polydipsia,
fever and gastrointestinal disturbances. Surgical ovariohysterectomy is
the safest and most effective treatment. For breeding animals with less
severe illness, purely medical treatments alternatives are possible.

Kristine Gonzales

This article provides an overview of some of the most common diseases
affecting the dam in the periparturient period, including disorders of lactation, inappropriate maternal behavior, mastitis, metritis, and eclampsia.
The dam experiences hormonal, physiologic, and physical changes during
pregnancy, parturition, and lactation. Obtaining a detailed history and

performing a thorough physical examination are essential for accurately diagnosing and treating the dam during this unique time. A particular challenge exists when identifying problems in the periparturient period, because all medications and aspects of management affect the health of both the dam and her offspring.

Robyn R. Wilborn

Although most veterinarians have been caring for neonates successfully for several years, it is often good to review our methods and aim to incorporate new practices that will increase survivability, especially of the weaker neonates. These tips are easy to incorporate and do not require radical change by the doctors or staff. Armed with some key pearls of neonatal knowledge and basic clinical skills, one can successfully prevent and treat the most common clinical presentations of neonatal puppies and kittens.

Bruce W. Christensen

 Video content accompanies this article at http://www.vetsmall. theclinics.com/.

All intact, male dogs experience benign prostatic hyperplasia and hypertrophy, usually by around 6 years old. Although these dogs are predisposed to prostatic infections, only a small subset actually develop infections or show clinical signs of discomfort or subfertility. Neutered male dogs have a higher incidence of neoplasia associated with the prostate. Updated diagnostic tests, including canine prostate-specific arginine esterase, are discussed. Castration is compared with medical treatment options. Updated treatment recommendations include reducing antibiotic exposure to 4 weeks for bacterial infections and use of nonsteroidal anti-inflammatory drugs for neoplastic disease.

Margaret V. Root Kustritz

Optimal age for ovariohysterectomy or castration has not been defined in the scientific literature. Bitches and queens are significantly less likely to develop mammary neoplasia, which has a high incidence and potentially high morbidity and mortality, if spayed when young. Tom cats exhibit undesirable behaviors that preclude them being good pets and should be castrated young. There is no compelling reason to castrate male dogs when young unless it is needed to control reproductive behaviors or prevent indiscriminate breeding. Alternatives to surgical sterilization that may be available in the future include intratesticular injection and immunization against gonadotropin-releasing hormone.

Cheryl S. Asa

Although surgical sterilization is the most common approach to reproductive management of dogs and cats in North America and many other places, there is growing interest in nonsurgical and reversible methods. This article summarizes the methods currently available for use as reversible contraception in dogs and cats, along with cautions about reported side effects. The products covered include synthetic steroid hormones, peptide hormone agonists, vaccines, and a barrier method.

Small Animal Theriogenology

VETERINARY CLINICS OF NORTH AMERICA: SMALL ANIMAL PRACTICE

RELATED INTEREST

Veterinary Clinics of North America: Exotic Animal Practice
May 2017 (Volume 20, Issue 2)
Reproductive Medicine
Vladimir Jekl, *Editor*

THE CLINICS ARE NOW AVAILABLE ONLINE!
Access your subscription at:
www.theclinics.com

Preface

Helping Miracles Happen

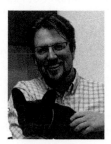

Bruce W. Christensen, DVM, MS
Editor

We are frequently asked what made us choose our career paths. I've always felt a bit sheepish about my answer because it seems so trite. But, though it smells of cliché, the truth is that I became a veterinarian because of an innate love of animals, and I specialized in reproduction and fertility because of a fascination with the miracle of life.

A miracle doesn't have to be inexplicable; a miracle just needs to be wondrous. It is fascinating to study how a sperm and ovum come together, fuse, develop, and eventually form autonomous life. And then there are the myriad mechanisms for delivering sperm to ovum, and the intricate, supportive environment needed for embryonic and fetal development in utero. Understanding the physiology does not lessen the wonder of it all. On the contrary, understanding enhances the miracle. The more you understand about how intricate the processes are that create and support developing life, the more you have to step back and marvel that it all works. And it does work. And has worked. Over and over, year in and year out for millennia in millions of organisms.

Well, it mostly works.

Sometimes something goes awry in those intricate processes and life falters. Sometimes miracles need a little assistance. And at other times we humans want to redirect those otherwise natural processes to cause a desired outcome that fits our husbandry goals. That we can take delicate processes that took millions of years to evolve, mess around with them, and create a desired product is also pretty miraculous. Fixing defective reproductive processes and manipulating normal reproductive pathways are what theriogenologists do. This issue offers some excellent, recent reviews of both fixing and manipulating fertility in small animal veterinary medicine.

I want to thank the authors who contributed so much of their time to produce these articles for the benefit of our profession. It was a pleasure to work with them, and

Vet Clin Small Anim 48 (2018) xi–xii
https://doi.org/10.1016/j.cvsm.2018.04.002
0195-5616/18/© 2018 Published by Elsevier Inc.

vetsmall.theclinics.com

I commend these articles to small animal practitioners striving to serve their dog- and cat-breeding clientele.

Bruce W. Christensen, DVM, MS
Kokopelli Assisted Reproductive Services
C/O Franklin Ranch Pet Hospital
10207 Franklin Boulevard
Elk Grove, CA 95757, USA

E-mail address:
kokopellivet@gmail.com

Been There, Done That

A Practical Primer for Veterinarians Considering Inclusion of Small Animal Theriogenology Services in Their Practice

Jane Barber, DVM, MS[a],*, Katherine Settle, DVM[b], Will Schultz, DVM[c]

KEYWORDS

• Theriogenology • Reproductive services • Dog • Bitch • Insemination

KEY POINTS

- Broadening your scope of practice to include theriogenology services offers a myriad of advantages.
- Theriogenology services are profitable, offer new revenue streams, and optimize use of support staff and hospital.
- Offering reproductive services sets your practice apart from competitor practices.
- Breeder clients are demanding but loyal and return for repeat services; they also request and follow recommendations for "high-end" services.

We sexagenarians (pun intended) with more than 100 years of combined clinical practice in small animal theriogenology pen this introductory article. Our goal is to impart a primer of useful experiential lessons and lagniappe to veterinarians considering the addition of small animal theriogenology services to their practice. Nothing in this article is referenced, nor can be accessed via search engines such as PubMed. However, we hope the reader will find the practical potpourri presented in this article just as useful as the researched and evidenced-based information to follow in accompanying articles.

With one voice, we attest that theriogenology is the most rewarding aspect of our practices. The clinical practice of theriogenology is interesting and evolving, and keeps us on our toes. Long-term relationships are forged between clients, colleagues, mentors, and mentees. Professional collaboration progresses to enduring friendship. We encourage you to join us and embark on your own journey into theriogenology practice. Bon voyage!

The authors have nothing to disclose.
[a] Veterinary Specialties at the lake, 1675 Mollys Backbone Road, Sherrills Ford, NC 28673, USA; [b] Sanford Animal Hospital, 200 West Seawell Street, Sanford, NC 27332, USA; [c] Schultz Veterinary Clinic, 2770 Bennett Road, Okemos, MI 48864, USA
* Corresponding author.
E-mail address: drjanebarber@aol.com

COMMITMENT

Theriogenology practice entails commitment. The commitment required is significant and should be duly considered before jumping in with both feet. Arguably, the commitment to practice small animal theriogenology is unparalleled in comparison with any other specialized area in veterinary medicine.

First and foremost, there is a commitment of time. Reproductive services often need to be provided at the whim of "Mother Nature." Bitches need to be bred when the time is right. And parturition often occurs during the wee hours of the night. It is unrealistic to presume that you will always be able to meet the needs of your breeder clients within the confines of your regular hours of operation. Truth be told, frequent are the impositions upon your personal time.

Once you agree to take on a case, you need to see it through to completion. Consider the following scenario. You have agreed with your breeder client to be on call for her bitch's whelping. It is Sunday afternoon and you have 30 relatives in your backyard for the annual family reunion. Your breeder client calls you with her bitch in dystocia. As inconvenient as it is, you leave the festivities to go do an emergency C-section, hopefully to rejoin your family in time for dessert. Alternatively, if you absolutely cannot fulfill your obligation, you must be able to discuss this with your client, prospectively plan for all possible contingencies, and then facilitate coordinated management of the case with a colleague.

A commitment to theriogenology also requires acquisition of a skill set and a mindset to lifelong learning and mentorship. We know so much more about reproduction in the dog and cat than we did 20 years ago. These advances in our understanding of small animal reproduction continue to lead to new treatments and techniques in managed reproduction. You need to educate your neophyte breeder clients and mentor them through the panoramic process that starts with preparing for breeding and ends with sending puppies off to their new homes. You need to reeducate some of your veteran clients on contemporary methodology for dog breeding. We cannot resist a twist on the old adage "you can't teach an old dog new tricks." Old dogs can learn new tricks; venerable but unsophisticated breeder clients can be educated and, in turn, can learn to embrace scientific breeding strategies. And your premier, well-educated clients will, in their efforts to refine and optimize their breeding programs, seek your counsel to help them eliminate genetic disease, maintain genetic diversity, and produce the preeminent individual of their breed.

The practice of small animal theriogenology often requires timely and frequent communication. Sometimes, dozens of communications are made between your office and all relevant parties involved in the breeding. There can be a lot of "cooks in the kitchen": the bitch owner(s), the bitch's handler, the dog owner(s), the dog's handler, the dog's collecting veterinarian, you, and your support team. Something as simple as a forgotten or delayed phone call can have dire consequences. Failure to make timely communication of a progesterone value can leave the dog owner insufficient time to take the dog to the collecting veterinarian's office to be collected in time to meet the courier service's pick-up deadline. A delayed shipment can potentially mean a lost opportunity for achieving pregnancy and the loss of a client.

"The job's not over until the paperwork is done." A mammoth commitment is needed to the never-ending task of completing paperwork generated in conjunction with providing theriogenology services. This paperwork goes far beyond just getting your medical records entered. In addition to your conventional medical record keeping and SOAPs, paperwork is required for a plethora of other services: puppy registration papers, verification of insemination, health certification, genetic testing, semen evaluation forms, semen cryopreservation forms, semen storage contracts, certificates and documentation required for international shipment of animals and semen, and the list goes on. The task can be tedious. Samples of the various forms are available.[1] A lack of attention to detail in completing forms can result in a mistake that can take double or triple the time and effort to remediate.

SCOPE OF SERVICES

Once you have made the commitment to offer theriogenology services, your next task is to decide the scope of the service offerings you will provide.

1. Basic theriogenology services. The most basic level of services to offer includes the following.
   - In the bitch, breeding management with full physical examination, brucellosis testing, ovulation timing, transvaginal artificial insemination and surgical artificial insemination.
   - In the dog, breeding management with full physical examination, collection, evaluation, and processing of dog semen for immediate insemination or chilled shipment.
2. Comprehensive theriogenology services. Comprehensive theriogenology practice includes the following.
   - Prebreeding management including genetic selection and breed-specific health screenings through organizations such as the Orthopedic Foundation for Animals (www.offa.org) and PennHIP (http://info.antechimagingservices.com/pennhip)
   - Seminars, presentations, and articles generated for breed groups, kennel clubs, and veterinarians.
   - Transcervical artificial insemination (TCI) performed with rigid endoscopy
   - Pregnancy diagnosis (relaxin assay, ultrasound examinations, radiography) and pregnancy management.
   - Routine and dystocia whelping management, postpartum management, and neonatal care from birth through weaning and beyond.
   - Elective and emergency caesarian delivery.
   - Traditional and nontraditional sterilization methods such as vasectomy, ovariectomy, ovary-sparing spay, and chemical sterilization.
   - Drug safety in breeding bitches and dogs.
   - Semen cryopreservation and storage.
   - Diagnosis and treatment of congenital abnormalities, sexual differentiation disorders, subfertility and infertility, and neoplasia in the dog and bitch.
   - Diagnosis and treatment of vulvovaginal abnormalities, abnormal estrus cycles, estrus induction, estrus suppression, misalliance, pyometra, pregnancy loss, gestational diabetes, pregnancy ketosis, dystocia, preterm labor, eclampsia, mastitis, agalactia, galactostasis, metritis, vaginitis, and ovarian remnant in the bitch.
   - Diagnosis and treatment of prostatitis, benign prostatic hypertrophy/hyperplasia, phimosis, paraphimosis, testicular degeneration, retrograde ejaculation, orchitis/epididymitis, and persistent frenulum in the dog.

GAINING PROFICIENCY

To be proficient, most practitioners of small animal theriogenology need to build on what they learned during their veterinary training. The journey to proficiency does not have to be solitary one. Small animal theriogenology practitioners are a small but growing community; we all know each other and are a tight-knit group. You are welcome to join our group. Help can be as easy as a phone call, text, or email.

There are many avenues available for continuing education (CE) in theriogenology and we encourage you take advantage of as many as possible.

Society for Theriogenology Membership

Join the Society for Theriogenology (SFT; www.therio.org) and take advantage of its many member benefits. The SFT offers opportunities to expand your knowledge and build professional relationships that will benefit you and your reproductive practice.

Website

The SFT website provides a wealth of information for members, including the membership directory, CE opportunities, career center for job opportunities, ability to search past copies of the *Clinical Theriogenology* journal, as well as society position statements and tools for the reproductive veterinarian. A "find-a-member" veterinarian/procedures search is available for the public to use in finding a reproductive veterinarian in their area.

Continuing education

At the annual Theriogenology Conference, you can stay on top of reproductive veterinary medicine by networking with your colleagues and hearing world-class speakers. You can also take advantage of SFT webinars. Held throughout the year, they give members an additional resource for getting their required CE hours and updates on the profession. Members receive reduced registration fees to the conference and receive the conference proceedings, regardless of attendance.

Society for TheriogenologySmall Animals listserv

Sign up for the SFT's small animal theriogenology listserv. This active, vibrant venue is how "we" talk to each other. Queries posted to the listserv may be as simple as a request for a source for the purchase of disposable supplies or as in depth as the management of a complicated clinical case. Often, listserv responses can give you reassurance and confidence in decision making regarding a diagnostic or therapeutic plan. The ability to solicit input and benefit from the experience of the collective is invaluable.

Access to Texas A&M University medical library

In a collaborative effort to enhance the access of veterinary practitioners to information and published evidence, the Medical Sciences Library at Texas A&M University and SFT have partnered, which allows SFT members access to the A&M Medical Sciences Library's electronic articles free of charge.

Webinars

Webinars are another free membership benefit. Past webinars are archived on the website.

Clinical Theriogenology journal

Clinical Theriogenology is the SFT's official publication. It is dedicated to keeping members informed on veterinary issues. Published quarterly, this journal brings members cutting edge research, plus items of interest and association news.

E-Newsletters

The SFT E-Newsletter is broadcast via email to keep you abreast of current issues.

Member "extra"

Attendance at the annual meeting and conference comes with a fortuitous extra. As estimable as the lecture sessions are, this opportunity takes place outside of the classroom and comes in the form of the tête-à-tête. This interaction allows you to put faces with the names of your colleagues. Conference attendees and speakers comprise some of the best minds in theriogenology in the world. They welcome you to introduce yourself and "rub elbows" with them at social events. Often a great tip or "pearl" of knowledge is shared over an evening of table talk.

Collaboration with a Mentor

Visiting a practice that is heavily involved in theriogenology can be invaluable to the neophyte. The hospital environment is ideal for "see it-do it" learning to build knowledge, acquire skills and gain confidence. Securing a mentor is easy—all you have to do is ask.

Become a Board-Certified Theriogenologist

The ultimate preparation for theriogenology practice is by formal training to become a specialist. Board certification by the American College of Theriogenologists can be achieved through traditional or alternate routes. With the traditional route, veterinarians enter a residency training program at an approved college of veterinary medicine for a period of 3 to 6 years. The alternate route allows veterinarians to devise a custom-tailored program of study while remaining in private practice. Guidelines and detailed information on both the traditional and alternate routes to becoming a diplomate can be found on the American College of Theriogenologists website (www.theriogenology.org).

Hire a Trained Associate

If you have the desire but lack the time, consider bringing the mentor to you. Hire an associate with the skill set you need.

Learn from Your Dog and Cat Breeder Clients

Your experienced breeder clients are a wealth of experiential knowledge. Although some breeder clients can present a challenge to your patience and intestinal fortitude, take a deep breath and remember that you may be the first breeder-friendly veterinarian that they have encountered. Do not take offense when they are demanding and insist on telling you what to do. Many of them know more about their breed than do you. Take advantage of what they can teach you about their breed-specific knowledge and experiences. The first step in earning their trust and respect is by listening to them.

A Reference Library Is Recommended

This concept may be generational, but we like our books—the kind with pages to turn and margins to annotate. The conundrum is that many of our "go-to" books are currently out of print. If you can get your hands on one, count yourself lucky. Here are a few of our favorites.

i. Feldman EC, Nelson RW. Canine and feline endocrinology and reproduction. 3rd edition. St Louis (MO): Saunders; 2004.
ii. Greco DS, Davidson AP. Small animal endocrinology and reproduction. Ames (IA): Wiley Blackwell; 2017.

iii. Greer M. Canine reproduction and neonatology. Jackson (WY): Teton New Media; 2015.

iv. Johnston SD, Root Kustritz MV, Olson PN. Canine and feline theriogenology. Philadelphia: W.B. Saunders; 2001.

v. Lopate C. Management of pregnant and neonatal dogs, cats, and exotic pets. Ames (IA): Wiley-Blackwell; 2012.

vi. Peterson ME, Kutzler MA. Small animal pediatrics, the first 12 months of life. St Louis: Elsevier Saunders; 2011.

vii. Root Kustritz M. Clinical canine and feline reproduction evidence-based answers. Ames (IA): Wiley-Blackwell; 2010.

viii. Root Kustritz M. Small animal theriogenology. St Louis (MO): Elsevier Science; 2003.

ix. Root Kustritz M. The dog breeder's guide to successful breeding and health management. St Louis (MO): Elsevier Science; 2006.

x. Senger P. Pathways to pregnancy & parturition. 3rd edition. Redmond (OR): Currents Conceptions, Inc; 2012.

Other Avenues to Proficiency

1. Attend CE conferences and meetings that have strong theriogenology content.
2. Attend industry-sponsored short courses and wet labs (MOFA Global, Minitube, Zoetis, ICSB, and Clone, for example).
3. Join the European Veterinary Society for Small Animal Reproduction. European meetings are enlightening and offer the opportunity for a fun-filled trip to interesting places (http://www.evssar.org).
4. Become a member of the International Veterinary Information Service (http://www.ivis.org/home.asp). Membership is free and there is a wealth of information to be gained.
5. Join the Canine and Feline Reproduction listserv (CAFEREPROD-L-request@cornell.edu) which provides stimulating discussions about small animal reproduction.
6. Attend seminars sponsored by various kennel, breed and event clubs.

EQUIPMENT

Much of the equipment needed in small animal theriogenology practice you already have in your general practice hospital. The list includes everything you need to operate a full-service general practice: tools needed to perform a general physical examination, in-house laboratory equipment, an operating room with inhalant anesthesia (we prefer sevoflurane), good anesthesia monitoring capability, and quality radiography equipment (digital preferred).

Comprehensive theriogenology practice also requires a good quality microscope (phase contrast optimally), rigid endoscopy system (for TCI, vaginoscopy, intrauterine procedures, etc), an ultrasound machine, equipment for semen processing and evaluation (variable speed centrifuge, water bath, automated or manual sperm cell counting equipment), semen cryopreservation and storage equipment, a puppy incubator (warmer with O_2 or an oxygen concentrator), and an in-house progesterone analyzer. You also need a gamut of reproduction-specific disposable supplies.

HELPFUL HINTS
Learn the Lingo

There is no faster way to sabotage your efforts to establish rapport with a new dog breeding client than to get the "deer in the headlights" look when he or she starts telling you about her champion dog. Test your knowledge with the following 3 questions. If you cannot answer them, you need to do some homework.

1. Your new client proudly introduces you to her new dog. What gender is it?

    In dog breeder talk, the word "dog" implies gender, and that gender is male. A canine is either a bitch or a dog. Avoid starting off on the wrong foot by calling her female a dog.

2. What are clearances?

    The term "clearances" when used by dog breeders refers to the health certifications recommended by the breed club to which the client belongs. The Orthopedic Foundation for Animals hip evaluation is the most recognized clearance. Clearance requirements are breed specific and are dictated by the common heritable problems encountered in a given breed. For example, clearances recommended for Labrador retrievers differ from those recommended for Cavalier King Charles spaniels.

3. What's a special?

    A special is the American Kennel Club reference to a dog or bitch who has achieved a champion title. To become a champion, he or she must have competed in American Kennel Club conformation shows and obtained 15 points with at least 2 majors. A major win is worth more points and means defeating a higher number of dogs or bitches.

Spend a day at an American Kennel Club or United Kennel Club dog show. In addition to expanding you dog breeding vocabulary, it will give insight into the show dog world.

Prepare for Reproductive Appointments

Have your receptionist get the complete signalment of the pet when the appointment is scheduled. If you are not familiar with the breed, look it up and take note of the breed standard (a description of the observable attributes of an ideal individual), common breed problems, and the clearances recommended.

Counsel Your Client to "Read the Fine Print" of Their Breeding Contract

Problems can arise if all parties to the contract do not have a clear understanding of their agreement. The contract should clearly state the number of chilled semen collections to be shipped, the number of puppies that constitute a litter, whether the number of puppies constituting a litter is determined by the number that are born alive or by the number surviving the first 3 days of life, options for rebreeding in the event that this breeding does not result in a litter and, if the bitch to be bred is not available to be rebred, whether the breeding may be used on another female of the bitch owner's choosing.

Counsel Your Bitch Owner Client to Have a Plan B

Despite prospective planning and preparation, unexpected events can undermine a breeding—the selected sire can succumb to sudden illness or simply fail to give a satisfactory collection on the day needed, the shipment may not arrive in a timely fashion, or the sperm cells may be dead on arrival when unpackaged. Advise your client to think about contingency plans, have a second choice option, and be ready to implement plan B should problems arise with plan A.

Troubleshoot Courier Shipments

With a reproductive practice, there will be many packages received and sent by FED EX, UPS, and so on. When expecting a delivery, always get the tracking number from the sender! When sending out a package, give the tracking number to the dog owner and the inseminating veterinarian. Remember, if your package is scheduled for a Saturday delivery, although "next day" is checked, "Saturday Delivery" must also be checked. Otherwise, your package will arrive on the next business day—Monday—and not as needed on Saturday.

Packages may need to be sent or delivered on weekends or holidays, so be sure to check the delivery company's schedule. Service is not the same for all locales. Some days have no pickups; others have no deliveries. In some of the larger cities, Sunday delivery options may be available, for a significant fee. Consideration should be given to any potential weather-related impact on the anticipated delivery date and time.

Preserve Client Confidentiality

Never discuss a client's visit with anyone. Ensure that all staff members are sensitive to the issue of client confidentiality. Preserve client anonymity when using a clinical case as a teaching example. Avoid scheduling disasters. Never schedule 2 clients who own the same dog breed with concurrent or sequential appointments. You do not want them meeting in your lobby or parking lot. They may be best friends, but neither may want the other to know about their visit. It is the client's prerogative, not ours, to divulge information about their dog to another dog breeder.

Train Reception Staff

In addition to dodging scheduling debacles, front staff need to be trained in the fine art (and it is a fine art) of answering calls and setting up appointments for theriogenology cases. Careful attention must be given to the appropriate date, time of day, and duration of the appointment. Consider the following scenarios by way of example.

Scenario 1

Unlike your typical general practice client who lives within 5 miles of your hospital, your breeder client may have to drive several hours to your hospital. Your receptionist should schedule this appointment at a time that provides a reasonable home departure time and avoids peak traffic times through metropolitan areas.

Scenario 2

Scheduling a pregnancy ultrasound examination at 10 days postovulation will not make for a happy client. Reception staff need to understand when routine pregnancy ultrasound and term gestation radiograph appointments should be scheduled. Charts modeled after a 63-day whelping chart can be made for scheduling pregnancy diagnosis ultrasound examinations and term radiography appointments. This empowers reception staff with a rapid and accurate method for determining the appropriate scheduling date without the need to manually count days on a calendar or ask other team members.

Delegate and Document All Client Communications

From a legal standpoint, "It did not happen if you did not write it down." Educate all staff members as to the importance of documenting all client communications—face-to-face conversations, phone calls, emails, and text messages. Consider having a mobile phone designated for client communications. Often, a text message is quicker and easier than a conversation. There will be times that a call is necessary for discussion, but the reporting of progesterone results and scheduling subsequent tests can best be delegated to a qualified assistant to handle by text messaging. Text messages provide permanent records of communications and can be added to a client's record. Emails can provide the same advantages. Do not communicate with clients via social (which means public) media such as Facebook.

Dedicate One Examination Room for Theriogenology Cases

If you can prospectively design this room, make it large. For a semen collection appointment, you may have a giant breed dog, a giant breed teaser bitch, and 3 or 4 humans in the room at one time. Put the theriogenology room in a quiet area of the hospital. Install a folding wall-mounted examination table (so you can get it out of the way when you are working with large and giant dog breeds). Have your semen evaluation equipment on the counter so clients can witness the sperm count determination and observe semen motility for themselves. Install an oxygen line hookup in the room (for preoxygenating bitches undergoing caesarian section delivery). Situate your theriogenology room adjacent to your operating room and install a viewing window so clients can witness the birth of their puppies without being in the way of your delivery team. But remember to install blinds on the operating room side of the window so you can control viewing of surgery.

Perform a Complete Physical Examination

Perform a complete physical examination on each patient. Remember that attached to each set of ovaries or testicles is the rest of the dog or cat. To be a satisfactory breeding candidate, the entire animal needs to be healthy.

Ask Permission Before You Shave

Ask permission before you shave hair for catheter placement, venipuncture, ultrasound examinations, and so on. The hair you shave may take months to grow back; this is a big deal for show dog clients. If shaving a leg is unavoidable, choose the "off side" (right) leg; it will be further away from the judge as the dog moves around the show ring.

Establish a Policy for Client Participation

Owners love to watch surgical inseminations, Cesarean sections, and participate in the puppy resuscitation. Formulate a hospital policy and follow it. Your clients know and talk to each other, and will be upset if they perceive that another client was permitted a greater level of participation than were they. If you do not allow the client into the viewing or resuscitation area, keep them updated frequently on how things are going. A major complaint from clients is that they are not being kept informed and updated on what is going on "behind closed doors."

Clinical Tips for the Male

- Ensure that nothing bad happens to the dog in the collection room. Perform venipuncture or digital prostate examinations elsewhere. Semen collection requires voluntary participation by the dog. This room is the "fun" room.
- The owner's presence may affect the semen collection process. Decide if it is better or not to have the owner in room. Drugs such as prostaglandin, gonadotropin-releasing hormone, and oxytocin can facilitate collection of hesitant males. For some males, collection outside yields a better result.
- For most dogs, the presence of an estrous teaser bitch optimizes semen collection. Collect and refrigerate or freeze panty liners or cotton balls containing secretions from bitches in estrus. These can be used when a teaser bitch is unavailable. Have a "Magic Carpet"—a nonskid rug containing estrus scent that is used exclusively for semen collection.

- Always label the semen collection tube with the dog's name and breed. It should never leave your hand without some form of identification. Include a copy of the semen evaluation and processing information with each shipment.
- Always document the address of shipment origin, whether paperwork was included, and if the semen-containing tube was labeled. Document lack of paperwork and/or tube labeling in the medical record.
- For shipped semen received, label and save the semen tube at least until the puppies are born. If the puppies do not look purebred or are not a possible color type, you have proof of paternity in the DNA of the residue contained in the semen tube.
- Before discharging a dog from your office, always verify that the penis is fully detumesced and retracted into the prepuce, and that the prepucial opening has not inverted during subsidence. An inverted prepuce is easily corrected by digital manipulation with a lubricated finger. As a cautionary note, the dog may experience a moment of discomfort with the process, so it is prudent to have an assistant restrain the head while it is being done.
- Educate clients on doing periodic testicular palpation. We are amazed at the number of owners of valuable breeding dogs who have never examined this part of their dog and have no clue as to what "normal" feels like.
- Do your due diligence in completing medical and legal documents generated for collecting, shipping, freezing, storing, and using canine sperm cells. Sample forms are available.[1]

Clinical Tips for the Female

- Invest in a progesterone analyzer as soon as it becomes feasible. The ability to get same-day results and perform same-day repeat analysis when problems arise will relieve a lot of headaches. When using a commercial laboratory for progesterone testing, it is imperative that results be reported the next day, even when the "next day" is a Sunday or holiday.
- Educate bitch owners on doing periodic examinations of both mammary chains.
- Instruct assistants to get an additional aliquot of blood at each blood draw for ovulation timing. Date and save the additional serum in the refrigerator or freezer. You may need it to repeat a progesterone test when a result just does not make sense or when you need to run a luteinizing hormone test or in the event the submitted sample becomes lost or destroyed.
- Luteinizing hormone and Brucellosis kits are available for in-house testing. Become familiar with the sensitivity and specificity of the rapid brucellosis test. Know what to do if you get a positive test result on a patient.
- You will be called on to manage ovulation timing remotely when your client lives afar. Proceed cautiously. You have relinquished autonomous control over a critical component in the timing process—namely, progesterone testing. Inherent to remote timing are more opportunities for communication, processing, and reporting errors. It is helpful to communicate directly with a team member from the hospital with which you will be working. Send an information sheet and blood collection tubes with the client so blood samples will be drawn correctly and, if desired, serum saved from each draw for retrospective luteinizing hormone testing. Ascertain how you will receive results. Often the progesterone test can be sent to a commercial laboratory on your hospital's account (so you may access results on Sunday and the collaborating hospital will not have to worry about retrieving and relaying results). The owner should expect to be charged for blood collection, processing, and sample submission

by the collaborating hospital. Always be respectful of your colleagues at other hospitals.

- If you have in-house testing capability, consider having the remote client send the serum samples to your clinic. Confidence in your own testing makes the process more accurate and timely.
- Remember to perform a digital vaginal examination on all bitches. Detection of a vestibulovaginal band, septum, or stricture is important. A septum may prevent intromission by the male during a natural service breeding and may lead to obstructive dystocia during parturition. These anatomic anomalies need to be dealt with in a timely fashion.
- Consider jugular or lateral saphenous venipunctures in lieu of cephalic veins for sample collection in breeding bitches. When you are called on to perform an emergency Caesarian section, you will be glad that intravenous catheter placement goes smoothly because the cephalic vein site is not riddled with scar tissue deposition resulting from multiple venipunctures at the very place you need to access.

Tips for Performing Transcervical Artificial Insemination

- The learning curve for TCI is long and steep for some practitioners. Hand–eye coordination is required, but with practice the procedure is rapid and has excellent success. Attendance at training courses or visiting clinics that have incorporated TCI into their practice is essential to the learning process.
- When mastering the TCI technique, consider performing TCIs on every case that comes in for vaginal insemination. Charge your client the same price as doing a vaginal insemination. Limit attempts at cervical catheterization to 5 to 10 minutes. Even if you are unable to catheterize the cervix, the semen is deposited at the external cervical os, resulting in an insemination that is as good or better than a simple vaginal insemination. When proficiency is achieved, the fees for the TCI may be increased.
- When advancing the TCI scope, insufflation of the vaginal vault with air will aid in maneuvering the scope to the external cervical os. To help keep the air inside the vagina, the scope can either be threaded through an "O" ring while holding the labia of the vulva closed, or an insufflation shunt can be placed in the caudal vagina with the cuff inflated. If the endoscope is resistant to advancement, releasing some of the air from the cuff of the shunt will make passage easier.
- If the external cervical os is ventrally or laterally situated, it can be difficult to access. Remove the scope, take the bitch outside to walk around and eliminate. Then try again. A full urinary bladder or colon can push the cervix laterally, making catheterization nearly impossible.
- If the entry angle seems too steep when advancing the scope, have an assistant gently push up on the ventral abdomen. This angle is especially steep in bulldogs.
- If, when passing the TCI scope, fluid is encountered in the cranial vagina, suction the fluid out. If the fluid is inflammatory, lavage the vaginal vault repeatedly with 0.9% saline solution until the effluent is clear. Then proceed with catheter placement through the external cervical os.
- Once the catheter is in place, deposit semen into the uterus slowly over at least 5 minutes. Observe the external cervical os and slow deposition if semen is observed leaking from the cervix.
- Rarely, a bitch will not stand for TCI. The administration of dexmedetomidine at one-half the manufacturer's recommended intravenous dose as given on the bottle will relax the bitch sufficiently to perform the procedure.

- Do not thaw frozen semen until you are ready to inseminate! What if you are unable to catheterize the cervix with a TCI? Make an initial assessment of the semen before insemination to validate and confirm that semen quality is the same as reported and acceptable for use. If it is dead or of very poor quality, you may need to thaw, with permission, additional breeding units or implement your client's plan B for the breeding. After insemination, you can evaluate motility again using the small amount of semen remaining in the hub of the needle. This confirms sperm cell viability and documents that no semen handling errors were made during the TCI procedure.

Tips for Surgical Artificial Insemination

- Deposit one-half of the volume of semen into each uterine horn while applying digital pressure for 1 to 2 minutes to the uterine horns at a point caudal to the semen deposition site. This maneuver helps to avoid immediate outflow of semen along the path of least resistance. Although single site intrauterine insemination of frozen semen in the bitch has been shown to not affect sperm distribution within the uterus, the number of viable spermatozoa used for insemination in this study was 3 times that often typically packaged in a breeding unit of frozen semen.[2]
- Keep the total volume to ≤ 2 mL for a large breed and 1 mL for small breeds. This will usually prevent overfilling of the uterus.
- Do not use needles or catheters smaller than 23-G for semen deposition.

Tips for Caesarian Delivery

- If you cannot be available for a required Caesarian delivery, inform your client well ahead of time and facilitate alternative arrangements.
- Familiarize yourself with Veterinary Perinatal Specialties Inc. (aka WhelpWise, www.whelpwise.com). Consider making your client aware of this service.
- Prepare your client and your team members for the surgery. Be mindful that you are performing surgery on more than 1 patient. Make decisions to ensure the safety of both the dam and the neonates. Have enough team members on hand for puppy resuscitation. We recommend having 1 staff member dedicated to assisting in surgery and monitoring anesthesia of the dam and 1 additional staff member for each 2 puppies to be delivered.
- Remind your client to bring all necessary items (puppy basket or container, heat source, blankets, etc) with them to the surgery appointment.
- Preoxygenate the bitch for 5 to 10 minutes before anesthetic induction. This is a great job to delegate, under supervision, to your client and works particularly well when you have an oxygen line available in your theriogenology room.
- If you are having difficulty exteriorizing the uterus through your laparotomy opening, lengthen your laparotomy incision. The additional time required to close the added length is far preferable to dealing with a rip in the uterus. If you still cannot get the uterus exteriorized, perform your hysterotomy without exteriorizing the uterus and deliver the first puppy. With the first puppy delivered, the uterine horn can often then be exteriorized.
- Perform hysterotomies midhorn. Palpate a puppy through the uterine wall and make hysterotomy incisions over the puppy's head or hindquarters. This will prevent incisure over placental sites and the resultant hemorrhage, which can be copious.
- Do not fumble the puppy! Wet puppies are slippery. It is challenging to transfer a puppy to an assistant without dropping it or incurring contamination of your

gloves or sterile surgical field. We recommend placing each puppy in a sterile towel and making a "puppy taco." The surgeon holds the top of the taco (both ends of the towel) and gently places the "U" portion of the taco (containing the puppy) into the upturned palms of the assistant. Towels are wrapped and autoclaved in packs of 6, then placed on a second mayo stand.

- If placental removal is difficult, consider gently teasing the attached chorionic membrane away from the umbilical cord. The placenta should then detach readily. If a placenta does not detach easily or if excessive hemorrhage is encountered, do not remove it. Leave this placenta in situ and exercise care to avoid incorporation of placental membranes in hysterotomy closures. Placentas will pass from the uterus and exit the body uneventfully. It is important to account for the passage of all placentas.
- Avoid passing suture through the mucosal layer and into the uterine lumen when closing hysterotomy sites.
- Yunnan baiyao, used in traditional Chinese medicine, may also be given if excessive hemorrhage continues postoperatively. An anectodally reported dose for yunnan baiyao is 2 tablets given twice daily by mouth for a 50- to 60-pound bitch.

MARKETING

Theriogenology practice constitutes a niche market; services are required by a small fraction of the companion animal population. Marketing efforts are best directed to your target audience, namely, dog and cat breeders. To that end, word-of-mouth marketing through the breeder clients is an excellent way to get your "name" out there. Go to dog and cat shows and performance events (Schutzhund, hunt tests, agility, search and rescue, etc) and mingle. You may purchase an advertisement page in the show catalog wishing the exhibitors good luck at the show and reminding them that your practice welcomes responsible breeders. Offer to come introduce yourself and present a seminar to area breed, kennel, and performance clubs. Ask clients to post litter birth announcements with pictures to your hospital Facebook page. In contrast with the situation with client case communications, social media is useful as a marketing tool. However, your hospital Facebook page must be constantly monitored for postings by that rare disgruntled client, so they can be dealt with promptly.

Reach out to your community of veterinary colleagues. Send a letter of announcement and brochures to area veterinary hospitals letting them know that you are offering theriogenology services. Do not forget to include regional emergency and referral hospitals. Odds are good that none of them offer, nor aspire to offer, theriogenology services. Hone your public speaking skills and offer to speak at local, regional, and state veterinary medical association meetings.

An informative, well-designed website explaining your reproductive services will educate prospective clients. Ask permission from current clients to post case reports and pictures of success stories and litter announcements. Remember, puppy "grandmothers" love to brag. Show a genuine interest in their puppies and you will be endeared. Also consider hosting an open house.

SUMMARY

Broadening your scope of practice to include theriogenology services offers a myriad of advantages. Theriogenology services are profitable, offer new revenue streams and optimize use of support staff and hospital. Offering reproductive services sets your practice apart from competitor practices. Breeder clients are demanding but loyal and return for repeat services; they also request and follow recommendations for "high-end" services. Your theriogenology clients often refer locally placed puppies and kittens to you for primary care and you gain new general practice clients. And it is fun!

Theriogenology is a rewarding addition to a veterinarian's repertoire. The ability to assist in creation of new life is amazing. And the new life you create goes on to benefit and enhance the wellbeing of people. The stories you hear from your clients about the puppies you "made" will be unbelievable but true: the Best in Show winner, the blood-hound who now is busy tracking down criminals on the streets of New York, the beagle who can tell her epileptic owner that a seizure is imminent, the golden retriever therapy dog for a veteran with posttraumatic stress disorder, and the sweet little puffball who is now a beloved family companion.

We invite new generations to join our community of veterinarians dedicated to small animal theriogenology. Together, we work toward preservation of species, solutions for pet population control, treatment of reproductive and heritable disease and mentorship of our clients in responsible breeding of purpose-bred dogs. You do not have to have it all figured out to jump in, just take the first step. . . and enjoy the journey.

REFERENCES

1. Greer ML. Forms useful in theriogenology practice. In: SFT Canine Seminar and Wet Lab Proceedings. 2016. p. 55–62. Available to SFT members on the SFT website www.therio.org.
2. Fukushima FB, Malm C, Henry M, et al. Site of intrauterine artificial insemination in the bitch does not affect sperm distribution within the uterus. Reprod Domest Anim 2010;45:1059–64.

Assisted Reproduction in the Male Cat

Aime K. Johnson, DVM

KEYWORDS

- Feline • Tom • Sperm collection • Electroejaculation • Cryopreservation

KEY POINTS

- Evaluation of the feline ejaculate is similar to evaluation in other species.
- A sperm sample can be obtained from most males in a clinic setting, but amount of sperm and volume obtained vary between techniques.
- Sperm cryopreservation is an excellent way to preserve genetics in valuable males; however, feline sperm perform better when appropriate ratios of extender components are used.

INTRODUCTION

Interest in the domestic cat examination, semen collection, evaluation, and use has increased in the past 10 years. Because the domestic cat can serve as a model for reproduction of exotic and endangered feline species, and as an animal model for human disease, research interest in assisted reproduction also has increased. Preserving the valuable genetics in purebred or research model catteries has increased the demand for quality reproductive management. Semen collection and evaluation are vital to diagnose and monitor progress for any reproductive problem in the tom. However, the process presents its own set of challenges unique to the cat due to the small volume and comparatively low sperm number produced in each ejaculate, as well as the decreased overall sperm quality seen in many exotic species or catteries. The demand for semen collection, evaluation, and subsequent use is growing as a way to preserve important or valuable genetic materials.

EXAMINATION

Before a reproductive examination, a good general physical examination should be performed to assess for any nonreproductive abnormality. This may include a minimum database, including blood work (complete blood count and serum chemistry). A thorough reproductive examination should consist of manual palpation of the

Disclosure Statement: The author has nothing to disclose.
Department of Clinical Sciences, Auburn University, 1500 Wire Road, Auburn, AL 36849, USA
E-mail address: akj0001@auburn.edu

Vet Clin Small Anim 48 (2018) 511–521
https://doi.org/10.1016/j.cvsm.2018.02.001
0195-5616/18/© 2018 Elsevier Inc. All rights reserved.

testicles, assessing for size, texture, and symmetry, followed by ultrasound to assess any irregularities within the testicular parenchyma. Measurements of the testicles should be taken to compare length, width, and height of each testicle. These measurements can be used to evaluate changes in testicular volume over time. The penis should be evaluated for any discoloration, discharge, and the presence of spines. Exteriorization of the penis may be difficult without sedation, so this portion of the examination might be best accomplished just before sperm collection when the tom is sedated or anesthetized.

Sperm collection in cats presents many challenges. First, the volume and total sperm number are extremely low when compared with other domestic animals such as the dog, bull, boar, ram, and stallion. The low volume alone makes routine semen evaluation a challenge by allowing enough of the ejaculate to be used for analysis, yet preserving enough sperm for insemination or cryopreservation. When the semen volume is often less than 50 to 100 µL, care must be taken to use the smallest number of sperm or volume necessary for analysis. Another challenge is the low sperm quality often encountered with feline breeding operations. Many of the catteries are purebred, and owners may have narrowed genetic lines in hopes of producing that perfect cat. Alternatively, research colonies often breed genetically similar animals either due to lack of genetic diversity within a closed colony, or to propagate a genetic trait desired for research. Last, nondomestic cat species have limited genetic diversity, which usually correlates with poor sperm quality. This impact has been demonstrated in the cheetah and Florida panther, whose population numbers crashed to fewer than 100 individuals before rallying again. However, the lack of genetic variation in these 2 species has resulted in a high proportion of abnormal sperm within the ejaculate (up to 70% for the cheetah[1] and 90% for the Florida panther[2]). It appears that despite the high degree of teratozoospermia, however, fertility can be maintained. It has been proposed that cats experiencing decreased numbers of normal spermatozoa may have a compensatory mechanism to overcome this fault and maintain fertility by increasing the number of copulations per female to increase the number of normal sperm available in the female.[3] It has also been shown that teratozoospermic cats experience an overall decrease in apoptosis during the first 2 meiotic divisions of spermatogenesis and produce 30% more spermatids per spermatocyte than normospermic cats.[4] Although fertility is maintained in natural breeding, the challenge of teratozoospermic animals is preserving the spermatozoal cells for future breeding. Pukazhenthi and colleagues[5] showed that in wild felids the primary factor negatively affecting sperm survival following cryopreservation was poor sperm morphology (**Fig. 1**). Therefore, cats that experience a high degree of teratozoospermia present their own challenges with successful cryopreservation.

SEMEN COLLECTION METHODS
Artificial Vagina

The best representative for semen analysis is an entire ejaculate collected during a natural ejaculation using an artificial vagina. The artificial vagina (AV) for the domestic cat is most commonly constructed using an Eppendorf tube and a rubber pipette bulb, as previously reported in literature.[6] The male is allowed to mount a queen in estrus, and the AV is slid over the penis as the male is thrusting. The AV is held in place by the collector's thumb and first finger to stimulate ejaculation. A second ejaculation can be obtained 5 to 10 minutes after the first using a clean AV. If the male has been adequately trained to the AV, or a queen in estrus is not available, the male may mount a gloved arm. The advantages of using an AV are that it can be performed readily in the

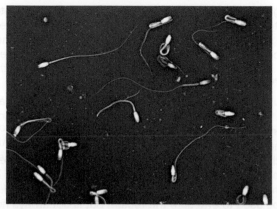

Fig. 1. An eosin-nigrosin sperm morphology stain showing common teratozoospermia in a tom cat. Note the numerous coiled tails and head and midpiece defects.

unanesthetized tom and allows a complete ejaculate to be obtained. Disadvantages are the requirement for training and a frequent necessity of a teaser queen. Often, weeks to months of conditioning and training are required before a tom is consistently producing ejaculates, and training may not be successful in all toms. Valiente and colleagues[7] worked with toms in their cattery 3 times weekly for 20 minutes and reported a mean of 3.9 months (1.5–5.5 months) before the first ejaculate was produced. With patience, collection using an AV is an excellent method for situations in which a single male or group of toms are collected on a regular basis, such as in a cattery or research colony, but is impractical for a single evaluation in a clinical setting using an untrained tom.

Electroejaculation

Electroejaculation (EEJ) has historically been the most common method of obtaining an ejaculate from a tom that is not trained to an AV. This method will consistently provide spermatozoa for evaluation and insemination, but the total sperm number obtained may vary greatly with each collection attempt. The advantage to this procedure is the ability to perform this in any tom and training is not required. This method is ideal for situations in which sperm is required from a tomcat for evaluation, preservation, or artificial insemination, and training to an AV is not feasible or practical. Disadvantages to this procedure are the requirements of general anesthesia, specialized equipment and technique are necessary, and ejaculates tend to be higher in volume and lower in concentration when compared with a collection obtained by urethral catheterization.[8] This author's preferred anesthesia protocol includes dexmedetomidine (30–40 µg/kg) and ketamine (3–5 mg/kg) in the muscle, followed by intubation and supplemental oxygen. Inhalant anesthesia (isoflurane) can be added if necessary, but the short procedure time generally does not require it. On occasion, electroejaculation using inhalation anesthetics may result in urination and contamination of semen samples. Zambelli and colleagues[9] compared the use of medetomidine alone with ketamine alone on the quality of ejaculates collected by electroejaculation. These researchers found that the use of an α_2-agonist (medetomidine in this study) produced higher numbers of spermatozoa in the ejaculate than using ketamine alone, and did not increase the incidence of retroejaculation. However, these researchers did not evaluate the use of these medications in combination. To prevent any perception of discomfort during the procedure, it is recommended that an anesthetic, such as keta-mine, be added to balance the sedative and analgesic effects of dexmedetomidine. Each tom should be monitored appropriately while under general anesthesia to mini-mize anesthetic complications.

Procedure for electroejaculation

- Electroejaculation is performed using a rectal probe 1 cm in diameter and 12 to 13 cm long. Appropriate electroejaculators for cats are available commercially (P-T Electronics, Boring, OR) (**Fig. 2**).
- Lubricate the rectal probe with nonspermicidal lubricant and insert the probe gently into the rectum approximately 5 to 7 cm. The electrodes should be oriented ventrally.
- If feces in the rectum prevent the placement of the probe, a lubricated gloved finger may be used to evacuate the rectum but is not always necessary.
- Manually extend the penis and clean with gauze moistened with saline (no alcohol or soap). Dry the penis with clean or sterile dry gauze.
- Place a sterile vial (Eppendorf) over the penis and direct the vial ventrally. This allows the ejaculate obtained to gravity flow into the tip of the tube and prevents the ejaculate from becoming lost in the hair surrounding the penis (**Fig. 3**).
- Turn on the ejaculator. Make sure the rheostat dial is set to zero before activating the power switch.
- Rotate the rheostat to provide a series of electrical stimuli by gradually turning the dial to the desired voltage for 2 to 3 seconds, then abruptly back to zero for 2 to 3 seconds. The stimuli should be administered in the following order:
  ○ Set 1: 10 times at 2 V, 10 times at 3 V, 10 times at 4 V, rest 3 to 5 minutes.
  ○ Set 2: 10 times at 3 V, 10 times at 4 V, 10 times at 5 V, rest 3 to 5 minutes.
  ○ Set 3: 10 times at 4 V, 10 times at 5 V, 10 times at 5 V (or 6 if needed, depending on previous response).
- The sample obtained between each electroejaculation set should be evaluated for the presence of sperm. This is usually readily evident, as an ejaculate contain-ing spermatozoa will be cloudy. Tapping the bottom of the vial on the table will facilitate the ejaculate to concentrate at the bottom tip of the Eppendorf. A new, sterile tube should be used between each set after collection to prevent contamination or loss of the sample. Tubes also can be changed within sets if a good sample of sperm is obtained. This preserves clean samples from the

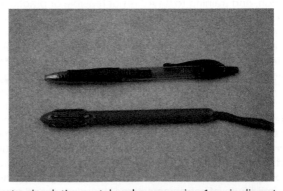

Fig. 2. A feline electroejaculation rectal probe measuring 1 cm in diameter and 12 to 13 cm long. Note the 3 linear electrodes that should point ventrally when in use.

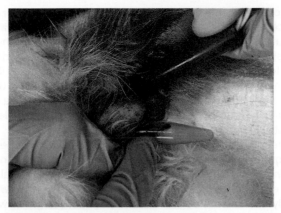

Fig. 3. For the electroejaculation technique, a sterile Eppendorf vial is placed over the erect penis and directed ventrally to collect the ejaculate as it is emitted. The handle of the rectal probe can be seen inserted into the rectum. Both testicles are also visible.

chance of possible urine contamination obtained during any future sets. However, because there is a loss of sperm with each transfer of the ejaculate, the fewest vials possible while still ensuring the ejaculate remains uncontaminated should be used.

- The volume of the ejaculate obtained in each set should be measured accurately using a pipette. Volumes range from as little as 5 μL to more than 50 μL for each set. Motility and sperm concentration can be performed on each set immediately after collection, or can be performed on the combination of all 3 sets. Approximate numbers obtained in our laboratory for samples obtained using electroejaculation (all 3 sets) are volumes of 10 to 150 μL (0.001–0.15 mL) and 0.05 to 100 million sperm per ejaculate.
- Addition of semen extender (50–100 μL) after each set is helpful in evaluating the low volume of semen obtained and preventing loss through evaporation of seminal plasma.

The tom's response to the stimuli should be monitored and the probe location adjusted accordingly. During the stimulation, both hind limbs typically would extend symmetrically. If they are not extending, or if one extends more than the other, confirm that the probe is in contact with the rectal wall, and that the electrodes are on ventral midline. If contraction of the hind legs is weak or not consistent with each set (strong, then weak, and so on), the probe can be adjusted cranially or caudally to ensure the electrodes are in the proper location over the prostate. If adjusting the probe is not effective, fecal material may be impeding the probe placement. Perform a digital examination, remove any fecal material, and replace the probe.

Urethral Catheterization

Because electroejaculation requires specialized equipment and some degree of operator training, collection using urethral catheterization has become very popular as a means to procure a sample for semen analysis. This procedure was first described by Zambelli and colleagues.[8] Male cats were heavily sedated with medetomidine (Domitor; Pfizer, Florham Park, NJ; 130–140 μg/kg, intramuscularly [IM]) for the procedure. Once heavy sedation was achieved, the penis was exposed and cleaned with saline. A tomcat urinary catheter (open-ended) was inserted into the urethra approximately 8 to 9 cm and removed. Care must be taken not to enter the bladder with the catheter. Once removed, the catheter was flushed with appropriate extender and the sample evaluated. Although the total sperm collected was lower than what was obtained by electroejaculation, these researchers were able to collect adequate numbers of spermatozoa for insemination or cryopreservation (mean of $21.0 \pm 18.1 \times 10^6$ sperm, as compared with electroejaculation with $33.6 \pm 34.5 \times 10^6$ total sperm).[8] This provides an excellent alternative method for semen collection in a practice setting. Because medetomidine is no longer available, a comparable dose of dexmedetomidine (Dexdomitor; Zoetis, Florham Park, NJ) would be 65 to 70 μg/kg IM.

Since this first reporting, several other anesthetic protocols have been evaluated. In 2015, this same group reported the results of using different doses of medetomidine (130 μg/kg used in the original study and 50 μg/kg, which is the typical clinical dose).[10] This group also evaluated catheterization technique. One group was catheterized once, immediately after the cat became sedate, the second group was catheterized 3 separate times 5 minutes apart starting with the onset of sedation, and the third was catheterized 20 minutes after the cat had reached adequate sedation. The results from this project showed that sperm were obtained following all methods, but the investigators' conclusions were that the best results (highest total sperm number) were obtained using the higher dose of sedation and a single catheterization performed right after the maximal sedation is achieved.[10]

A second study evaluating an injectable anesthetic protocol for this procedure used premedication with methadone (0.2 mg/kg) and a much lower dose of dexmedetomidine (5 μg/kg) in the muscle followed by induction with propofol intravenously.[11] This protocol gives an option for those patients who may not tolerate the cardiovascular side effects that manifest with a high dose of an α_2-agonist. Using this protocol, similar sperm numbers were obtained when compared with the previous study. A greater volume of ejaculate was obtained (200–400 μL), but all other parameters evaluated were similar, making this anesthesia protocol a viable alternative to dexmedetomidine alone.

In the author's experience, waiting 20 minutes after the administration of dexmedetomidine, placing an open-ended tomcat catheter 9 cm into the urethra (therefore avoiding the bladder), and allowing it to sit for 1 to 2 minutes before slowly removing it provides the most consistent results in obtaining a sample.

Other Techniques

As an alternative to an ejaculate, sperm collection by epididymal flushing or mincing after castration or postmortem followed by cryopreservation has been widely described.[12–14] The research performed in the domestic cat has provided a model for the technique in endangered feline species in attempts to preserve valuable genetics.[15] As a note, one report showed that sperm motility and membrane integrity were decreased when the cat was euthanized with pentobarbital before epididymal collection when compared with induction of general anesthesia.[16] Therefore, if an animal is undergoing epididymal sperm collection followed by euthanasia, it is advised to anesthetize the cat for castration, and then administer the euthanasia agent after the testicles are removed. If cryopreservation is not feasible in the clinical setting, epididymal sperm recovery can be performed, processed, cooled to 5°C, and shipped overnight to a facility for freezing. Cooling for 24 hours did not affect the post-thaw motility.[17]

If collection directly from the male is not possible, spermatozoa for evaluation may be collected by aspiration or lavage of the queen's vaginal vault following mating. Collection by this method may be useful to rule out azoospermia, but there may be a higher rate of morphologic defects in this sample because normal sperm should be moving out of the vaginal vault and into the uterus very quickly following breeding. Because retroejaculation is a common occurrence in the tom, cystocentesis and analysis of the urine sediment after ejaculation may yield enough sperm cells for a limited analysis. However, both sperm motility and morphology are likely to be compromised. This method is typically used only to rule in or out the presence of sperm. Because cystocentesis can usually be performed in an unsedated animal, this would allow sperm collection without the use of sedatives and offers a quick check of the presence of sperm after a natural mating.

SEMEN EVALUATION

Following collection of semen, the volume of the ejaculate is recorded, and the sample is extended at least 1:1 immediately with suitable media. If a low volume is obtained, increasing the volume with extender to a more workable amount is helpful. For example, if 10 μL are obtained, adding 100 μL of extender increases the volume and decreases the concentration (and therefore using too many sperm cells) for sample analysis. The ratio of extension will depend on what the ejaculate will be used for after collection. If the sample will be used for insemination or analysis immediately, this author uses Ham's F-10 (Thermo Fisher Scientific, Waltham, MA) with 25 mM Hepes, 1 mM pyruvate and glutamine, penicillin/streptomycin/neomycin, and 5% fetal bovine serum. If the sample will be cryopreserved, the sperm can be directly extended into TES-Tris-egg yolk extender (TEST) refrigeration medium (Refrigeration Medium; Irvine Scientific, Santa Ana, CA).

Motility (total and progressive) should be recorded by estimation under low-power microscopy on a warmed microscope slide, or using a computer assisted analysis calibrated for feline spermatozoa. Concentration can be obtained using a hemocytometer at a 1:100 dilution or Nucleocounter (ChemoMetech, Allerod, Denmark).

SPERM CRYOPRESERVATION

Successful pregnancies following cryopreservation of ejaculated feline semen were first reported in 1978 by Platz and colleagues[18] with a conception rate of 10.6% (6/56 attempts) following intravaginal insemination. Two inseminations of 50 to 100 × 10⁶ sperm each were inseminated into the vaginal canal on days 2 and 3 after induction of ovulation. Litter sizes ranged from 1 to 4 (average 2) kittens. Since this time, a myriad of freezing semen extenders and insemination techniques have been studied in cats with varying results. Among the most popular are Tris-egg yolk based, TES-Tris-egg yolk extender (TEST), and TEST-soybean lecithin extenders. For the domestic cat, TEST yolk buffer composed of TES buffer, Tris lactose, and 20% egg yolk is an effective extender and is commercially available.[19,20] However, comparative research using many available semen extender options is lacking in cats, likely due to the difficulty of performing these studies on a single ejaculate with the low volume and sperm number obtained from cats.

One subject for research has been the glycerol concentration for cryopreservation in the tomcat. Villaverde and colleagues[21] evaluated sperm survival rates in glycerol concentrations of 3%, 5%, and 7%. Their results showed that the 3% glycerol had a lower post-thaw motility than either the 5% or 7%. The 7% glycerol concentration showed higher acrosomal membrane damage when compared with the 5%. Their conclusion was, when comparing these 3 percentages, the 5% glycerol concentration resulted in the best sperm preservation. Since this time, a 4% glycerol concentration has become popular, and this is the concentration used by the author.

Various sperm dilution methods have been evaluated to determine the best outcome for cryopreservation. A 1-step dilution method occurs when the extender containing the glycerol is added directly to the post-centrifuged sample before cooling. A 2-step dilution method is where the sample is cooled in nonglycerol-containing extender and the cryoprotectant extender is added slowly in a stepwise fashion immediately before freezing. Buranaamnuay[22] recently evaluated a 1-step compared with a 2-step freezing process with epididymal sperm. In this study, the 2-step process produced better overall sperm quality after cryopreservation. This is consistent with this author's observations, especially when working with teratozoospermia or lower-quality sperm.

Appropriate cooling rates also optimize post-thaw sperm quality. Using an ultra-rapid (14°C/min) or a rapid (4°C/min) cooling rate from room temperature to either 0 or 5°C caused a significant decrease in the number of intact acrosomes, thereby affecting the post-thaw semen quality in teratozoospermic cats. This effect was diminished when a slower cooling rate of 0.5°C/min was used.[5] A comparison of 5 freezing rates in another study indicated that a rate of 3.85°C/min from 5°C to −40°C resulted in the greatest post-thaw motility and lowest number of damaged acrosomes. In this study, the samples were cooled to 5°C at a rate of 0.2°C/s before freezing.[23]

Many different cryopreservation protocols for feline semen have been described in different situations.[20] This author uses a protocol previously described with a slow-cool, 2-step dilution method because of the high degree of teratozoospermia observed in most cats in breeding colonies where external breeding has been limited either due to choice (valuable genetics) or necessity (breeding for a genetic trait or defect for research).[24]

- Following collection, the collected ejaculate is immediately extended 1:1 in Ham's F-10 with Hepes or directly into TEST refrigeration medium (Refrigeration Medium; Irvine Scientific).
- Sample is then centrifuged at 300g for 8 minutes.
- The supernatant is removed and the resulting sperm pellet is resuspended in a quantity of TEST refrigeration medium sufficient to achieve a concentration of 100 to 120 × 10^6 motile sperm/mL (no fewer than 50 × 10^6 motile sperm/mL).
- The sperm and an equal volume of diluted 8% glycerol TEST-Freezing Medium (12% glycerol undiluted) are placed in a room temperature water bath and cooled for several hours in a cold room.
- Once the sample is at 5°C, an equal volume of this 8% glycerol medium is added to the sperm solution in a 3-step process:
  ○ Add one-fourth of the total volume to the ejaculate.
  ○ Wait 5 minutes.
  ○ Add another one-fourth of the total volume.
  ○ Wait 5 minutes.
  ○ Add the remaining volume. This results in a final glycerol concentration of 4%, and a final concentration of approximately 50 to 60 million spermatozoa/mL.
- The ejaculate is loaded into 0.25-mL straws and sealed.
- If loading less than 0.25 mL in a straw, a small amount of TEST medium with 4% glycerol can be loaded first, followed by an air bubble, then the sperm suspension to ensure a proper freezing rate for that straw.

When a programmable freezer is not available, freezing in a 2-step process yields the best post-thaw survival when working with fragile or low-fertility feline sperm. The straws are placed on the upper tier of a metal holding rack, 7.5 cm above the liquid nitrogen (−30°C) for 1 minute. The straws are then lowered to a second rack 2.5 cm above the liquid nitrogen (−130°C) and held there for an additional 1 minute before

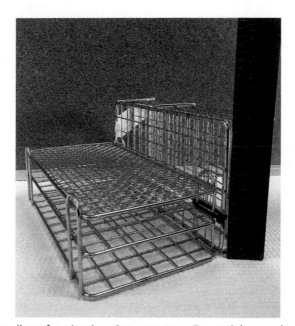

Fig. 4. This setup allows freezing in a 2-step process. Two stainless steel test-tube racks of appropriate size, 1 placed on side and 1 placed flat, are secured together with plastic ties. Adequate liquid nitrogen is added into Styrofoam box to a depth of 3 cm. The test-tube rack apparatus is placed inside. The lid is replaced and the system is allowed to equilibrate. The straws are placed on the upper tier of a metal holding rack, 7.5 cm above the liquid nitrogen (−30°C) for 1 minute. The straws are then lowered to a second rack, 2.5 cm above the liquid nitrogen (−130°C) and held there for an additional 1 minute before plunging into the liquid nitrogen.

plunging into the liquid nitrogen and transferred to canes for long-term storage (**Fig. 4**). To thaw, straws are removed from liquid nitrogen storage, held in the air for 10 seconds, and transferred to a 37°C water bath for 30 seconds. Immediately following thawing, the straws are thoroughly dried, opened, and the semen placed in a vial. The thawed semen is diluted in a drop-wise fashion with an equal volume of warmed Ham's F-10 medium with Hepes buffer and 5% fetal calf serum. Following dilution, the sample is centrifuged at 300g for 8 minutes. The supernatant containing the egg yolk, glycerol, and diluent is immediately removed, and the pellet resuspended in 100 to 200 μL of the Ham's F-10 medium before insemination.

If the sperm to be cryopreserved are epididymal sperm, the same procedures should be followed. Post-thaw motilities following cryopreservation of epididymal sperm will depend on pre-freeze quality, but have been recorded as high as 32% (54% fresh).[25]

A comparison of post-thaw characteristics of sperm collected by urethral catheterization and epididymal sperm was performed by Prochowska and colleagues.[26] Sperm from male cats were collected by urethral catheterization as described previously. A second sample of sperm from the same cat was obtained by epididymal mincing following castration. Both sperm samples were cryopreserved using the same methods. Post-thaw sperm characteristics of the 2 collection methods were not different, indicating that either method will provide a viable option for sperm cryopreservation.[26]

SUMMARY

In conclusion, collection of semen from the domestic cat can be accomplished with the necessary equipment. Evaluation of the ejaculate is similar to evaluation in other species. The cat often has a higher incidence of teratospermia due to the reduced genetic pool available in many catteries, research colonies, and exotic species. In natural breeding situations, cats appear to compensate for teratospermia by increased numbers of matings per estrus. Spermatozoal defects adversely affect the quality of the semen following cryopreservation, but epididymal sperm has resulted in viable pregnancies. By adjusting the process for each individual cat, most cats can undergo successful sperm collection and cryopreservation to preserve genetics.

REFERENCES

1. Pukazhenthi BS, Wildt DE, Howard JG. The phenomenon and significance of teratospermia in felids. J Reprod Fertil Suppl 2001;57:423–33.
2. Roelke ME, Martenson JS, O'Brien SJ. The consequences of demographic reduction and genetic depletion in the endangered Florida panther. Curr Biol 1993;3(6):340–50.
3. Pukazhenthi BS, Neubauer K, Jewgenow K, et al. The impact and potential etiology of teratospermia in the domestic cat and its wild relatives. Theriogenology 2006;66(1):112–21.
4. Franca LR, Godinho CL. Testis morphometry, seminiferous epithelium cycle length, and daily sperm production in domestic cats (Felis catus). Biol Reprod 2003;68(5):1554–61.
5. Pukazhenthi B, Santymire R, Crosier A, et al. Challenges in cryopreserving endangered mammal spermatozoa: morphology and the value of acrosomal integrity as markers of cryo-survival. Soc Reprod Fertil Suppl 2007;65:433–46.
6. Tanaka A, Kuwabara S, Takagi Y, et al. Effect of ejaculation intervals on semen quality in cats. J Vet Med Sci 2000;62(11):1157–61.
7. Valiente C, de la Sota PE, Arauz S, et al. Ejaculation training, seminal alkaline phosphatase and semen preservation through cooling in a milk-based extender in domestic cats. J Feline Med Surg 2014;16(4):312–6.
8. Zambelli D, Prati F, Cunto M, et al. Quality and in vitro fertilizing ability of cryopreserved cat spermatozoa obtained by urethral catheterization after medetomidine administration. Theriogenology 2008;69(4):485–90.
9. Zambelli D, Cunto M, Prati F, et al. Effects of ketamine or medetomidine administration on quality of electroejaculated sperm and on sperm flow in the domestic cat. Theriogenology 2007;68(5):796–803.
10. Cunto M, Kuster DG, Bini C, et al. Influence of different protocols of urethral catheterization after pharmacological induction (Ur.Ca.P.I.) on semen quality in the domestic cat. Reprod Domest Anim 2015;50(6):999–1002.
11. Pisu MC, Ponzio P, Rovella C, et al. Usefulness of an injectable anaesthetic protocol for semen collection through urethral catheterisation in domestic cats. J Feline Med Surg 2017;19(10):1087–90.
12. Tebet JM, Martins MI, Chirinea VH, et al. Cryopreservation effects on domestic cat epididymal versus electroejaculated spermatozoa. Theriogenology 2006;66(6–7):1629–32.
13. Toyonaga M, Sato Y, Morita M, et al. The qualities of cryopreserved epididymal sperm collected from feline epididymides stored at low temperature. J Vet Med Sci 2010;72(6):777–80.

14. Siemieniuch MJ, Woclawek-Potocka I. Assessment of selected quality parameters of epididymal cat (*Felis catus* s. domestica, L. 1758) sperm using flow cytometry method and computer assisted sperm analyser. Reprod Domest Anim 2008; 43(5):633–7.

15. Pukazhenthi B, Comizzoli P, Travis AJ, et al. Applications of emerging technologies to the study and conservation of threatened and endangered species. Reprod Fertil Dev 2006;18(1–2):77–90.

16. Jimenez E, Perez-Marin CC, Millan Y, et al. Influence of anaesthetic drugs on the epididymal sperm quality in domestic cats. Anim Reprod Sci 2011;123(3–4): 265–9.

17. Martins JL, Villaverde AI, Lima AF, et al. Impact of 24-h cooling prior to freezing on the survival of domestic cat (*Felis catus*) epididymal sperm. Reprod Domest Anim 2009;44(Suppl 2):366–8.

18. Platz CC, Wildt DE, Seager SW. Pregnancy in the domestic cat after artificial insemination with previously frozen spermatozoa. J Reprod Fertil 1978;52(2): 279–82.

19. Luvoni GC. Gamete cryopreservation in the domestic cat. Theriogenology 2006; 66(1):101–11.

20. Buranaamnuay K. Protocols for sperm cryopreservation in the domestic cat: a review. Anim Reprod Sci 2017;183:56–65.

21. Villaverde AI, Fioratti EG, Penitenti M, et al. Cryoprotective effect of different glycerol concentrations on domestic cat spermatozoa. Theriogenology 2013;80(7): 730–7.

22. Buranaamnuay K. Determination of appropriate cryopreservation protocols for epididymal cat spermatozoa. Reprod Domest Anim 2015;50(3):378–85.

23. Zambelli D, Caneppele B, Castagnetti C, et al. Cryopreservation of cat semen in straws: comparison of five different freezing rates. Reprod Domest Anim 2002; 37(5):310–3.

24. Johnson AK, Pukazhenthi B. Semen collection, evaluation, and cryopreservation in the domestic feline. Clin Ther 2010;2(3):233–8.

25. Cocchia N, Ciani F, El-Rass R, et al. Cryopreservation of feline epididymal spermatozoa from dead and alive animals and its use in assisted reproduction. Zygote 2010;18(1):1–8.

26. Prochowska S, Nizanski W, Partyka A. Comparative analysis of in vitro characteristics of fresh and frozen-thawed urethral and epididymal spermatozoa from cats (*Felis domesticus*). Theriogenology 2016;86(8):2063–72.

Assisted Reproduction in the Female Cat

Aime K. Johnson, DVM

KEYWORDS

- Feline • Queen • Ovulation induction • In vitro fertilization • Cryopreservation
- Embryo transfer

KEY POINTS

- There have been great advances in assisted reproduction in the female cat in the past 10 to 20 years.
- Consistent ovulation induction and artificial insemination are vital to any assisted reproduction program.
- Many of these techniques developed in the domestic cat can be used to assist in the conservation efforts of the non-domestic cat.

INTRODUCTION

As a general reminder of the cat's reproductive cycle, the female cat is a seasonal polyestrus-induced ovulator. The queen requires more than one mating to achieve enough stimulation for the luteinizing hormone surge necessary for ovulation. Ovulation occurs in approximately 50% of queens after one mating, but approaches 100% of queens allowed to mate 4 or more times.[1] Observation of breeding episodes is helpful to evaluate the number of times the tom attempts to copulate and also to evaluate the female for the classic "after reaction" that confirms copulation took place. If the after reaction does not occur, penetration of the penis into the vagina was unlikely. Appropriate breeding management is often the key to good fertility in a cattery. Minor changes in procedures may have an enormous impact on pregnancy rate and litter size. When presented with a queen or cattery, a detailed history and observation of protocol are as essential as a complete physical examination. Because the queen is a long day breeder, maintaining the animals under artificial lighting for at least 14 hours per day reduces seasonal variation, but in the author's experience, even cats maintained under this lighting system experience a decrease in pregnancy rates during the shorter days of the year. A queen will typically show estrus within 1 to 2 months after initiating an artificial lighting period.

Disclosure Statement: The author has nothing to disclose.
Department of Clinical Sciences, Auburn University, 1500 Wire Road, Auburn, AL 36849, USA
E-mail address: akj0001@auburn.edu

Vet Clin Small Anim 48 (2018) 523–531
https://doi.org/10.1016/j.cvsm.2018.02.002
0195-5616/18/© 2018 Elsevier Inc. All rights reserved.

When presented a specific queen for breeding management, a general and reproductive physical examination (with blood chemistries and endocrine testing when indicated) should be performed to rule out obvious causes of infertility dealing with physical limitations (vaginal stricture) or generalized diseases (such as renal disease, diabetes, or hyperthyroidism). If physical/genital abnormalities are present or if there is no other obvious cause for the infertility, a karyotype of one or both members of the breeding pair may be necessary to confirm the genetic makeup of the animal is normal.

Use of a high-quality ultrasound unit will allow imaging of the uterus by starting at the bladder and moving cranially. The uterus should be evaluated for size, symmetry of the horns, the presence of thickened endometrium (**Fig. 1**) or cystic structures, and fluid within the lumen (**Fig. 2**). Ovaries can usually be detected immediately caudal to the kidneys and can be evaluated for the presence of follicles or cysts (**Fig. 3**).

Because cats are induced ovulators, successful induction of ovulation is critical for any assisted reproduction technique. One group has shown consistent results inducing estrus and ovulation using a combination of equine chorionic gonadotropin (eCG) and human chorionic gonadotropin (hCG) in a timed artificial insemination protocol.[2] Treatment is initiated in nonestral, nonluteal queens as determined by observing for behavioral estrus and a serum progesterone level less than 1 ng/mL. Queens received an initial injection of eCG (100 IU intramuscularly [IM]) followed by an injection of hCG (75 IU IM) 85 hours later. Insemination is performed 31 to 33 hours after the hCG injection, and ovulation is expected between 25 to 30 hours after hCG. Using this protocol, 100% of queens ovulated with a 75% pregnancy rate (6/8 queens) when inseminated with either laparoscopic intrauterine or laparoscopic oviductal inseminations.[2] This protocol can be modified to substitute porcine luteinizing hormone (pLH) for hCG. The estrus induction method used by this author is directly adapted from Conforti and colleagues.[2] Cats must be nonluteal and not in estrus before beginning the induction protocol (low progesterone and <50% cornified on vaginal cytology). Alternatively, cats can be placed on supplemental altrenogest (Regumate; 0.088 mg/kg orally) once daily for 38 days. After a withdrawal period of 5 days, the cats receive 100 IU eCG followed by pLH 85 hours later. Insemination should occur 30 to 33 hours later.

An alternate method is to allow the queen to come into a natural estrus and administer hCG intravenously twice daily on days 2 to 4 of estrus. The ovulation rate using this protocol was 95.6% (43/45 queens).[3] In this study, queens were inseminated at

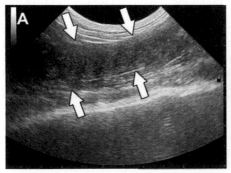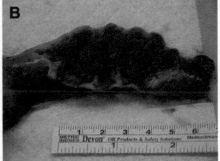

Fig. 1. (*A*) A longitudinal ultrasound image of the uterine horn in a 7-year-old queen. Note the light and dark linear striping along the uterus indicating thickened endometrium. The margins of the uterus are marked by arrows. (*B*) The same uterus after removal. Note the thickened folds of the endometrium.

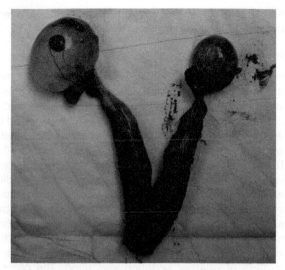

Fig. 2. Gross image of bilateral ovarian cysts in an infertile queen.

15, 20, and 30 hours after the last hCG injection. Ovulation is expected to occur between 25 and 27 hours after administration of hCG.

One concern with insemination protocols is the effect of anesthesia on ovulation. Howard and colleagues[4] reported that queens inseminated (laparoscopic intrauterine) after ovulation produced more corpora lutea and embryos and had a higher pregnancy rate than those inseminated before ovulation (50% vs 14.3% pregnancy rate). A mean of 6.6×10^6 motile sperm were used in both groups. Because of the concern that anesthesia may inhibit ovulation, many researchers elect to inseminate after ovulation

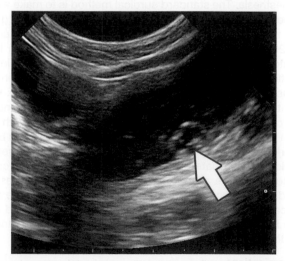

Fig. 3. An ultrasound image of the uterus. This uterus is fluid filled (*black hypoechoic area*) with an endometrial cyst present (*arrow*). This queen had a history of infertility and was eventually spayed. Cystic endometrial hyperplasia with a mucometra was confirmed on histopathology.

has occurred (28–40 hours). However, others have not found an effect of anesthesia on ovulation rate with slightly higher doses of hCG.[3]

Vaginal Insemination

When frozen semen was used for vaginal insemination, the pregnancy rate was low (10.7% or 6/56 attempts).[5] Vaginal insemination is therefore best reserved for cases in which a large amount of fresh or good-quality cooled transported semen is available. This procedure may be performed by inserting an open-ended tomcat catheter approximately 1 to 2 cm into the vaginal vault in the nonanesthetized queen, depositing the semen, and elevating the hind quarters for approximately 10 minutes to prevent backflow. This technique is difficult in many queens because of a less than compliant nature and the violent after reaction associated with breeding/vaginal stimulation. Most researchers have better success using a deep vaginal insemination technique under heavy sedation or general anesthesia. In the sedated queen, the vaginal vault is initially dilated with a 2-mm-diameter probe. The insemination pipette is then inserted 3 to 4 cm into the vaginal canal; the semen is deposited, and the hind quarters are elevated after insemination. Ovulation induction is still required after transvaginal insemination regardless of whether sedation was used. The pregnancy rate after vaginal insemination was 77.8% when 80×10^6 fresh motile sperm were used. The pregnancy rate decreased to 33.3% using 40×10^6 motile spermatozoa and 6.6% with 20×10^6 motile spermatozoa. The use of at least 80×10^6 motile spermatozoa when performing a vaginal insemination is commonly recommended.[3]

Intrauterine Insemination

The main advantage of intrauterine insemination in the queen is the reduction in insemination dose compared with vaginal insemination. In fact, a pregnancy rate of 80% was achieved using only 8×10^6 motile sperm (10% of the recommended vaginal dose) when inseminated surgically into one uterine horn,[6] and lower doses have also been successful. Intrauterine insemination is performed surgically with the queen under general anesthesia. The standard surgical method is to make a midline incision on the ventral abdomen. Both uterine horns are located and examined for signs of abnormality before insemination. Following visual examination, one uterine horn is isolated. A 22- to 20-gauge intravenous catheter is inserted through the uterine wall (mid horn) and into the lumen. The catheter is advanced off the needle into the uterine horn in the direction of the ovary. The needle is removed. The semen (approximately 20–50 μL) is infused through the catheter and into the uterine horn. Care should be taken not to contaminate the abdomen with the sperm sample. Once insemination is complete, the catheter is removed, and a gauze pad is placed with direct pressure over the insertion site to control bleeding. If desired, the process can be repeated into the opposite uterine horn with a fresh catheter. If both horns are inseminated, half of the semen should be inseminated into each horn. This procedure can also be performed laparoscopically. The advantage is that this technique is less invasive. The uterus is grasped with atraumatic forceps and stabilized against the abdominal wall. An intravenous catheter is inserted through the abdominal wall and guided into the proximal uterine horn toward the ovary. The needle is removed, and the semen is infused through the catheter into the uterine horn.

Transcervical insemination

Transcervical insemination is widely performed in the bitch. Although not as commonly performed in the queen, it was first described in 1988 by Hurlbut and colleagues.[7] Modifications on the technique were made and, in 2001, Zambelli and Cunto[8] showed promise with a narrower catheter. Placement through the cervix was accomplished with assistance through rectal digital manipulation, and placement was confirmed via ultrasound. More recently, Zambelli and Cunto[8] described an endoscopic trans-cervical technique. Queens were placed under general anesthesia in sternal recumbency with the hind end slightly elevated. An endoscope (120 mm in length, 1.1 mm in diameter, 0° view) was inserted until the dorsal vaginal fold was visualized. A specialized catheter with a rounded tip needle was passed alongside the endoscope and through the cervix. This technique was successful in 12 of 14 queens. In the 2 unsuccessful queens, failure was due to a narrowed vaginal canal that did not allow manipulation of the catheter and the scope at the same time. With the right equipment, this technique allows nonsurgical placement of the sperm into the uterus.

Laparoscopic oviductal insemination

Laparoscopic oviductal insemination is becoming more available, especially for nondomestic cats.[2,9] This procedure has produced successful pregnancies with much lower sperm numbers, as low as 1×10^6 motile sperm in 5 μL in each oviduct. Using this small amount of motile sperm allows the opportunity to achieve successful pregnancies with valuable, limited, or low-quality sperm. A disadvantage to this technique is that it can be challenging and requires specialized equipment. Using laparoscopic equipment for manipulation and visualization, the ovaries are identified and evaluated for response (number of corpora lutea [CLs] present) (**Fig. 4**). Specialized atraumatic forceps are used to identify and grasp the craniomedial edge of the ovarian bursa. An intravenous catheter is inserted through the abdominal wall, and a blunted 22-gauge needle is inserted through the catheter and into the oviductal opening. Five to 10 μL of semen is infused approximately 2 cm into the oviductal opening (**Fig. 5**). When using very small amounts of semen, placing the sample in the distal end of the needle will minimize loss of the inseminate.

Embryo transfer

Embryo transfer in the cat has lagged behind other domestic species such as the horse and cow. Nevertheless, the first successful embryo transfer procedure was first described in cats in the late 1970s.[10] In the late 1980s, Goodrowe and colleagues[11] evaluated the quality of embryos recovered after a natural or induced estrus. The recovery rate and number of embryos recovered were not different between groups;

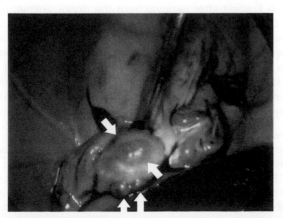

Fig. 4. A laparoscopic image of the ovary before oviductal insemination. Note the CLs present on the ovary (*arrows*).

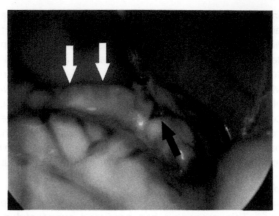

Fig. 5. The oviductal opening is exposed (*black arrow*). The oviduct can be seen to the left of the picture (*white arrows*). The blunted needle would be inserted approximately 1.5 to 2 cm into the oviductal opening toward the oviduct.

however, only 43% of embryos were of transferrable quality in the induced group compared with 79% in the natural group. After this time, work concentrated on improving hormonal induction protocols, and in the late 1980s, it was determined that a lower dose of follicle-stimulating hormone produced more viable embryos.[12] In 2000, Tsutsui and colleagues[13] described successful embryo transfer in the non–breeding season. Embryos (morulae) were collected 6 days after ovulation induction from the oviducts and proximal uterine horn after removal from the donor queen. Five embryos were transferred fresh into the uterine horn of the recipient that had the greatest number of CLs. Conception rate after transfer was 94.4% with a 68% embryo survival rate. In this study, pregnancy was maintained by a long-acting progestogen. A mention in this study was that 57.7% of the queens failed to deliver and required a cesarean section. In 2010, Yu and colleagues[14] evaluated the dose of eCG on the efficacy of superovulation and embryo production in the queen. In this study, varying doses of eCG were administered. One hundred hours after administration of eCG, 100 IU of hCG was administered. Cats were inseminated (surgical intrauterine) 30 hours after administration of hCG. Seven days later, the oviducts and uterine horns were flushed after removal from the donor animal. In this study, the mean number of blastocysts collected per cat, and the percentage of cats that produced embryos was highest for the 200 IU eCG dose group, but was still low at 1.5 blastocysts recovered per cat and 31.8% (21 of 66) of cats producing embryos. The in vivo collection of embryos is best accomplished after removal of the oviducts and uterus from the donor female, which serves as a disadvantage when the desire is to preserve genetics from valuable individuals. Therefore, in vitro fertilization (IVF) has become more widely accepted in the valuable queen.

In vitro fertilization

In the cat, oocytes are ovulated in metaphase II making IVF much easier than in the bitch. Goodrowe and colleagues[15] first reported the birth of kittens after transfer of IVF embryos in 1988. These researchers aspirated in vivo matured oocytes directly from the follicles of gonadotropin-treated queens, fertilized them in vitro, and transferred resulting 2- to 4-cell embryos into the oviducts of recipient queens. Five of the 6 cats receiving embryos became pregnant. Six to 18 embryos were transferred resulting in the birth of litters ranging from 1 to 4 kittens. In 1997, Pope and colleagues[16] reported the birth of kittens that resulted from the collection of immature oocytes matured and fertilized completely in vitro. Over the past decades, culture conditions have been modified with improved success with in vitro produced embryos. Currently, blastocysts are surgically transferred between days 4 and 6 into the uterus of recipients, corresponding with the approximate time when the embryos would enter the uterus naturally. Reports show blastocyst rates up to 50% to 80% on days 6 to 8.[17–19]

An advantage to in vitro production of embryos is the ability to aspirate the oocytes laparoscopically from the donor queen without damaging or removing the reproductive tract. Pope and colleagues[20] reported an average of 24 mature oocytes per aspiration session after treatment with gonadotropins. The number of oocytes recovered decreased over time in individual cats with the average number of oocytes recovered from aspirations 1 to 6 ranged from 30 to 40, but decreasing to 20 to 30 recovered oocytes for aspiration sessions 7 to 12. The interval between gonadotropin treatments in this laboratory averaged 7 to 8 months. Interestingly, more oocytes were recovered during the first aspiration of a donor cat's life when that aspiration occurred at 6 or 7 months of age (54 and 47 oocytes, respectively) rather than starting at 9 to 12 months (26–29 oocytes).

GAMETE PRESERVATION

To advance the genetics of valuable animals and especially the non-domestic feline species, cryopreservation of the female gametes would be beneficial. Feline oocytes and embryos contain a high level of fatty acids and therefore do not freeze well. The first litters born after embryo cryopreservation were reported in 1988.[21] The embryos were cryopreserved using techniques described in other species. Once thawed, they were incubated overnight before being transferred into recipients. Since this time, standard cryopreservation techniques have been replaced with vitrification in several species. Vitrification is a process that eliminates intracellular ice formation, but in doing so, exposes the embryo to osmotic changes and high levels of cryoprotectants that may be toxic to the embryo. In the cat, this technique has shown promise. Recently, a study examined the survival rate of embryos when vitrified at different stages of development. The conclusion was that embryos containing at least 4 cells through the compact blastocyst stage showed the highest survivability after thawing. For expanded blastocysts, reducing the blastocyst cavity before vitrification improved expansion rates after thawing. None of these embryos were transferred into recipients.[22] Cryopreservation of oocytes has been described, but is still considered experimental in most feline species. Recently, a study was performed evaluating 2 commercial vitrification kits and survivability of feline oocytes. Following vitrification, the oocytes underwent fertilization using intracytoplasmic sperm injection (ICSI) and in vitro maturation to assess survivability. However, even with the best conditions in this study, the highest rate of morula formation was low, with only 3 morula formed from 143 oocytes vitrified (35 oocytes matured, 10 cleaved after ICSI).[23]

SUMMARY

In conclusion, feline assisted reproduction has made great advances in the last few decades. In clinical practice, ovulation induction and surgical insemination are attainable with good success. Techniques such as embryo transfer and gamete cryopreservation are still limited to the research and endangered species setting, but with work, can become more commonplace in clinical medicine as techniques become more refined.

REFERENCES

1. Concannon P, Hodgson B, Lein D. Reflex LH release in estrous cats following single and multiple copulations. Biol Reprod 1980;23(1):111–7.
2. Conforti VA, Bateman HL, Schook MW, et al. Laparoscopic oviductal artificial insemination improves pregnancy success in exogenous gonadotropin-treated domestic cats as a model for endangered felids. Biol Reprod 2013;89(1):4.
3. Tanaka A, Takagi Y, Nakagawa K, et al. Artificial intravaginal insemination using fresh semen in cats. J Vet Med Sci 2000;62(11):1163–7.
4. Howard JG, Barone MA, Donoghue AM, et al. The effect of pre-ovulatory anaesthesia on ovulation in laparoscopically inseminated domestic cats. J Reprod Fertil 1992;96(1):175–86.
5. Platz CC, Wildt DE, Seager SW. Pregnancy in the domestic cat after artificial insemination with previously frozen spermatozoa. J Reprod Fertil 1978;52(2):279–82.
6. Tsutsui T, Tanaka A, Takagi Y, et al. Unilateral intrauterine horn insemination of fresh semen in cats. J Vet Med Sci 2000;62(12):1241–5.
7. Hurlbut SL, Bowen MJ, Kraemer DC. The feasibility of trans-cervical catheterization and nonsurgical embryo collection in the domestic cat (Felis-catus). Theriogenology 1988;29(1):264.
8. Zambelli D, Cunto M. Transcervical artificial insemination in the cat. Theriogenology 2005;64(3):698–705.
9. Swanson WF. Laparoscopic oviductal embryo transfer and artificial insemination in felids–challenges, strategies and successes. Reprod Domest Anim 2012;47(Suppl 6):136–40.
10. Kraemer DC, Flow BL, Schriver MD, et al. Embryo transfer in the nonhuman primate, feline and canine. Theriogenology 1979;11(1):51–62.
11. Goodrowe KL, Howard JG, Wildt DE. Comparison of embryo recovery, embryo quality, oestradiol-17 beta and progesterone profiles in domestic cats (Felis catus) at natural or induced oestrus. J Reprod Fertil 1988;82(2):553–61.
12. Dresser BL, Sehlhorst CS, Wachs KB, et al. Hormonal-stimulation and embryo collection in the domestic cat (Felis-catus). Theriogenology 1987;28(6):915–27.
13. Tsutsui T, Yamane I, Hattori I, et al. Feline embryo transfer during the nonbreeding season. J Vet Med Sci 2000;62(11):1169–75.
14. Yu XF, Cho SJ, Bang JI, et al. Effect of equine chorionic gonadotropin on the efficiency of superovulation induction for in vivo and in vitro embryo production in the cat. Theriogenology 2010;73(4):413–20.
15. Goodrowe KL, Wall RJ, O'Brien SJ, et al. Developmental competence of domestic cat follicular oocytes after fertilization in vitro. Biol Reprod 1988;39(2):355–72.
16. Pope CE, McRae MA, Plair BL, et al. In vitro and in vivo development of embryos produced by in vitro maturation and in vitro fertilization of cat oocytes. J Reprod Fertil Suppl 1997;51:69–82.
17. Freistedt P, Stojkovic M, Wolf E. Efficient in vitro production of cat embryos in modified synthetic oviduct fluid medium: effects of season and ovarian status. Biol Reprod 2001;65(1):9–13.
18. Freistedt P, Stojkovic P, Wolf E, et al. Energy status of nonmatured and in vitro-matured domestic cat oocytes and of different stages of in vitro-produced embryos: enzymatic removal of the zona pellucida increases adenosine triphosphate content and total cell number of blastocysts. Biol Reprod 2001;65(3):793–8.

19. Karja NW, Otoi T, Murakami M, et al. Effect of protein supplementation on development to the hatching and hatched blastocyst stages of cat IVF embryos. Reprod Fertil Dev 2002;14(5–6):291–6.
20. Pope CE. Aspects of in vivo oocyte production, blastocyst development, and embryo transfer in the cat. Theriogenology 2014;81(1):126–37.
21. Dresser BL, Gelwicks EJ, Wachs KB, et al. First successful transfer of cryopreserved feline (Felis catus) embryos resulting in live offspring. J Exp Zool 1988; 246(2):180–6.
22. Ochota M, Wojtasik B, Nizanski W. Survival rate after vitrification of various stages of cat embryos and blastocyst with and without artificially collapsed blastocoel cavity. Reprod Domest Anim 2017;52(Suppl 2):281–7.
23. Fernandez-Gonzalez L, Jewgenow K. Cryopreservation of feline oocytes by vitrification using commercial kits and slush nitrogen technique. Reprod Domest Anim 2017;52(Suppl 2):230–4.

Evaluation of Canine Sperm and Management of Semen Disorders

Kara A. Kolster, DVM

KEYWORDS

- Male • Dog • Sperm • Fertility

KEY POINTS

- A thorough assessment of semen quality in the dog includes evaluation of sperm motility, concentration, morphology, and membrane integrity.
- The use of computer-assisted sperm analysis tools allows consistent, objective, repeatable analyses.
- Pharmacologic therapy and dietary supplements may improve fertility.
- Proper husbandry and stud dog management maximizes fertility.

INTRODUCTION

The stud dog is half the equation when evaluating potential causes of infertility in a canine breeding. Assessing male fertility is often the first step because of the ease of obtaining a semen sample for analysis. Unfortunately, the results of routine laboratory tests may not always correlate with actual fertility. The most accurate method of assessing male fertility is insemination of a fertile female; however, this is time consuming and not practical for small breeding operations. The realistic evaluation is completed with an appropriate assortment of laboratory tests.

The three main areas to consider in evaluation of canine semen quality are (1) total sperm count; (2) viability, assessed as motility, progressive motility, live/dead ratio, and acrosomal membrane integrity; and (3) morphology. Once a problem has been identified, appropriate management and intervention may help to improve fertility in a particular stud dog.

OVERVIEW OF SEMEN ABNORMALITIES

Quality of semen reflects the health of the seminiferous tubules, epididymis, prostate, and the dog's general health. Sperm morphology, in particular, is determined by the seminiferous tubules and to a lesser extent by the epididymis.[1]

The author has nothing to disclose.
Springfield Veterinary Center, 4416 Springfield Road, Glen Allen, VA 23060, USA
E-mail address: karakolster@gmail.com

Vet Clin Small Anim 48 (2018) 533–545
https://doi.org/10.1016/j.cvsm.2018.02.003   vetsmall.theclinics.com

Spermatogenesis is the process through which spermatogonial stem cells undergo mitotic and meiotic divisions to become spermatids. This process occurs in the seminiferous epithelium. Spermiogenesis is the process, occurring in the lumen of the seminiferous tubules, through which spermatids undergo multiple cytologic transformations and mature into spermatozoa. The stages of spermatogenesis and spermiogenesis occur at specific locations within the seminiferous tubule. Aberrations of the testicular environment at any of these stages can result in the production of abnormal sperm and possible infertility (**Table 1**).

Significant maturational changes also occur as sperm pass through the efferent ductules and epididymis. It is in these areas that sperm develop the capacity for motility, the acrosomal membrane forms, the cytoplasmic droplet migrates distally and is shed, and some defective sperm are eliminated.[1] The most important functional changes occur in the efferent ductules and caput epididymis; sperm collected from these areas are not capable of fertilization. Sperm obtained from the cauda epididymis are capable of fertilization.[1] Sperm are stored and remain viable for a period of time in the cauda epididymis before ejaculation.

PHYSICAL EXAMINATION

Complete physical examination of the stud dog should be performed, to include palpation of testicular consistency, measurement of testicular width, visual examination of the penis and prepuce, palpation of the prostate per rectum, and ultrasonography of the prostate and testes, if indicated. Normal testicular consistency approximates a peeled, hard-boiled egg. It is common for one testis to be slightly larger than the other. A typical testis-to-epididymis size ratio is appreciated with experience; change in this ratio may indicate testicular atrophy or epididymal swelling. Any heat, swelling, pain, or dermatitis associated with the testes and scrotum should be noted.

LABORATORY EVALUATION OF SEMEN

Accurate semen analysis requires knowledge of the appropriate tools and tests to use, and evaluation of as many parameters as possible. Instructions for performing common procedures, such as semen collection, slide preparation for bright field microscopic motility and morphology evaluation, and use of a Neubauer hemacytometer, are not described. The reader is referred to previously published literature for details of these techniques.[2,3]

Semen evaluations have traditionally been performed manually; however, more recently computer-assisted sperm analysis (CASA) systems have become popular.[4] CASA systems are automated systems combining computer and microscope hardware and software to provide objective analysis of semen parameters. The initial development of CASA systems nearly 40 years ago was driven by the needs of commercial breeding operations and research laboratories to reduce the influence of human variability in semen analysis.[5] CASA systems offer rapid and accurate assessment of total motility; progressive motility; multiple other velocity parameters; concentration; and, in some systems, morphology.

The earliest CASA systems, CellSoft (CRYO Resources Ltd, New York, NY) and Hamilton-Thorne (Hamilton Thorne, Beverly, MA), and, more recently, SpermVision (MOFA Global, Verona, WI), are photometers. They function by obtaining multiple digital images of a field of sperm cells in rapid succession, identifying individual sperm cells, and tracking those sperm across frames to assess motility.[5] Semen samples are analyzed at a standard dilution, allowing the CASA system to calculate concentration of the raw sample.

Table 1
Common morphologic sperm abnormalities in the dog

Name	Primary/ Secondary	Major/ Minor	Description	Negative Effect on Fertility
Sperm head defects				
Knobbed acrosome	Primary	Major	Doubled over acrosomal membrane; may have knobbed, folded, or dented appearance	Yes
Pyriform or tapered head	Varies	Varies	Narrowing in distal portion of head (pyriform) or entire head (tapered)	Unknown
Microcephaly	Primary	Major	Excessively small head	Yes/unknown
Macrocephaly	Primary	Minor	Excessively large head	Unknown
Nuclear vacuoles (diadem defect)	Primary	Major	Crater-like appearance at equatorial or apical region of sperm head	Suspected
Detached heads	Secondary	Minor	Sperm head free from midpiece and tail	Yes
Midpiece defects				
Distal midpiece reflex	Primary	Major	Typically 180° bend at distal edge of midpiece; often cytoplasmic droplet at center of bend; double bend gives coiled appearance	Yes
Dag defect	Primary	Major	Fractured, coiled, or split midpiece	Yes
Segmental aplasia of mitochondrial sheath	Primary	Major	Narrowed area of midpiece, prone to fracture	None known
Proximal droplets	Primary	Major	Retained cytoplasmic droplet appears as focal swelling at proximal midpiece	Suspected
Distal droplets	Secondary	Minor	Retained cytoplasmic droplet appears as focal swelling at distal midpiece	None known
Pseudodroplet	Primary	Major	Abnormal distribution of mitochondrial sheath causes focal swelling that mimics cytoplasmic droplet	Unknown
Bowed midpiece	Secondary	Minor	Curved/rounded appearance of midpiece	Yes
Principle piece (tail) defects				
Bent principle piece	Secondary	Minor	180° bend of distal tail; likely stain artifact	None known
Coiled principle piece	Secondary	Minor	Tight coil of distal tail	Unknown

(continued on next page)

Table 1 *(continued)*				
Name	**Primary/ Secondary**	**Major/ Minor**	**Description**	**Negative Effect on Fertility**
Abaxial and multiple tails	Secondary	Minor	Tail attachment offset from center of head; multiple tails	None known
Other defects				
Teratoid forms	Primary	Major	Severe morphologic aberrations, may not be easily recognizable as sperm	Yes

Adapted from Barth AD, Oko RJ. Abnormal morphology of bovine spermatozoa. Ames (IA): Iowa State University Press; 1989; and Chenoweth PJ. Genetic sperm defects. Theriogenology 2005;64:130–279; with permission.

There are other semen analyzers available that are not part of a CASA system. The Sperma-Q (MOFA Global) is a photometer that can measure concentration, but not motility, of a semen sample. Densimeters, such as the ARS Densimeter (Animal Reproduction Systems, Chino, CA), are instruments that measure semen concentration based on transmittance of light through the sample as compared with a standard buffer.

All photometers and densimeters are calibrated to a certain concentration range; therefore, samples outside this range must be diluted for accurate measurement. Additionally, the parameters by which a CASA system identifies and analyzes sperm cells vary by species, instrument, and settings. Differences in the technical settings of these instruments can vary the results obtained.[6] This is an important consideration when comparing results between laboratories, and in fresh versus chilled or cryopreserved semen containing egg yolk extender.

Newer CASA systems, such as SpermVision and NucleoCounter SP-100 (Chemo-Metec, Allerod, Denmark), can evaluate sperm viability, defined as membrane integrity, by fluorescent labeling. This is an important advancement because viability, along with total and progressive motility, sperm morphology, DNA quality, concentration, and total sperm number, are correlated with fertility.[7–9] The Nucleocounter SP-100 measures viability by comparing two samples from the same ejaculate. The first sample is diluted in a buffer that lyses cell membranes. The lysate is loaded into a sample cassette prefilled with propidium iodide (PI), which stains the free nuclei. A green light is passed through the sample chamber, causing the PI-labeled nuclei to fluoresce red and allowing the cells to be counted by the instrument. The second sample is diluted in phosphate-buffered saline, which does not alter cell membranes. PI does not penetrate intact cell membranes. When the second sample is loaded into the PI-filled cassette, only the nuclei of cells with damaged membranes are labeled with PI. This sample is also analyzed by fluorescence. The difference between the lysate and nonlysed samples is used to calculate the percent viability, or percent of membrane-intact sperm in the original sample.[10,11]

Fluorescence microscopy was previously only available in university and research settings. Advancement of CASA systems is making this technology more widely available. Additionally, CASA systems with reagents in prefilled, disposable cassettes reduce human exposure to potentially hazardous DNA dyes. Work has begun using fluorescent markers to correlate fertility parameters in a population of know fertile male dogs.[12]

Normal sperm count is directly correlated to body size and testicular volume.[2] The total volume of the ejaculate is highly dependent on the amount of prostatic fluid, or third fraction, of ejaculate collected. The second, sperm-rich, fraction is the most important sample for evaluation. Semen concentration is determined using a hemocytometer, a CASA system, other photometer or densimeter, or fluorescent markers. Concentration per milliliter is multiplied by ejaculate volume to obtain the total sperm count. Correct dilution in any methodology is vital to obtain an accurate result. This is done using calibrated laboratory pipettes, a commercial leukocyte dilution system (LeukoChek, Biomedical Polymers, Gardner, MA), or diluents appropriate to a specific CASA system. CASA systems exhibit lower variability than human-derived (eg, hemocytometer) measurements of semen concentration.[13,14] However, accuracy of a CASA system may vary depending on sample concentration and inclusion or exclusion of background debris from measurement.[5,14] CASA systems that exclude background debris from measurement are useful for measuring sperm concentration in semen extended with egg yolk.

Without the aid of a CASA system, total motility and progressive motility are evaluated subjectively on wet mount by bright field microscopy. Live/dead ratio is subjectively evaluated using bright field microscopy and a vital stain, such as eosin-nigrosin. The intact sperm membrane is not permeable to certain stains. Cells that exclude stain are considered live. Cells that take up the stain have a permeable membrane and are likely dead. The Nucleocounter SP-100 has significantly lower variability in evaluating sperm membrane integrity compared with human-analyzed tests, such as live/dead staining.[15]

Sperm membrane integrity is also evaluated by the hypo-osmotic swelling test. When exposed to a hypo-osmotic environment, sperm cells with intact membranes allow fluid to enter the cell to balance the osmotic gradient. The influx of fluid causes the sperm cell to swell. This is most evident as curling of the tail, which is seen on wet mount under bright field microscopy. Hypo-osmotic swelling test results in fresh semen samples are positively correlated with progressive motility and normal morphology.[16]

Sperm morphology is perhaps one of the most commonly misused tests in semen analysis. Accurate evaluation requires appropriate stains, quality bright field, phase-contrast, or differential interference contrast microscopy, and knowledge and experience in identifying sperm abnormalities. Canine sperm morphology is commonly evaluated using an eosin-nigrosin stain or a modified Giemsa stain.[17] Spermac stain (Conception Technologies, San Diego, CA) is also useful, particularly for evaluation of acrosomal membranes.[18] When using a quick preparation modified Giemsa stain, immersion at each step for 5 minutes is recommended[3]; this is significantly longer than manufacturer recommendations. Rapid drying of the slide minimizes staining artifacts.[2] Phase-contrast microscopy uses light to produce a high contrast image of transparent cells, therefore eliminating the need for stain. A minimum of 200 sperm should be counted, and percentage of normal and abnormal sperm calculated.[3] Some CASA systems have the ability to evaluate morphology; however, this is generally limited to analysis of the sperm head and is highly dependent on the software settings of a particular instrument.[6]

There are several systems for categorizing sperm morphologic abnormalities. In one of the more common classification systems, primary abnormalities are considered those that develop during spermatogenesis or spermiogenesis and are caused by pathologic processes in the seminal epithelium, and secondary abnormalities are considered those that originate after sperm has left the testes and are caused by abnormal epididymal function. Abnormalities that occur because of rough handling after ejaculation are artifactual changes and should be differentiated as such. Another system classifies sperm with major abnormalities as those with severe aberrations that are generally believed to be incapable of fertilization, and minor abnormalities as those that are less likely to cause changes in fertility.[1] This creates some confusion because there is often not detailed knowledge of the effect on fertility of specific morphologic abnormalities in the dog.

Serum hormone measurements may be useful in further characterizing infertility in dogs. Male dogs with at least 12 months duration of infertility showed lower basal testosterone levels than dogs of normal fertility.[19] Increased follicle stimulating hormone (FSH) can be a marker of primary testicular failure.[2,20] This occurs because of decreased negative feedback from inhibin, which is normally produced by the Sertoli cells.[2] Increased FSH in the face of declining semen quality or azoospermia carries a poor prognosis because the testicular changes are likely irreversible.[21] These tests should be performed by a laboratory with validated assays for the dog.

Alkaline phosphatase is used to indicate patency of the ductus deferens in the dog. Nearly all of the alkaline phosphatase present in a normal ejaculate is contributed by the second, sperm-rich, fraction.[22] The cutoff of 5000 U/L is generally used to indicate a complete ejaculate. It is useful to analyze a suspected second fraction and a known third fraction sample for comparison. Low alkaline phosphatase in an azoospermic sample, particularly in both the suspected second and known third fractions, can indicate bilateral epididymal obstruction or incomplete ejaculation.[22] High alkaline phosphatase in an azoospermic ejaculate, or alkaline phosphatase significantly higher in the second versus third fraction, indicates failure of spermatogenesis and carries a poor prognosis for future fertility. Dogs with one functional testis have lower alkaline phosphatase levels in the presence of an ejaculate containing sperm than normal intact males.[22]

Anti-Müllerian hormone is produced in the male exclusively by the Sertoli cells. It is used as a diagnostic tool for determining gonadectomy status in a suspect cryptorchid dog.[23] Recent evidence has indicated anti-Müllerian hormone may be a biomarker for testicular atrophy and Sertoli cell tumor in the dog.[24–26]

Ultrasonography is an important tool in evaluation of stud dog fertility. It has been used for some time in evaluation of prostatic disease and testicular tumors. More recently, B-mode and Doppler ultrasonography have been correlated to current fertility in the dog.[19,27] Increased echogenicity of the testes was associated with fewer morphologically normal sperm.[27] Conversely, a study in bulls showed that hypoechoic testes were associated with poor morphology.[28] It is possible that both increased and decreased echogenicity may represent changes in the testicular architecture that lead to decreased semen quality. The rate of blood flow through the testicular artery is positively correlated to current semen quality, likely because it represents a marker of the rate of spermatogenesis.[19,29] Testicular echogenicity may correlate to future change in semen motility. No ultrasound parameters have been correlated to future change in total sperm output or total morphologically normal sperm.[29] Testicular size and total sperm output are positively correlated with body weight in the dog; however, in dogs of comparable body weight, testicular volume, as measured by ultrasonography, has not been shown to be a reliable indicator of fertility.[2,19]

PHARMACOLOGIC TREATMENTS

Numerous dietary supplements have been used by veterinarians and dog owners to improve semen quality in stud dogs. Data supporting these uses in most cases are sparse and frequently conflicting. All dietary supplements should be administered cautiously, especially when no beneficial effects are proven and detrimental effects are possible.

Fish oil or other fatty acid supplements have been evaluated in multiple studies with results ranging from no effect to varied beneficial effects in boars,[30–32] turkeys,[33] rams,[34] rats,[35] and stallions.[36] A recent study in normospermic dogs supplemented with fish oil showed significantly increased percent motility, total sperm count, total sperm viability, and a trend toward increased percent morphologically normal sperm.[37] The sperm membrane contains large amounts of phospholipids. It is possible that supplementing fatty acids may increase flexibility of the sperm membrane and thus improve flagellar motion and observable motility. Evidence in rams suggests that fish oil supplementation increases sperm concentration because of an acceleration of spermatogenesis.[34]

Vitamin E supplementation of dogs classified with poor semen quality increased their percent motile sperm and total sperm count to levels similar to normospermic dogs.[38] Increased serum testosterone and levels of superoxide dismutase were also observed.[38] Testosterone drives Leydig cell function and thus higher levels may improve semen quality. Superoxide dismutase is an important antioxidant and free radical scavenger; it is normally produced in the testes, prostate, and epididymis. Low superoxide dismutase is associated with poor sperm quality.[38] The risk of oxidative damage within the testes may be Increased by fatty acid supplementation. Some of the conflicting results in studies evaluating fish oil supplementation on sperm quality may be caused by lack cosupplementation with vitamin E or other antioxidants.[37,39]

Selenium acts indirectly as an antioxidant in the testes. Cosupplementation of selenium and vitamin E increases the percent of morphologically normal sperm in dogs. However, excessive selenium supplementation should be avoided because that can actually increase sperm damage.[39]

Zinc in prostatic fluid helps to protect against infection and stabilize sperm DNA. Low zinc levels have been associated with decreased fertility in dogs.[40] Zinc supplementation at low doses Is harmless but high doses may cause toxicity.

Glucosamine and glycosaminoglycans, most commonly chondroitin sulfate, have been anecdotally reported to improve semen quality in multiple species. It is a component of several nutritional supplements marketed for male dogs and recommended by some veterinarians.[41] However, there is no documentation of beneficial effect. There are no known adverse effects of supplementation.[42]

Carnitine is involved in fatty acid transport into the sperm cell, which is then used to produce energy and allow for sperm motility. It may also have a role in sperm maturation, and as an antioxidant and free radical scavenger. No specific reproductive studies have been performed in dogs but it has been examined in sport dogs and cardiac patients, and reproductive evidence from humans and laboratory species is promising. Significantly lower levels of L-carnitine were found in the seminal fluid of infertile men compared with fertile men.[43] In another study, carnitine levels in semen were positively correlated to total sperm count, percent motility, and percent morphologically normal sperm.[44] Addition of L-carnitine to culture media improved the motility and chromatin quality of mouse sperm.[45] In mice, carnitine supplementation hastened recovery from experimentally induced testicular damage.[46–48] Supplemental carnitine is used in certain cases of cardiomyopathy in the dog, and was found to have beneficial effects on body temperature, respiratory rate, and inflammatory cytokines in heavily exercised dogs, such as search and rescue dogs.[49] The recommended dose is 50 mg/kg daily.[50] Carnitine is naturally high in meat and milk, so dogs eating foods high in animal protein likely do not need additional supplementation. There are no documented toxicity studies in dogs.

Benign prostatic hyperplasia (BPH) is another cause of oxidative stress to the testes and developing sperm. Sperm are particularly susceptible to oxidative damage because of their reduced cytoplasm content and limited amount of natural antioxidants. Reactive oxygen species can accumulate in the prostatic fluid of dogs with BPH, causing increased number of sperm with fragmented DNA, increased percentage of morphologic defects, and decreased mitochondrial activity, which affects the ability of sperm to penetrate the zona pellucida.[40,51] Increased prostatic fluid pH in dogs with BPH may also contribute to sperm damage.[40,52] Interestingly, no change was seen in sperm motility between healthy dogs and dogs with BPH, suggesting that the damage may not be evident on cursory semen evaluation.[51] Standard medical treatment with a 5-α reductase inhibitor (eg, finasteride) and antibiotics, if prostatitis is also present, may improve semen quality in dogs with BPH by reducing the amount of oxidative sperm damage and normalizing characteristics of prostatic fluid.

Gonadotropin-releasing hormone may be used to temporarily increase testosterone and luteinizing hormone in male dogs when no definitive cause for infertility has been identified.[53] This treatment increased the semen quality of three oligozoospermic dogs sufficient to produce litters.[54] Multiple protocols exist with none clearly superior.[2,55] Gonadotropin-releasing hormone should not be used chronically because the subsequent down-regulation of FSH and luteinizing hormone causes cessation of spermatogenesis.[55,56]

NONPHARMACOLOGIC TREATMENTS

Normal spermatogenesis occurs at temperatures 3° to 5° lower than body temperature. Increased scrotal temperature is known to cause temporary testicular dysfunction and sperm abnormalities in multiple livestock species. Generally, minimal to no change is seen in the first 10 days after heat insult because sperm ejaculated during that time were nearly mature and in transit through the epididymis when hyperthermia occurred.[57] Depending on the intensity and duration of the insult, sperm abnormalities may be seen for the length of one or more spermatogenic cycles (62 days in the dog). Dogs may be less sensitive than other studied species to heat stress. No significant changes were seen in the semen quality of dogs exposed to moderate, short-term scrotal hyperthermia.[58] The effects of higher temperatures or longer duration hyperthermia on canine semen have not been studied. Anecdotally, some individual dogs seem more susceptible to heat stress than others. Frostbite and contact with irritating disinfectants or rough kennel surfaces are a source of heat stress secondary to scrotal dermatitis, and systemic illness causing fever and obesity can also increase scrotal temperature. Management of living conditions and general health to reduce the risk of heat stress may be beneficial to some dogs. This can include planning collections for semen freezing during the cooler months of the year.

Dog owners and inseminating veterinarians often request multiple semen collections over a short period of time (eg, two collections in the same day) and popular stud dogs may have multiple bitches to breed in quick succession. Frequency of semen collection has a significant effect on the number of sperm obtained. In dogs collected every 2 to 3.5 days, the total number of sperm obtained per collection did not change. When collection frequency was increased to once or twice daily, the number of sperm per collection decreased rapidly, presumably until daily sperm output was reached. The amount of sperm obtained over a given period of time was not significantly changed regardless of collection frequency, that is, daily collections for 7 days resulted in the same total number of sperm as two semiweekly collections.[59] Another study showed that a second collection in one day produced 70% more total sperm than one collection.[60] When semen collection is repeated on subsequent days, sperm numbers drop to reflect the daily sperm output. Thus, there is no long-term benefit in total sperm number with increased collection frequency. There is no evidence of significant change in semen motility or percent of morphologically normal sperm with increased frequency of collection in normospermic dogs.[59,60] This suggests that in dogs with normal fertility, there is no benefit to a "clean out" collection frequently requested by owners. However, in dogs exhibiting asthenoteratospermia, increased collection frequency was thought to stimulate secretory function of the epididymal epithelial cells, and to normalize pH and sodium/potassium ratio in seminal plasma. This may help maintain acceptable semen quality in these dogs.[61]

Assisted-reproductive technologies, such as intracytoplasmic sperm injection, which can aid conception using poor-quality sperm in other species, are not yet available in canine theriogenology. One available technique that may prove useful is sperm separation by density-gradient centrifugation. This process separates viable, motile sperm from nonmotile sperm. It can also remove certain contaminants, such as red blood cells.[62] Multiple commercial products are available. Several have been shown to increase the percentage of progressively motile sperm, sperm viability, membrane integrity, and in vitro oocyte penetration rate of treated ejaculates.[63–65] Although it is not likely to be indicated for most dogs, sperm separation may increase breeding success in certain cases of subfertility and when using epididymal sperm.[65]

PROGNOSIS

Transitory insults to sperm production are expected to improve with time, a minimum length of one complete spermatogenic cycle from resolution of the underlying cause. Therefore, repeat semen evaluations are recommended at approximately 2-month intervals. The recommendation is the same to evaluate response to any dietary supplements or husbandry modifications. Serial evaluations provide the best prognostic information.

Some conditions may cause irreversible testicular changes, and thus a guarded prognosis for future fertility. It is wise to caution owners of such dogs that, if any viable sperm are being produced, they may be fertile but likely not consistent producers. Continued inclusion of subfertile males is often dependent on the goals of the breeding program, and whether that male's genetic value outweighs the breeder's need to reliably achieve pregnancies.

SUMMARY

Fertility evaluation of the male dog should start with thorough a physical examination and assessment of total sperm count, viability, and morphology. Adjunct tests, such as ultrasonography and serum hormone levels, may help identify the cause of abnormal semen parameters. Some cases of infertility may resolve with treatment of the underlying cause. In cases that are not expected to improve, owners are counseled in their breeding decisions.

Thorough and accurate evaluation of a male dog's potential fertility, and interpretation of findings and counsel based on results, is a valuable service that veterinarians can provide to dog breeders and owners.

REFERENCES

1. Barth AD, Oko RJ. Abnormal morphology of bovine spermatozoa. Ames (IA): Iowa State University Press; 1989.

2. Johnston SD, Root Kustritz MV, Olson PNS. Canine and feline theriogenology. Philadelphia: W.B. Saunders; 2001.
3. Root Kustritz MV. The value of canine semen evaluation for practitioners. Theriogenology 2007;68:329–37.
4. Amann RP, Waberski D. Computer-assisted sperm analysis (CASA): capabilities and potential developments. Theriogenology 2014;81:5–17.
5. Amann RP, Katz DF. Reflections on CASA after 25 years. J Androl 2004;25: 317–25.
6. Rijsselaere T, Van Soom A, Maes D, et al. Computer-assisted sperm analysis in dogs and cats: an update after 20 years. Reprod Domest Anim 2012;47(Suppl 6):204–7.
7. Fraser L, Gorszczaruk K, Strzezek J. Relationship between motility and membrane integrity of boar spermatozoa in media varying in osmolality. Reprod Domest Anim 2001;36:325–9.
8. Love CC, Thompson JA, Brinsko SP, et al. Relationship between stallion sperm motility and viability as detected by two fluorescence staining techniques using flow cytometry. Theriogenology 2003;60:1127–38.
9. Love CC, Noble JK, Standridge SA, et al. The relationship between sperm quality in cool-shipped semen and embryo recovery rate in horses. Theriogenology 2015;84:1587–93.
10. NucleoCounter SP-100 user's guide, revision 1.5. Allerod (Denmark): ChemoMetec A/S; 2006. Available at: https://chemometec.com/cell-counters/sperm-cell-counter-sp-100-nucleocounter/. Accessed December 2, 2017.
11. Viability testing with NucleoCounter SP-100, addendum to user's guide, revision 1.3. Allerod (Denmark): ChemoMetec A/S; 2006. Available at: https://chemometec.com/cell-counters/sperm-cell-counter-sp-100-nucleocounter/. Accessed December 2, 2017.
12. Hesser A, Darr C, Gonzales K, et al. Semen evaluation and fertility assessment in a purebred dog breeding facility. Theriogenology 2017;87:115–23.
13. Scofield DB, Baumber-Skaife J, Loomis PR. Improvements in equine semen processing techniques that aid optimal fertility. Clinical Theriogenology 2016;8: 465–9.
14. Hansen C, Vermeiden T, Vermeiden JPW, et al. Comparison of FACSCount AF system, improved Neubauer hemocytometer, corning 254 photometer, SpermVision, UltiMate and NucleoCounter SP-100 for determination of sperm concentration of boar semen. Theriogenology 2006;66:2188–94.
15. Daub L, Geyer A, Braun J, et al. Sperm membrane integrity in fresh and frozen-thawed canine semen samples: a comparison of vital stains with the Nucleo-Counter SP-100. Theriogenology 2016;86:651–6.
16. Karger S, Geiser B, Grau M, et al. Prognostic value of a pre-freeze hypo-osmotic swelling test on the post-thaw quality of dog semen. Anim Reprod Sci 2016;166: 141–7.
17. Kruger TF, Ackerman SB, Simmons KF, et al. A quick, reliable staining technique for human sperm morphology. Arch Androl 1987;18:275–7.
18. Goericke-Pesch S, Failing K. Retrospective analysis of canine semen evaluations with special emphasis on the use of the hypoosmotic swelling (HOS) test and acrosomal evaluation using Spermac. Reprod Domest Anim 2013;48:213–7.
19. de Souza MB, England GB, Mota Filho AC, et al. Semen quality, testicular B-mode and Doppler ultrasound, and serum testosterone concentrations in dogs with established infertility. Theriogenology 2015;84:805–10.

20. Douglas RH, Umphenour N. Endocrine abnormalities and hormonal therapy. Vet Clin North Am Equine Pract 1992;8:237–49.
21. Kelsey TW, McConville L, Edgar AB, et al. Follicle stimulating hormone is an accurate predictor of azoospermia in childhood cancer survivors. Schlatt S. ed. PLoS One 2017;12(7):e0181377.
22. Tornelli A, Arauz M, Baschard H, et al. Unilateral and bilateral vasectomy in the dog: alkaline phosphatase as an indicator of tubular patency. Reprod Domest Anim 2003;38:1–4.
23. Themmon APN, Kalra B, Visser JA, et al. The use of anti-mullerian hormone as diagnostic for gonadectomy status in dogs. Theriogenology 2016;86:1467–74.
24. Giudice C, Banco B, Veronesi MC, et al. Immunohistochemical expression of markers of immaturity in Sertoli and seminal cells in canine testicular atrophy. J Comp Pathol 2014;150:208–15.
25. Banco B, Veronesi MC, Giudice C, et al. Immunohistochemical evaluation of the expression of anti-mullerian hormone in mature, immature and neoplastic canine Sertoli cells. J Comp Pathol 2012;146:18–23.
26. Holst BS, Dreimanis U. Anti-mullerian hormone: a potentially useful biomarker for the diagnosis of canine Sertoli cell tumours. BMC Vet Res 2015;11:166.
27. Moxon R, Bright L, Pritchard B, et al. Digital image analysis of testicular and prostatic ultrasonographic echogenicity and heterogeneity in dogs and the relation to semen quality. Anim Reprod Sci 2015;160:112–9.
28. Arteaga AA, Barth AD, Brito LFC. Relationship between semen quality and pixel-intensity of testicular ultrasonograms after scrotal insulation in beef bulls. Theriogenology 2005;64:408–15.
29. England G, Bright L, Pritchard B, et al. Canine reproductive ultrasound examination for predicting future sperm quality. Reprod Domest Anim 2017;52(Suppl 2): 202–7.
30. Rooke JA, Shao CC, Speake BK. Effects of feeding tuna oil on the lipid composition of pig spermatozoa and in vitro characteristics of semen. Reproduction 2001;121:315–22.
31. Castellano CA, Audet I, Bailey JL, et al. Effect of dietary n-3 fatty acids (fish oils) on boar reproduction and semen quality. J Anim Sci 2010;88:2346–55.
32. Yeste M, Barrera X, Coll D, et al. The effects on boar sperm quality of dietary supplementation with omega-3 polyunsaturated fatty acids differ among porcine breeds. Theriogenology 2011;76:184–96.
33. Blesbois E, Douard V, Germain M, et al. Effects of n-3 polyunsaturated dietary supplementation on the reproductive capacity of male turkeys. Theriogenology 2004;61:537–49.
34. Samadian F, Towhidi A, Rezayazdi K, et al. Effects of dietary n-3 fatty acids on characteristics and lipid composition of ovine sperm. Animal 2010;4:2017–22.
35. Sebokova E, Garg ML, Wierzbicki A, et al. Alteration of the lipid composition of rat testicular plasma membranes by dietary (n-3) fatty acids changes the responsiveness of Leydig cells and testosterone synthesis. J Nutr 1990;120:610–8.
36. Brinsko SP, Varner DD, Love CC, et al. Effect of feeding a DHA-enriched nutraceutical on the quality of fresh, cooled and frozen stallion semen. Theriogenology 2005;63:1519–27.
37. Risso A, Pellegrino FJ, Relling AE, et al. Effect of long-term fish oil supplementation on semen quality and serum testosterone concentrations in male dogs. Int J Fertil Steril 2016;10:223–31.

38. Kawakami E, Kobayashi M, Hori T, et al. Therapeutic effects of vitamin E supplementation in 4 dogs with poor semen quality and low superoxide dismutase activity in seminal plasma. J Vet Med Sci 2016;77:1711–4.
39. Kirchoff KT, Kailing K, Goericke-Pesch S. Effect of dietary vitamin E and selenium supplementation on semen quality in Cairn Terriers with normospermia. Reprod Domest Anim 2017;52(6):945–52.
40. Krakowski L, Wachocka A, Brodzki P, et al. Sperm quality and selected biochemical parameters of seminal fluid in dogs with benign prostatic hyperplasia. Anim Reprod Sci 2015;160:120–5.
41. Hess M. Documented and anecdotal effects of certain pharmaceutical agents used to enhance semen quality in the dog. Theriogenology 2006;66:613–7.
42. Bhathal A, Spryszak M, Louizos C, et al. Glucosamine and chondroitin use in canines for osteoarthritis: a review. Open Vet J 2017;7:36–49.
43. Ahmed SD, Karira KA, Jagdesh, et al. Role of L-carnitine in male infertility. J Pak Med Assoc 2011;61:732–6.
44. Matalliotakisi I, Koumantaki Y, Evageliou A, et al. L-carnitine levels in the seminal plasma of fertile and infertile men: correlation with sperm quality. Int J Fertil Womens Med 2000;45:236–40.
45. Aliabadi E, Soleimani Mehranjani M, Borzoei Z, et al. Effects of L-carnitine and L-acetyl-carnitine on testicular sperm motility and chromatin quality. Iran J Reprod Med 2012;10:77–82.
46. Amendola R, Bartoleschi C, Cordelli E, et al. Effects of L-acetylcarnitine (LAC) on the post-injury recovery of mouse spermatogenesis monitored by flow cytometry. 1. Recovery after X-irradiation. Andrologia 1989;21:568–75.
47. Amendola R, Cordelli E, Mauro F, et al. Effects of L-acetylcarnitine (LAC) on the post-injury recovery of mouse spermatogenesis monitored by flow cytometry. 2. Recovery after hyperthermic treatment. Andrologia 1991;23:135–40.
48. Ramadan LA, Abd-Allah AR, Aly HA, et al. Testicular toxicity effects of magnetic field exposure and prophylactic role of coenzyme Q10 and L-carnitine in mice. Pharmacol Res 2002;46:363–70.
49. Clero D, Feugier A, Driss F, et al. Influence of pre and per-exercise nutritional supplementation on working dogs biological markers evolution during a standardized exercise. EC Veterinary Science 2015;1(1):10–25.
50. Pelletier B. L-carnitine or vitamin B6 of interest in the dog. Action Veterinaire 1992;1210:19.
51. Flores RB, Angrimani D, Rui BR, et al. The influence of benign prostatic hyperplasia on sperm morphological features and sperm DNA integrity in dogs. Reprod Domest Anim 2017;52(Suppl 2):310–5.
52. Fontbonne A. Infertility in male dogs: recent advances. Rev Bras Reprod Anim, Belo Horizonte 2011;35:266–73.
53. Purswell BJ, Wilcke JR. Response to gonadotrophin-releasing hormone by the intact male dog: serum testosterone, luteinizing hormone and follicle-stimulating hormone. J Reprod Fertil Suppl 1993;47:335–41.
54. Kawakami E, Hori T, Tsutsui T. Changes in plasma luteinizing hormone, testosterone and estriadiol-17 beta levels and semen quality after injections of gonadotropin releasing hormone agonist and human chorionic gonadotropin in three dogs with oligozoospermia and two dogs with azoospermia. Anim Reprod Sci 1997;47:157–67.
55. Goericke-Pesch S. Long-term effects of GnRH agonists on fertility and behavior. Reprod Domest Anim 2017;52(Suppl 2):336–47.

56. Ramaswamy S, Weinbauer GF. Endocrine control of spermatogenesis: role of FSH and LH/testosterone. Spermatogenesis 2014;4:e996025.

57. England GCW. Physiology and endocrinology of the male. In: England GCW, von Heimendahl A, editors. BSAVA manual of canine and feline reproduction and neonatology. Gloucester (England): British Small Animal Veterinary Association; 2010. p. 13–22.

58. Henning H, Masal C, Herr A, et al. Effect of short-term scrotal hyperthermia on spermatological parameters, testicular blood flow and gonadal tissue in dogs. Reprod Domest Anim 2014;49:145–57.

59. Boucher JH, Foote RH, Kirk RW. The evaluation of semen quality in the dog and the effects of frequency of ejaculation upon semen quality, libido, and depletion of sperm reserves. Cornell Vet 1958;48:67–86.

60. England GB. Semen quality in dogs and the influence of a short-interval second ejaculation. Theriogenology 1999;52:981–6.

61. Kawakami E, Hori T, Tsutsui T. Changes in semen quality and in vitro sperm capacitation during various frequencies of semen collection in dogs with both asthenozoospermia and teratozoospermia. J Vet Med Sci 1998;60:607–14.

62. Phillips TC, Dhaliwal GK, Verstegen-Onclin KM, et al. Efficacy of four density gradient separation media to remove erythrocytes and nonviable sperm from canine semen. Therlogenology 2012;77:39–45.

63. Dorado J, Alcaraz L, Duarte N, et al. Change in the structures of motile sperm subpopulations in dog spermatozoa after both cryopreservation and centrifugation on PureSperm® gradient. Anim Reprod Sci 2011;125:211–8.

64. Dorado J, Alcaraz L, Duarte N, et al. Centrifugation on PureSperm® density gradient improved quality of spermatozoa from frozen-thawed semen. Theriogenology 2011;76:381–5.

65. Hishinuma M, Sekine J. Separation of canine epididymal sperm by Percoll gradient centrifugation. Theriogenology 2004;61:365–72.

Breeding Soundness Examination of the Bitch

Carla Barstow, DVM*, Robyn R. Wilborn, DVM, MS, Aime K. Johnson, DVM

KEYWORDS

- Canine • Bitch • Breeding soundness evaluation (BSE) • Fertility

KEY POINTS

- A thorough physical examination done at the beginning of a bitch's breeding career may help identify any abnormalities that may cause a problem in the future.
- Obtaining an accurate history is important to guide diagnostic testing and future breeding management.
- Interpret diagnostic results with respect to the patient. Results should be examined as a whole and not as individual parts.

INTRODUCTION

The breeding soundness examination (BSE) is performed to identify animals that may have a challenge with fertility. A BSE, however, represents a limited point in time, during which they are considered either fertile or subfertile, and that status may fluctuate throughout the year. A BSE provides a minimum database of information to assist clinicians in making a judgment about an animal's future fertility.[1] These examinations are routinely performed in male dogs, because it is relatively easy to collect a semen sample for analysis and examine the testicles and prostate. BSEs are infrequently performed in bitches largely due to the inability to easily examine most of the reproductive organs. A BSE, however, can provide valuable information to guide future breedings and can assist in maximizing future fertility. A limited BSE can be performed at any time of a bitch's cycle; however, if the goal is to obtain diagnostic samples from the uterus, then the stage of the cycle must be taken into consideration when planning the BSE.

Although infertility in the bitch is not the scope of this article, some problems that may cause infertility are briefly discussed as well as some of the diagnostic tools that can allow clinicians to better asses a female's future reproductive potential.

The authors have nothing to disclose.
Department of Clinical Sciences, Auburn University, 1220 Wire Road, Auburn, AL 36849, USA
* Corresponding author.
E-mail address: clb0085@auburn.edu

Additional information regarding infertility can be found in "Clinical Approaches to Infertility in the Bitch."[2] The true testament of fertility is pregnancy and the birth of live offspring.

HISTORY/SIGNALMENT

The female is responsible for achieving and maintaining a pregnancy as well as rearing the puppies until weaning age. It is ideal to look critically at the female both prior to the start of her breeding career as well as after any problems may have occurred during pregnancy or parturition. It is important to ensure that a thorough and accurate history is taken.

Age

Younger bitches are likely to be more fertile than older bitches. Thomassen and colleagues[3] found that bitches older than 6 years had a lower whelping rate than younger ones. Females are born with all the oocytes they will ever have. Whereas males can continually make new spermatozoa, females do not have the luxury of replacing aged oocytes. As females age, the incidence of cystic endometrial hyperplasia increases and thereby decreases their future fertility.[4] Litter size has also been shown to decrease with age.[5] It is recommended, however, to wait until a bitch reaches musculoskeletal maturity before beginning her breeding career.

Breeding History

See **Boxes 1** and **2** for lists of questions to discuss with owners. Progesterone timing, coupled with vaginal cytology and vaginoscopy, ensures that the bitch is bred in her most fertile window to maximize conception rates. Using an unproved stud dog adds another variable to potential infertility. *Brucella canis* can cause infertility and abortion[6] and should be ruled out early in the BSE process. Information on the cycle length from an owner gives insight as to if the cycles have occurred at the expected time or if the time between each cycle has been shorter or longer than expected.

Breeding Plans

If breeding an older maiden bitch or one that has had trouble conceiving in the past, then using unproven, irreplaceable frozen semen may not be the best option. Instead, recommend choosing fresh semen from a young male with recent reproductive successes.

Box 1
History questions to ask an owner

Has the bitch ever been bred before?
- What type of semen was used?
- What method of insemination was used?
- How and when was pregnancy diagnosed?
- Did she become pregnant and carry the litter to term?
- Was progesterone timing used?
- Was a proved stud used?

Does she have any familial history of infertility or early pregnancy loss?
- Any familial history of reduced litters sizes?

When was the last brucellosis test?

Lifestyle

Raw diets have been shown anecdotally to reduce litter size and conception rates.[7] Few medications are labeled safe for pregnant and nursing bitches. It is ideal that they are current on vaccines before coming into heat.

Box 2
Additional questions to ask breeder

- How often does she come into heat?
- Do her cycles progress regularly?
- Does she have a history of clinical false pregnancies?
- How many litters are you expecting her to have?
- How are you planning to breed her?
- What is she currently being fed?
- Is she currently on any medications/supplements (prescribed or over the counter)?
- What heartworm and flea prevention is she taking?
- Is she up to date on her vaccinations?
- What is her daily activity level?

Genetic Testing

Genetic testing is an integral component to a responsible breeding program. The appropriate testing or clearances for each particular breed should be completed prior to breeding. The Canine Health Information Center (caninehealthinfo.org) is a good reference for which tests are required for each individual breed. The tests listed for a particular breed are based on the recommendations from each parent club. Veterinarians need to assist owners with interpretation of the results and how best to plan future breedings.[8] Some of these diagnostic tests are as simple as performing venipuncture or taking radiographs and may be performed by a general practitioner, whereas others require further training and equipment, such as brainstem auditory evoked response (BAER) testing, ophthalmic evaluations, and echocardiograms.

A clinician's job is not to refuse to breed a dog if it has a genetic defect but rather to educate the owner on the severity of that disease and what it means for the health of the dog and its future offspring. If dogs that are simply carriers for diseases are no longer being bred, then the gene pool will become even more severely limited than it already has become in some breeds. Greer[9] grouped different genetic diseases based on the impact on quality of life to both owner and animal. Those groups can then help guide breeding decisions to maximize the health of the animals while preserving the gene pool. For example, dogs with hip dysplasia, a disease that can be impactful on quality of life, are in the highest ranked group and should be bred only with extreme caution and only because of other highly desirable traits that they possess.

Diet/Supplementation

It is important to discuss not only what diet a female is currently fed and but also what will be fed while she is pregnant and lactating. Anecdotally, females have been unable to achieve pregnancy or have lost litters when fed raw diets. Although this was not directly proved a cause of the infertility, most clinicians agree that raw diets during pregnancy and lactation are not worth the potential risk to the dam and neonates.[10]

Also, raw diets can be formulated incorrectly, causing a deficiency or excess of essential nutrients necessary for pregnancy and lactation.[11] It is ideal to transition breeding females to a high-quality commercial kibble diet when they are going to be bred. The daily caloric intake does not need to be increased until the third trimester of pregnancy; otherwise the excess calories can lead to over-conditioning.

As long as a bitch is fed a commercially available diet, she should not need supplementation of any kind.[12] Supplementation can lead to toxic amounts of vitamins and minerals being given, and the excess amount may inhibit the function of normal body systems. A few of the most popular supplements are discussed along with their implications for brood bitches.

Calcium

Calcium homeostasis is tightly controlled. When excess calcium is given via supplementation, the constant high levels of calcium negatively feed back to stop the production of parathyroid hormone. Parathyroid hormone is responsible for regulation of calcium and, once the mechanism has been down-regulated, alternative stores of calcium are unavailable when needed (ie, labor and lactation). Calcium is necessary for muscle contractions, and low ionized calcium during labor may lead to a decrease in uterine contractility, which may lead to dystocia.[13] Calcium supplementation during pregnancy may also lead to eclampsia during lactation.[14] Thus, calcium should never be supplemented to breeding females unless medically indicated.

Folic acid

The reports in regard to folic acid supplementation in dogs are conflicting. One study indicated a significant decrease in the occurrence of cleft palates[15]; however, the incidence of cleft palates was not known prior to the start of the study. Recently a gene mutation was found in Nova Scotia duck tolling retrievers that is responsible for cleft palate formation.[16] No amount of supplementation is able to correct an underlying genetic abnormality. Administration of folic acid to brood bitches seems to cause no harm but is of questionable value at this time for the prevention of birth defects.

Red raspberry tea leaves

Red raspberry tea leaves have been touted to strengthen the uterus, reduce labor pain, and ease delivery. They contain a variety of vitamins, minerals, and calcium. Despite these claims, however, when given to a pregnant bitch they can disrupt implantation and cause premature labor, due to uterine irritability.[17] Karen Copley of WhelpWise stated during an interview that they have noted an increased fetal mortality rate of 33% when pregnant bitches were supplemented with red raspberry tea leaves during pregnancy compared with an average of 5% to 7% in nonsupplemented bitches; however, a formal study has not been published.[18] Breeding females should not be given any supplement that contains this ingredient.

Omega-3 fatty acids

Dogs are incapable of producing omega-3 fatty acids on their own and must receive them through their diet; therefore, these are considered essential fatty acids. Omega-3 fatty acids are required for pregnancy and lactation. They help support proper development of the fetal brain and retina during gestation. Deficiency in these essential fatty acids has been associated with poor placental development and smaller litter sizes.[12] These fatty acids are included, however, in all high-quality commercial dog foods; additional supplementation is likely not harmful but is also not necessary.

PHYSICAL EXAMINATION

The physical examination is the most important part of any BSE. Although the reproductive organs are pivotal, the rest of the body systems that support those organs cannot be forgotten. Not every body system is discussed, just the more essential ones (in the authors' opinion) in regard to the reproductive success of the bitch.

Body Condition Score

Underweight and overweight bitches can have irregular cycles and have trouble conceiving and maintaining pregnancy to term.[19] Underweight bitches (body condition score 1 or 2 of 9) do not have enough body fat stores to adequately support pregnancy and lactation. Overweight dogs (body condition score 8 or 9 of 9) are more prone to developing respiratory compromise.[20] Also, excessive fat is stored in the muscles, including the muscles of the uterus. This decreases muscle tone, making a bitch more prone to uterine inertia and consequent dystocia.[5,20]

Respiratory

Particularly in brachycephalic breeds, the upper airway should be evaluated for obstruction, including stenotic nares. Oxygen delivery to the tissues, including the uterus, is partially dependent on hemoglobin saturation[21]; any compromise in ventilation has an impact on uterine oxygenation. Any preexisting obstruction is exacerbated when a bitch is heavily pregnant.

Cardiovascular

Pregnant bitches can experience a dilutional anemia. The volume of blood increases during gestation, without a subsequent increase in red blood cells.[22] The extra volume of dilute blood can create turbulent blood flow, leading to a low-grade functional murmur In humans.[23] Many small animal cardiologists agree that these murmurs can also occur in pregnant bitches; however, the authors are unaware of any reports in the literature. Breeding animals should be carefully evaluated before breeding, to ensure that cardiac problems neither are present nor likely to arise when pregnant.

Musculoskeletal

It is important that a bitch be structurally sound before achieving pregnancy, because the added weight of the gravid uterus can affect how she carries herself and exacerbate any skeletal abnormalities. Bitches that are acutely lame due to an injury may be bred if a veterinarian believes that the lameness is mild enough and will resolve before she enters the third trimester. Bitches that are chronically lame should be bred with caution, ensuring that she will be physically able to carry the litter without additional pain or discomfort and that she has been screened for possible genetic defects that may be the source of the lameness, which may then be passed to her offspring (eg, hip or elbow dysplasia).

Endocrine

Several canine endocrinopathies have been shown to have a heritable basis, including hypoadrenocorticism,[24] congenital hypothyroidism,[25] and autoimmune thyroiditis.[25] Testing for these diseases should occur prior to breeding, if a diagnostic test is available.

Integumentary

Although the skin is not vital for achieving and maintaining pregnancy, it holds an important function because dermatopathies can alert a clinician to other underlying conditions. For example, females that have been diagnosed with generalized demodicosis should not be bred, because it is potentially heritable.[26] Dogs with chronic allergies and atopy should be used with caution in a breeding program.

Nervous

Canine idiopathic epilepsy and other epilepsy-like diseases (neuronal ceroid-lipofuscinoses and episodic falling syndrome) are believed heritable and may appear in family lines of certain breeds. There are many ongoing studies looking for candidate genes for genetic testing.[27] Discretion should be exercised when breeding dogs with a known family history of epilepsy.

Reproductive

Although the nongravid uterus is rarely discernible, abdominal palpation should still be performed to rule out other pathology. Some bitches are overly tense and do not allow for an adequate impression. Examine the length of the mammary chain by individually palpating every gland to ensure that there are not any masses present within. Mammary neoplasms are more likely to occur in older intact bitches. Confirm that the nipples are not inverted and that none are missing. Supernumerary teats are usually nonfunctional. Inspect the vulva for any conformational defects, such as being hooded, tipped, or rotated. If abnormal vulvar anatomy is present, this may present a unique challenge for the male to be able to breed her by natural cover.

Abnormalities of the clitoris

Clitoral hypertrophy may occur due to anabolic steroid administration. Mibolerone is available via compounding pharmacies and is used to keep females out of heat during competitions. Varying degrees of clitoral hypertrophy are reported to occur in 15% to 20% of female dogs treated with mibolerone at the recommended dose.[28] Alternatively, clitoral hypertrophy may also be seen with masculinization of the female puppy as a result of progesterone or altrenogest (a weak androgen) given to the dam when pregnant.[29] Although not as common, it is possible for a female to have an enlarged clitoris, and even the presence of an os clitoris, due to an intersex condition (**Fig. 1**). This may occur in cases of a dog appearing otherwise phenotypically female. In these types of cases, the enlarged clitoris usually becomes evident at the time of puberty and never regresses.

Abnormalities of the vagina

The cervix and cranial vagina are formed from the paramesonephric ducts, whereas the caudal vagina and vestibule originate from the urogenital sinus.[30] The area where these tissues meet is known as the vestibulovaginal junction, or cingulum. The hymen forms here, just cranial to the urethral papilla, and should normally be open at birth. Incomplete separation of these tissues may lead to a varying degree of severity of vaginal septums or strictures (**Fig. 2**). Normal bitches have a narrowing in this region, which should not be confused with an anomaly.[31]

Digital examination of the vaginal vault is best done during proestrus and estrus, because a bitch may resent vaginal manipulation when in anestrus. The edema that is commonly present with proestrus and estrus may potentially alter her conformation, thereby minimizing the effect that any anomaly may have on a bitch's breeding career.

Prior to a digital examination, it is important to collect any samples needed for culture or cytology (discussed later), because this examination may contaminate the vaginal cavity. When a digital vaginal examination is performed, any masses or strictures should be noted. As a gloved finger is introduced into the vulva, the clitoris and

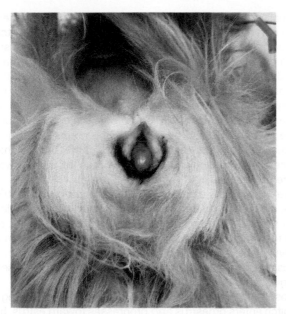

Fig. 1. Os clitoris in a 10-month-old poodle mix. No known history regarding the dam's use of hormones. She had been previously spayed elsewhere and notations were not made regarding any abnormalities found at surgery. An intersex condition was assumed. Owner declined karyotyping.

clitoral fossa should be located. A finger should be guided dorsally and then horizontally. The opening to the urethra sits ventrally to the urethral tubercle, which can be palpated along the ventral floor of the vaginal vault. Once over the shelf in the vagina, feel circumferentially, noting any masses, strictures, or septa.

As discussed previously, it is not uncommon to find a small remnant band of tissue or a circumferential stricture located at the vestibulovaginal junction. The true incidence of a pathologic stricture is unknown, however, because a majority of the population may be asymptomatic and a problem may not be noted until they are bred.[31]

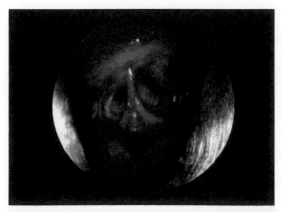

Fig. 2. Endoscopic image of a vaginal septum. (*Courtesy of* Margaret Root Kustritz, University of Minnesota, St Paul, MN.)

Sometimes vaginal septa are small and thin enough that they can be digitally broken down, but others may need sedation/surgery to be corrected. If a bitch is asymptomatic and is not going to be bred, then there is no medical reason to surgically correct the problem. If a bitch has a more extensive septum, surgical correction is usually required. Depending on the extent of the defect, however, surgical correction may not always be possible.[31] As a consequence to a persistent septum or stricture, the male may be unable to penetrate the vaginal canal during a natural breeding; these females require an assisted breeding. It is also possible that the anomaly may cause a dystocia at the time of whelping by inhibiting the normal passage of the puppies through the vaginal canal. In a retrospective study of 453 bitches that presented for an emergency cesarean section, 10% of them had at least 1 vaginal anomaly, including stricture or stenosis.[32]

Digital vaginal examination is usually diagnostic in most cases of strictures or septa, because they are most often located just cranial to the urethral papilla, which is easily palpated in most bitches. Palpation may be difficult in small bitches, however, due to the small size of their vaginal canal. It is also possible that the lesion is located more cranially than what is able to be felt via digital palpation.[31] Vaginoscopy may then be performed in those cases to fully evaluate the vaginal canal (discussed later). It is unclear if these vaginal anomalies are heritable.

Vaginal prolapse (hyperplasia) occurs more commonly in younger, large breed bitches. As the bitch enters proestrus and progresses toward estrus, high levels of estrogen are mitotic and vasoconstrictive, creating hyperplasia and edema within the vaginal tissues, causing the vaginal mucosa to prolapse out the vulva in some bitches (**Fig. 3**). This disease has a familial predisposition, which suggests that it may be hereditary,[31] and, therefore, using affected bitches for breeding should be discouraged. Bitches with a prolapse may need to be bred via artificial insemination. The prolapse should reduce naturally because estrogen levels decline during estrus. It is possible, however, for the prolapse to continue during diestrus before reducing. Estrogen levels rise again at the end of pregnancy and the prolapse may reoccur. This may lead to an obstructive dystocia; thus, planned cesarean sections are a good choice for any bitch with a prolapse that does not reduce during diestrus/pregnancy. Vaginal prolapse is likely to reoccur with subsequent heat cycles[31] and may increase in severity.

If the prolapse is occurring for the first time in an older bitch, then vaginal neoplasia should be suspected. Vaginal and vulvar neoplasia are uncommon in the bitch, accounting for only 3% of all canine tumors.[33] The most common vaginal/vulvar neoplasm in the dog is the benign leiomyoma.[31]

Transmissible venereal tumor has worldwide distribution and is most common in tropical and subtropical urban areas containing large populations of free roaming

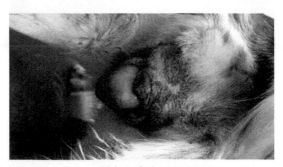

Fig. 3. Vaginal prolapse in a 6-year-old beagle in proestrus.

dogs.[31] Transmission occurs via transfer of neoplastic cells onto vaginal mucosa during coitus and onto nasal and oral mucosa by licking of affected genitalia of self or other dogs. The tumors appear as single or multiple firm, small gray to red nodules early in the course of the disease, progressing to widely pedunculated, cauliflower-like or multilobar hemorrhagic or ulcerated masses that may exceed 10 cm in diameter.[34] Transmissible venereal tumor is an important consideration for any mass involving the vulva or caudal vagina and is usually easily diagnosed by gross appearance and histologic presence of round cells from an impression smear.

DIAGNOSTICS
Brucellosis

Brucellosis can lead to infertility and abortion in the bitch and orchitis in the male. It is also possible that an animal may not show any clinical signs.[6] Therefore, *B canis* should be screened for at every breeding. In the bitch, this means testing on a semi-annual to annual basis, depending on how often she is being bred. This disease is zoonotic and also highly contagious between dogs. Dogs need not have sexual contact to contract brucellosis. It is shed in every bodily fluid and is easily transmitted from dog to dog via ingestion or inhalation. A canine brucellosis test should be a routine part of every BSE for both male and females.

Ultrasound

Ultrasound is a noninvasive way to look closely at the structure of the ovaries and uterus. Ultrasound can identify cysts (**Fig. 4**) and tumors that may be present on the ovary. A skilled ultrasonographer can identify the approximate number of follicles and/or corpora lutea (CL) that are present on the ovaries. Although it is possible to perform daily ultrasounds to pinpoint ovulation, this is not practical in the bitch. Follicles in the bitch range from 6 mm to 9 mm (0.6 cm–0.9 cm) prior to the luteinizing hormone surge and can increase to 9 mm to 12 mm (0.9 cm–1.2 cm) prior to ovulation.[35] Ovarian cysts can range in size from 0.2 cm to 4 cm with a median of

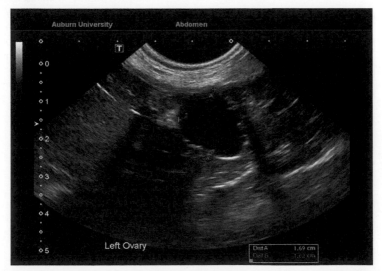

Fig. 4. Abdominal ultrasound image of an ovarian cyst in a 12-year-old Cavalier King Charles spaniel.

0.5 cm.[36] Because it is possible for the size of cysts and follicles to overlap, it is important to use the history along with the clinical findings to reach a diagnosis. Most bitches with ovarian cysts have had a prolonged estrus cycle or vaginal discharge outside the normal estrus cycle.[36]

During anestrus, it is expected that the ovaries are small and nonproductive (**Fig. 5**). In proestrus and estrus, the presence of follicles should be noted on the ovaries. In diestrus, CL should be visible on the ovaries (**Fig. 6**). Bitches usually have more CL than puppies; it is unclear if these extra CL are the result of unfertilized oocytes or embryo loss.[37] In **Fig. 7**, this image shows only 2 CL on the right ovary and there was none visible on the left ovary. This bitch was diagnosed with hypoluteoidism (documented with serial progesterone concentrations during pregnancy of <2 ng/mL) and was medically managed to carry 6 puppies to term.[38]

The uterus can be looked at critically for evidence of cystic endometrial hyperplasia (**Fig. 8**) and any masses that might be present. The uterus is expected to be small and difficult to follow during anestrus (**Fig. 9**). The uterus should not contain fluid in the lumen at any stage of the estrus cycle.

Vaginoscopy

Vaginoscopy can be used to visualize any abnormality that could be palpated during digital examination or diagnose any that occur further cranial than a digital examination would reach. The vaginal canal in the bitch is long and is impossible to fully examine via digital palpation alone. Vaginoscopy can be performed using a vaginoscope, an otoscope, or an endoscope. The otoscope works well for smaller bitches. The rigid endoscope offers the advantage of visualizing the entire vaginal canal, as well as having ports that allow passage of instruments for collection of samples for uterine culture and biopsy. Vaginoscopy can be performed during any time in the cycle; however, a bitch is usually more accepting of the procedure if she is in proestrus or estrus. Under the influence of estrogen during proestrus, the vaginal mucosa is edematous and pink, whereas during estrus, the mucosa becomes paler and more crenulated as the edema wanes[39] (**Fig. 10**).

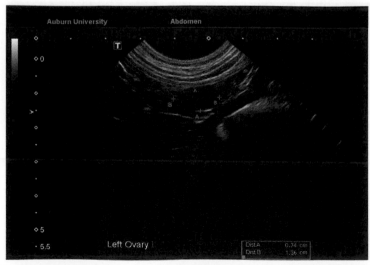

Fig. 5. Abdominal ultrasound image of an anestrus ovary of a 2-year-old basset hound. There is no follicular activity present.

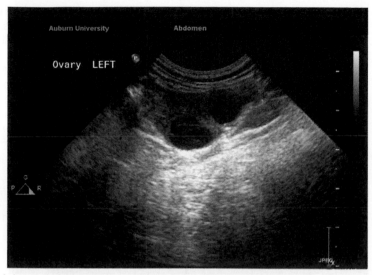

Fig. 6. Abdominal ultrasound image of an ovary with corpora lutea from a 4-year-old Labrador retriever a couple days after ovulation.

Vaginal Culture

Vaginal cultures in a normal bitch are of questionable diagnostic value and are not recommended as part of routine BSE. If a bitch is having malodorous vaginal discharge or trouble conceiving, however, then a culture may be warranted. If a clinician requests a vaginal culture, then this sample should be taken first before any other diagnostics or vaginal examinations are performed.[40] This helps minimize

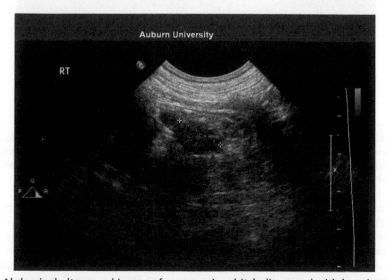

Fig. 7. Abdominal ultrasound image of an ovary in a bitch diagnosed with hypoluteoidism. Only 2 CL (*red arrows*) were visible on the right ovary. The other ovary had no CL present. With medical management, she was able to carry 6 puppies to term.

A

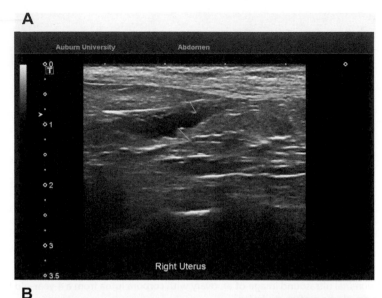

B

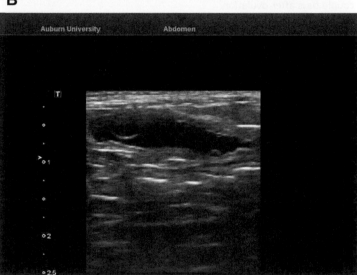

Fig. 8. Abdominal ultrasound image of a cystic endometrial hyperplasia. The endometrial lining is uneven due to cyst formation (A) is from a 12-year-old Cavalier King Charles spaniel. The endometrial lining is thickened (*white lines*). (B) is from a 6-year-old Pomeranian. There is less cyst formation in the younger bitch.

contamination and makes results easier to interpret. A double-guarded swab (**Fig. 11**) should be used to prevent contamination of the sample with contents from the vulva and caudal vagina. The vagina is not a sterile environment; therefore, it is expected to have growth of normal bacterial flora. Some normal flora that may be found include *Escherichia coli*, *Streptococcus* spp, *Pasteurella* spp, *Staphylococcus* spp, *Bacillus* spp, *Enterococcus* spp, and *Proteus* spp.[41] If a pure culture with heavy growth is seen and inflammatory cells noted on cytology (details later), then therapy should be instituted. Vaginal cultures are best taken at the beginning

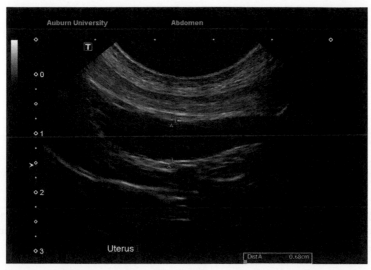

Fig. 9. Abdominal ultrasound image of an anestrus uterus. The endometrium is smooth, because there is no evidence of cystic endometrial hyperplasia in this 2-year-old basset hound.

of proestrus, so that results can be obtained and treatment initiated before breeding occurs.[41]

Vaginal Cytology

Depending on the stage of the estrus cycle, different cell types are present on vaginal cytology (**Table 1**). Neutrophils may be seen in proestrus (**Fig. 12**) and in the early stages of diestrus (**Fig. 13**) but should not be seen during estrus (**Fig. 14**). There may or may not be bacteria seen on the cytology. If no concurrent inflammation is present, this can be a normal finding because the vagina is not a sterile environment. Vaginal cytology should be performed to determine the stage of the cycle when a bitch is presented for breeding. Cytology should be done any time there is abnormal vaginal discharge (**Figs. 15** and **16**) or if a culture has been taken. If cytology indicates inflammation and a positive culture is obtained with heavy growth, this certainly warrants further investigation and treatment.

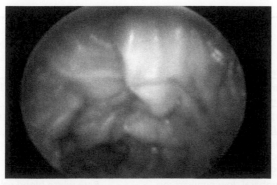

Fig. 10. Appearance of the vaginal mucosa during estrus as viewed through an endoscope. The mucosa is pale in color and crenulated in appearance.

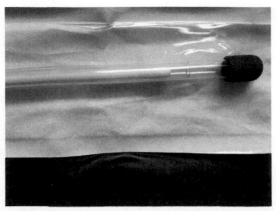

Fig. 11. Double-guarded swab used for collecting samples from the cranial vagina. The outer guard protects the swab from contaminates when traveling through the vulva and caudal vagina. (*Courtesy of* MOFA Global, Verona, WI.)

Uterine Culture

The uterus should be a relatively sterile environment, although normal flora from the vagina may be found in the uterus during proestrus and estrus. Completely sterile uterine cultures may be obtained via a surgical approach, because it is not currently possible to pass a guarded instrument through the cervix.[40] Adequate samples, however, may be obtained via nonsurgical methods. A cranial vaginal culture taken during proestrus or estrus may be an adequate substitute, because this contains uterine fluid, which has passed through the cervix and can be used to diagnose a uterine infection.[42] An alternate technique to obtain a uterine culture during proestrus or estrus is to perform a low-volume uterine lavage. Using a rigid endoscope, a catheter is passed through the cervix and into the uterine horns. A small amount of saline is infused and aspirated. The fluid is centrifuged and the sediment is submitted for culture and cytology.[43]

Uterine Cytology

A uterine cytology should be acquired any time a uterine culture is taken to correlate the growth of any bacteria with the presence of inflammatory cells. A uterine cytology

Table 1
Vaginal cytology

Stage of Estrous Cycle	Major Epithelial Cell Types Seen	Other Cells
Proestrus	Parabasal and intermediate, increasing amounts of cornification	Few white blood cells, red blood cells
Estrus	Superficial and anuclear, completely cornified cells	Red blood cells may or may not be present
Diestrus	Superficial and parabasal, 50% cornified on day 1 of cytologic diestrus	Many white blood cells seen for the first couple days
Anestrus	Parabasal, low numbers, no cornification	Rare white blood cell

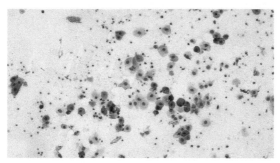

Fig. 12. Proestrus cytology. There are few cornified cells, occasional white blood cells, and numerous red blood cells present (Diff-Quik stain, original magnification × 100).

can be obtained surgically or nonsurgically. Nonsurgically, a cytology brush (Endoscopy Support Services, Brewster, New York) may be passed through the cervix using a rigid endoscope and endometrial cells can be collected when the bitch is in proestrus or estrus. A uterine cytology may also be collected, as described previously, using low-volume uterine lavage and examining the sedimented pellet.

Results from uterine culture should be interpreted in light of the cytologic findings. Normal bacterial flora from the vagina may be present in the uterus. If there is a pure culture with inflammatory cells noted on cytology, then appropriate bacterial therapy should be implemented.

Uterine Biopsy

Uterine biopsies are helpful in determining the presence and extent of cystic endometrial hyperplasia, inflammation, and infection. Biopsies should be submitted to a reproductive pathologist for best interpretation. Currently, there is not a universal system in place for grading canine uterine biopsies as there is in the mare.

Uterine biopsy, surgical approach

The surgical approach allows better visualization of the uterus and ovaries, safeguarding that any other underlying pathology does not become overlooked. This approach is similar to an ovariohysterectomy, using a small midline incision to exteriorize the uterus and ovaries. The entire reproductive tract should be palpated for pathology. A uterine biopsy may be obtained via a small wedge or punch biopsy

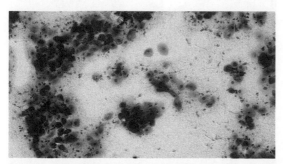

Fig. 13. Diestrus cytology. Some cells are still cornified, but there is a greater amount of noncornified cells present, plus an influx of neutrophils seen (Diff-Quik stain, original magnification × 100).

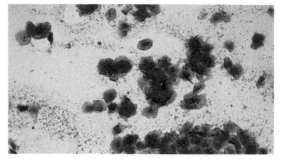

Fig. 14. Estrus cytology. Note that all the cells are cornified and the absence of white blood cells (Diff-Quik stain, original magnification × 100).

from one or both of the uterine horns. It is imperative that a full-thickness biopsy, including endometrial tissue, is obtained in the sample otherwise the sample may be nondiagnostic.[42] A uterine culture or cytology may be obtained through the same opening as the biopsy. The uterus is then closed with an inverting stich using absorbable suture. Surgical uterine biopsies can be obtained at any stage in the estrous cycle[43]; however, it is important to ensure that suture is not introduced into the lumen, because this can serve as a nidus for the development of cystic endometrial hyperplasia, if performed during diestrus.[44] Biopsy at any stage of the cycle may result in local endometritis, which in turn may develop into pyometra, so bitches should be treated with antibiotics prophylactically for 7 days after the procedure.[45]

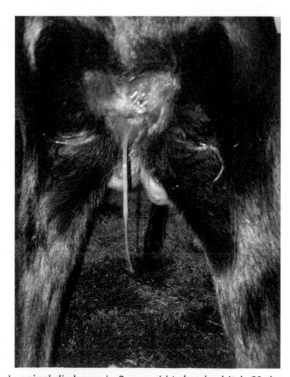

Fig. 15. Abnormal vaginal discharge in 3-year-old Labrador bitch 60 days in gestation.

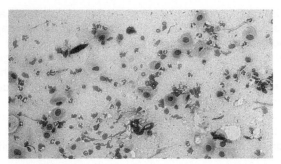

Fig. 16. Vaginitis in a 4-month-old puppy. Note the excessive amount of neutrophils that are present (Diff-Quik stain, original magnification × 200).

Uterine biopsy, nonsurgical approach

The nonsurgical approach offers the option of being able to obtain diagnostic samples without general anesthesia and a surgical incision into the abdomen. The rigid endoscope is passed vaginally and the biopsy instrument (**Fig. 17**) can be passed down the port and through the cervix. Due to the small sample size obtained, multiple blopsy samples should be taken to provide a more representative sample of the uterus. Biopsies obtained with the endoscope are comparable to full-thickness biopsy samples.[46] Biopsies taken this way should be procured in proestrus, estrus, or early anestrus, so as to not breach the cervix during diestrus and risk the transfer

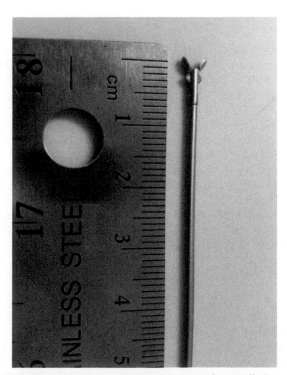

Fig. 17. Transcervical uterine biopsy instrument. Due to the small size, multiple biopsies should be taken to ensure that a representative sample is acquired.

of vaginal bacteria into the uterus, which may lead to a pyometra[45] as well as create any disturbances to the diestrual endometrium, because this may induce cystic endometrial hyperplasia.[44] The vaginal tissues are much thinner during diestrus and anestrus and it is easier to cause a perforation during this stage of the cycle.[43] The most valuable information from biopsies can be attained when there is increased glandular tissue from increased endocrine activity, which occurs during proestrus, estrus, or very early anestrus, after progesterone has returned to baseline.[43] Caution has been expressed by some investigators, that, if samples are obtained during proestrus or estrus, then the bitch should not be bred on that cycle, in case accidental uterine perforation has occurred, which may result in sperm peritonitis at the time of breeding.[43]

SUMMARY

It is important to have an honest conversation with owners regarding their expectations for a particular brood bitch. With a thorough physical examination, obtaining an accurate history, and performing appropriate diagnostics when warranted, a clinician can greatly enhance a bitch's future reproductive potential.

ACKNOWLEDGMENTS

The authors would like to thank their technician, Maureen Henderson, LVT, for her assistance in helping to obtain the photographs and to the American Kennel Club Canine Health Foundation (Grant number: 02282-E) for sponsoring their theriogenology residency.

REFERENCES

1. Purswell BJ, Althouse G, Root MV. Guidelines for using the canine breeding soundness evaluation. Theriogenology Handbook. Hastings (NE): Society for Theriogenology; 1992.
2. Wilborn R, Maxwell H. Clinical approaches to infertility in the bitch. Vet Clin Small Anim 2012;42:457–68.
3. Thomassen R, Sanson G, Krogenæs A, et al. Artificial insemination with frozen semen in dogs: a retrospective study of 10 years using a non-surgical approach. Theriogenology 2006;66:1645–50.
4. Moxon R, Whiteside H, England GCW. Prevalence of ultrasound-determined cystic endometrial hyperplasia and the relationship with age in dogs. Theriogenology 2016;86(4):976–80.
5. Kelley RL. Canine reproductive management: Factors influencing litter size. Proceedings of the Society for Theriogenology Annual Meeting. Colorado Springs (CO), August 7–11, 2002. p. 291–301.
6. Hollett, RB. Update on canine brucellosis. Proceedings of the Society for Theriogenology Annual Meeting. Albuquerque (NM), August 25–29, 2009. p. 287–295.
7. Morley P, Strohmeyer R, Tankson J, et al. Evaluation of the association between feeding raw meat and Salmonella enterica infections at a Greyhound breeding facility. J Am Vet Med Assoc 2006;228(10):1524–32.
8. Traas AM, Casal M, Haskins M, et al. Genetic counseling in the era of molecular diagnostics. Theriogenology 2006;66:599–605.
9. Greer M. Canine reproduction and neonatology. Jackson (MS): Teton New Media; 2015.

10. Greco, D. Misconceptions about canine nutrition. Proceedings of the Society for Theriogenology Canine Breeder Symposium. St. Louis (MO), August 16, 2008. p. 31–33.

11. Schlesinger D, Joffe D. Raw food diets in companion animals: a critical review. Can Vet J 2011;52(1):50–4.

12. Greco D. Nutritional supplements for pregnant and lactating bitches. Theriogenology 2008;70(3):393–6.

13. Hollinshead FK, Hanlon DW, Gilbert RO, et al. Calcium, parathyroid hormone, oxytocin and pH profiles in the whelping bitch. Theriogenology 2010;73(9): 1276–83.

14. Root Kustritz M. Practical matters: do not institute calcium supplementation during canine pregnancy. DVM360 2008.

15. Domosławska A, Jurczak A, Janowski T. Oral folic acid supplementation decreases palate and/or lip cleft occurrence in Pug and Chihuahua puppies and elevates folic acid blood levels in pregnant bitches. Pol J Vet Sci 2013;16(1):33–7.

16. Wolf Z, Leslie E, Arzi B, et al. A LINE-1 Insertion in DLX6 Is responsible for cleft palate and mandibular abnormalities in a canine model of pierre robin sequence. PLoS Genet 2014;10(4):e1004257.

17. Barnes J, Anderson L, Phillipson JD. Herbal medicines. 3rd edition. London: Pharmaceutical Press; 2007.

18. Copley, Karen. Comparison of Traditional Methods for Evaluating Parturition in the Bitch Versus Using External Uterine and Fetal monitors. Proceedings for the Society for Theriogenology Annual Conference. Colorado Springs, CO, August 7–11, 2002.

19. Davidson A. Breeding soundness examination of small animals. MSD Veterinary Manual. 11th edition. Kenilworth (NJ): Merck publishing group; 2016.

20. Zoran D. Obesity in dogs and cats: a metabolic and endocrine disorder. Vet Clin North Am Small Anim Pract 2010;40(2):221–39.

21. West J. Pulmonary pathophysiology: the essentials. 8th edition. Philadelphia: Wolters Kluwer; 2013.

22. Lozano M. Updates on anesthesia for non-obstetric and obstetric surgery during pregnancy. Clin Theriogenology 2013;5(3):190–200.

23. Tsiaras S, Poppas A. Normal changes in cardiovascular hemodynamics in pregnancy. In: medical care of the pregnant patient. 2nd edition. Philadelphia: ACP Press; 2008. p. 311–8.

24. Klein S, Peterson M. Canine hypoadrenocorticism: Part 1. Can Vet J 2010;51: 63–9.

25. Lathan P. Canine hypothyroidism. Clinicians brief 2012;25–8.

26. It V, Barrientos L, Lopez Gappa J, et al. Association of canine juvenile generalized demodicosis with the dog leukocyte antigen system. Tissue Antigens 2010;76: 67–70.

27. Hülsmeyer V, Fischer A, Mandigers P, et al. International Veterinary Epilepsy Task Force's current understanding of idiopathic epilepsy of genetic or suspected genetic origin in purebred dogs. BMC Vet Res 2015;11:175.

28. Concannon PW, Meyers-Wallen VN. Current and proposed methods for contraception and termination of pregnancy in dogs and cats. J Am Vet Med Assoc 1991;198:1214–25.

29. Curtis EM, Grant RP. Masculinization of female pups by progestogens. J Am Vet Med Assoc 1964;144:395–8.

30. Senger PL. Pathways to pregnancy and parturition. 3th edition. Redmond (WA): Current Conceptions Inc; 2015.

31. Johnston S, Root-Kustritz M, Olson P. Canine and feline theriogenology. Philadelphia: Saunders; 2001.
32. Ayers S, Thomas P. Population characteristics of 453 bitches undergoing 510 cesarean section procedures between 1999 and 2009–a retrospective study. Clin Theriogenology 2010;2(4):451–65.
33. Cotchin E. Neoplasia in the dog. Vet Rec 1954;66:879–85.
34. Cohen D. The canine transmissible venereal tumor: a unique result of tumor progression. Adv Cancer Res 1985;43:75–112.
35. Concannon P. Reproductive cycles of the domestic bitch. Anim Reprod Sci 2011; 124:200–10.
36. Knauf Y, Bostedt H, Failing K, et al. Gross pathology and endocrinology of ovarian cysts in bitches. Reprod Domest Anim 2014;49:463–8.
37. Marinellia L, Rotab A, Carnierc P, et al. Factors affecting progesterone production in corpora lutea from pregnant and diestrous bitches. Anim Reprod Sci 2009;114: 289–300.
38. Shumack B, Wilborn R, Johnson AK, et al. Management of a high-risk pregnancy in a Portuguese water dog. Clin Theriogenology 2017;9(3):486.
39. Levy X. Videovaginoscopy of the canine vagina. Reprod Dom Anim 2016; 51(Suppl. 1):31–6.
40. Threlfall W. Canine: breeding soundness examination of the bitch. CVC in Kansas City Proceedings 2008.
41. Root Kustritz M. The dog breeder's guide to successful breeding and health management. St Louis (MO): Saunders; 2006.
42. Root Kustritz M. Collection of tissue and culture samples from the canine reproductive tract. Theriogenology 2006;66(3):567–74.
43. Lopate, C. Endometrial culture, cytology and biopsy: Procedure, interpretation and tips. Canine seminar and wet lab conference proceedings. Society for Theriogenology Annual conference. Asheville (NC), July 27, 2016.
44. Nomura K. Histological evaluation of canine deciduoma induced by silk suture. J Vet Med Sci 1995;57(1):9–16.
45. Gunzel-Apel AR, Wilke M, Aupperle H, et al. Development of a technique for transcervical collection of uterine tissue in bitches. J Reprod Fertil Suppl 2001; 57:61–5.
46. Christensen BW, Schlafer DH, Agnew DW, et al. Diagnostic value of transcervical endometrial biopsies in domestic dogs compared with full thickness uterine sections. Reprod Domest Anim 2012;47(Suppl 6):342–6.

Current Review of Artificial Insemination in Dogs

Stuart J. Mason, MANZCVS

KEYWORDS

- Transcervical • TCI • Norwegian catheter • Artificial insemination • Bitch
- Breeding management

KEY POINTS

- Poor timing of breeding/insemination is the most common cause for failed pregnancy.
- There is no one good test for staging a bitch's cycle; a combination of tests needs to be used.
- A minimum of 150 to 200 $\times$ 10^6 live normal sperm are recommended for insemination.
- Transcervical insemination has a higher pregnancy rate than vaginal insemination with fresh semen.
- Transcervical insemination has a higher pregnancy rate than laparotomy insemination with frozen semen.

INTRODUCTION

Artificial insemination (AI) is the collection of semen from the male and the subsequent insertion of the collected semen into the female. AI in dogs has come a long way since the first successfully reported vaginal insemination with fresh semen performed by Fr Abbé Lazzaro Spallanzani in Italy, in 1780, resulting in the birth of 3 puppies.[1] From fresh semen inseminations wherein breeders are unable to achieve a natural mating, through to the international movement and insemination of frozen thawed semen, knowledge and technologies of both bitch timing techniques and insemination techniques have undergone dramatic change.

AIs may be requested for several reasons, including request of breeder, failure to achieve a successful mating (including slip matings), inability to achieve a mating (conformational), or due to the use of fresh chilled or frozen semen. A successful natural mating requires full intromission of the dogs' penis into the vagina, with the bulb of the penis being locked into the vagina by the cingulum. The male must turn by lifting one hind leg over the rump of the bitch with the penis locked in the vagina, resulting in both animals facing away from each other in the 'tie' position. The animals must

Disclosure Statement: The author has nothing to disclose.
Monash Veterinary Clinic, 1662 Dandenong Road, Oakleigh East, Victoria 3166, Australia
E-mail address: drstuartmason@gmail.com

Vet Clin Small Anim 48 (2018) 567–580
https://doi.org/10.1016/j.cvsm.2018.02.005
0195-5616/18/© 2018 Elsevier Inc. All rights reserved.

vetsmall.theclinics.com

remain tied for a minimum of 10 minutes in order to achieve a successful breeding with maximal pregnancy rates, with anything less than 10 minutes being termed a slip-mating.[2] Slip matings are commonly the result of an *outside tie* (the bulbus glandis engorges outside the vulva). Conception rates of *outside tie* breeding may be improved by elevating the hind quarters of the bitch for 5 minutes.[3] It is during the tie that large volumes of prostate fluid are deposited into the bitches vagina/uterus, which due to being instilled after the semen-rich fraction, is thought to aid in the passage of sperm to the oviduct of the female for fertilization.[4]

For an AI to be most successful it is important that the procedure be performed at the appropriate stage of the bitches' cycle, that semen of adequate quality is used, and that the procedure is performed appropriately with a good understanding of the success rates of the different insemination procedures.

Five forms of insemination of the bitch have been described, with only the first 4 being commonly performed today:

1. Vaginal insemination
2. Endoscope-assisted transcervical insemination (EIU)
3. Non-EIU (Norwegian catheter)
4. Laparotomy insemination (surgical insemination, surgical implant)
5. Laparoscopic insemination

BREEDING MANAGEMENT AND TIMING OF INSEMINATION
Ovarian Endocrinology Summary

A good understanding of the cycle of the bitch is imperative for maximizing pregnancy rates, as poor timing of insemination is the most common cause of pregnancy failure in the bitch.[3] Bitches spontaneously ovulate; ovulating a primary oocyte arrested in prophase I of the second stage of meiosis.[5,6] The developing follicles (which secrete estrogen) on the ovary of the bitch undergo preluteinization after the preovulatory luteinizing hormone (LH) surge, which occurs approximately 2 days before ovulation.[7,8] The LH surge stimulates luteinization of the granulosa cells to secrete progesterone before ovulation, possibly to aid in the resumption of meiosis of the oocytes.[6] After ovulation, 36 to 50 hours after the LH surge, the corpus luteum forms from luteinization of the thecal and granulosa cells. The corpus luteum secretes progesterone, with progesterone being solely responsible for pregnancy maintenance in the bitch. Six days after ovulation the bitch enters into diestrus.[9] Bitches are unique in that there is no maternal recognition of pregnancy; all bitches have an obligatory diestrus period of 9 to 10 weeks. Following regression of the corpus luteum at the end of diestrus, the bitch enters a phase of hormonal quiescence (anestrus). At the end of the anestrus period (3 or more months), there is an increase in follicle stimulating hormone and LH, which is responsible for the induction of the next estrous (heat) period.

Laboratory Tests for Staging the Bitches Cycle

Luteinizing hormone assay
LH may be measured by a quantitative or qualitative assays. LH levels will remain undetectable until the point of the LH surge. Unfortunately the LH surge length is quite varied in the bitch (24–60 hours), so daily serum analysis is required to detect the LH surge. There is an increasing phase of up to 12 to 24 hours and then a decline over 12 to 36 hours.[10] Qualitative LH tests are the only tests readily available today, and give a positive result greater than 1 ng/mL. Because the LH levels vary (4–14 ng/mL[10,11]) at the peak of the LH surge, coupled with slow increase and

decrease, even with daily testing it is possible to not detect the LH surge in some bitches. On average the LH surge occurs 5 days before the point of the oocyte being ready to be fertilized; however, with a range of 3 to 8 days after the LH surge,[11] and the possibility of anovulatory cycles, its usefulness alone is questionable.

Progesterone assay

Progesterone levels increase from the LH surge, and their detectable levels can be used as an indirect indicator of ovulation. Progesterone continues to increase through estrus and early diestrus, with the cervix closing under the influence of increasing progesterone. Cervical closure is thought to occur at progesterone levels of approximately 60 to 90 nmol/L (20–30 ng/mL) with one publication citing cervical closure at levels greater than 68.9 ± 15.4 nmol/L (21.67 ± 4.81 ng/mL)[12] and another at levels greater than 81.2 ± 12.3 nmol/L (25.5 ± 3.87 ng/mL).[13] Cervical closure is thought to help protect the uterus from infection and help provide an ideal environment for fertilization.[12] If insemination is required after cervical closure, then an intrauterine technique should be used. Progesterone is most commonly measured today by chemoluminescence with serum being recommended rather than plasma.[14] Collection of blood for progesterone is best done on a fasted sample. Samples should not be refrigerated for the first 2 hours after collection, as refrigeration during this time will reduce the measured level of progesterone.[14] The serum should be separated immediately following collection of blood if the sample will be refrigerated within the first 2 hours.[14]

It is generally accepted that the LH surge occurs around 6 nmol/L (2 ng/mL) and ovulation at 15 to 25 nmol/L (4–8 ng/mL), with ovulation being deemed complete with values greater than 30 nmol/L (10 ng/mL).[15] In the author's opinion there is no magical value of progesterone at which fertility is ideal as advocated by some; it is important to look for changes in values and develop a feel for the cycle and time of ovulation in each individual bitch. It is also imperative to understand that different analytical machines (especially some smaller, in-house machines) will give differing values of progesterone and it is important to establish a normal range of values for each machine.

Vaginal cytology

In addition to progesterone changes during the estrus cycle of the bitch, the cytology of the vagina changes as a result of changing estrogen levels. Increasing estrogen levels from the developing follicle during proestrus result in hyperplasia of the vagina of the bitch, with this being represented by increasing cornification evident on vaginal cytology samples. As the vagina undergoes hypertrophy, the surface cells of the vaginal mucosa become further away from the blood supply of the submucosa, resulting in reduced oxygenation and death of the surface cells. As a result of reduced oxygenation, there is increasing enlargement of the cytoplasm, nuclear pyknosis, and cornification of the surface cells.[16] The percentage of anuclear cells increases to 50% of the cornified cells by the start of estrus. Six days after ovulation, the end of the fertile period (estrus) is indicated by the influx of neutrophils and parabasal cells reducing the percentage of cornified vaginal epithelial cells.[9] Vaginal cytology alone is a poor indicator for the ideal time to breed[9]; however, in conjunction with progesterone assays and vaginoscopy, it aids in the determination of the phase of the cycle (proestrus, estrus, diestrus, or anestrus) and the appropriateness of different insemination methods.[12,17] Samples are collected using a moistened cotton swab into the vagina, and then the cells are rolled onto a microscope slide and stained with Diff-Quik (most commonly).

Vaginoscopy

Vaginoscopically the vagina changes dramatically through estrus. The procedure is performed using a 25-cm-long, 11-mm diameter WelchAllyn sigmoidoscope. Deep edematous folds of proestrus, begin to flatten out and reduce under the influence of reducing estrogen and rising progesterone levels after the LH surge. As estrogen levels continue to reduce and progesterone continues to increase through estrus, the hypertrophy and hyperplasia of the vagina reduces, resulting in a cobblestone appearance of the vagina (crenulation) indicating ovulation is complete and the bitch is in the fertile period. By the start of diestrus the vagina returns to a flat state with no significant folds in the mucosa.[18]

A combination of (or all of) progesterone assay, LH assay, vaginal cytology, and vaginoscopy is used to stage the cycle of the bitch and determine the appropriate breeding time.[17] Although good-quality fresh sperm may survive in the bitches' reproductive tract for up to 7 to 10 days, ovulation should be confirmed in all forms of AI to maximize both pregnancy rate and litter size. In the case of frozen semen, accurate assessment that the bitch is in the fertile period is imperative, as frozen-thawed dog spermatozoa has a reduced survival time after thaw. It has been shown that insemination of the bitch at least 3 days after ovulation will maximize whelping rates with frozen-thawed dog semen[19]; however, insemination should be performed before the onset of diestrus to maximize pregnancy rates[20] and remove the risk of an intrauterine insemination inducing cystic endometrial hyperplasia/pyometra.[21–24] There is a 48-hour window at which time crenulation is maximal,[18] and this is thought to correspond to the maximal fertile period of the bitch.[25,26]

Although some operators promote insemination in the early stages of diestrus, published reports pertaining to pregnancy results with fresh, chilled, and frozen semen support the insemination being performed in estrus not diestrus.[19,20,25–32] Canine ova have been shown to be fertilizable up to 8 to 9 days after ovulation (5–6 days after cervical closure),[13,33] which leads some operators to push bitches into early diestrus for insemination. It must be noted, however, that it has been shown, using fresh semen via intrauterine insemination, that there is a declining pregnancy rate and litter size with increasing days of insemination after cervical closure.[13,33] Tsutsui and colleagues[34] obtained pregnancy rates with fresh semen of 100% (5 of 5) 6 days after ovulation, 71% (5 of 7) 7 days after ovulation, 38% (3 of 8) 8 days after ovulation, and 0% (0 of 7) 9 days after ovulation; Verstegen and colleagues[13] achieved pregnancy rates of 60% (3 of 5) 7 days after ovulation, 60% (3 of 5) 8 days after ovulation, and 20% (1 of 5, 1 puppy) 9 days after ovulation. These results show a trend for reducing pregnancy rates with increasing day of insemination after cervical closure, likely due to aging ova and an unfavorable uterine environment of metestrus and early diestrus.[13,20,33] These results were obtained using fresh semen, so it would be prudent to expect pregnancy rates to be lower when using frozen semen in this same manner due to the reduced viability of frozen semen compared with fresh semen.

ANATOMY OF THE BITCH

Understanding the anatomy of the bitch is important to ensure the process of AI is done successfully for each of the different methods of insemination. The external genitalia of the female begins at the vulva, which is the entrance to the vestibule. The vestibule contains the clitoris and the urethral opening. The vestibule is quite short with the lumen heading at approximately a 45° angle from horizontal toward the lumbar vertebrae of the bitch. The vestibule terminates at the cingulum (a narrowing), which has its function to lock around the bulb of the penis to maintain erection during a tied mating. From the cingulum the vagina extends forward approximately parallel to the lumbar spine. The vagina of the bitch is quite long and extends to the level of the cervix. Just caudal to the cervix are 3 folds in the dorsal wall of the vagina (dorsomedial folds), which consist of 3 components: the caudal, middle, and cranial tubercles. The cranial vagina ends at the cervix, which protrudes caudally into the vagina creating a cavity between the opening of the cervix (cervical os) and the cranial-most portion of the vagina known as the fornix. The cervical lumen extends cranially from the cervical os, and in most cases the cervical os faces toward the floor of the vagina. From the cervix, the uterus extends cranially from its short body in 2 distinct horns to the uterine tubes and the ovaries. The uterus of the bitch is bicornuate.

SEMEN COLLECTION AND EVALUATION

The semen to be used for insemination is collected by digital manipulation of the stud dog. Different sterile/new collecting receptacles may be used depending on the operator: latex artificial vagina with sterile plastic centrifuge tubes, glass vials, or funnels with plastic centrifuge tubes. It is important that during digital manipulation of the dog that the prepuce is retracted back over the bulb of the penis before the penis is erect as occurs in a natural mating.[27,35] Erection and collection of the stud dog within the prepuce will not only cause significant pain for the male but it will also provide a negative stimulus for future collections/breeding and will likely result in the collection of poorer-quality semen. The semen should be collected in the presence of the estrus bitch to be inseminated.

The male dog ejaculates in 3 fractions, so it is recommended to collect the semen into these separate fractions as it is ejaculated. The first fraction while the male is attaining an erection and thrusting is the first, prostate fraction. Once a full erection is attained and thrusting usually ceases, the second, semen-rich fraction (SRF) is ejaculated. The SRF is a small volume most commonly 0.5 to 1.5 mL[2]. Once the color of the ejaculate is noting to clear, the collecting receptacle must be changed to collect the third prostate fraction. The first prostate fraction is generally discarded, as it contains a lot of cells (smegma) and bacteria and, if the ejaculate was correctly fractioned, should contain few sperm. Should fractionation be poor it is recommended to centrifuge (700 g, 6 minutes) and wash the semen in an appropriate artificial extender.[27] Collecting the semen into one receptacle and mixing all 3 fractions together for insemination is thought to reduce fertility.[36]

All semen should be evaluated for morphology, motility, and total counts before insemination using microscopy.[27] Pregnancy rates are expected to be maximized by only using semen with more than 60% normal sperm cells[37] and 70% progressive motility (fresh semen)[27,28] and 40% progressive motility (frozen semen).[19,29] It is recommended to inseminate a total of 150 to 200 $\times$ 10[6] live, morphologically normal spermatozoa for best pregnancy rates.[25,28,38] It is most commonly recommended that samples containing blood or pus should be discarded and either another sample collected later or another stud dog be used. Although there are published reports of using semen separation media (most commonly single-layer centrifugation) that show favorable results for separating erythrocytes from sperm,[39] and improving motility, morphology, and viability results for fresh, frozen, or chilled semen,[40–43] there are not, to the author's knowledge, any published reports of improved fertility (notably pregnancy rates) from use of such techniques with hemospermic or poor-quality semen samples.

ARTIFICIAL INSEMINATION TECHNIQUES
Vaginal Insemination

The aim of a vaginal insemination is to deposit the semen at the cervical os. During a natural mating it is thought that the penis will align with the cervical os depositing the semen into the uterus,[35] which may explain the lower reported pregnancy rates with vaginal insemination than natural mating. In all cases the lubricated catheter is passed into the vagina by passing through the dorsal commissure of the vulva at a 45° angle from horizontal toward the lumbar spine. Once resistance is felt, then the angle of the catheter is changed to be parallel to the lumbar spine and the catheter is gently advanced forward until resistance is felt while palpating the cervix through the abdominal wall.[27] The catheter should be at the level of the cervix, however, often may only be at the level of the caudal tubercle of the dorsomedial fold.

Several devices exist for performing vaginal inseminations in bitches:

Osiris catheter
The Osiris is a rigid catheter with an inflatable cuff near the distal opening (**Fig. 1**). It is approximately 25 cm long and 5 mm in diameter. Once appropriately positioned, the cuff is blown up through the external valve, which results in vaginal distension aiding in preventing backflow of semen around the catheter. The semen is instilled through the lumen, and the syringe should be left attached to prevent backflow through the catheter. The Osiris catheter is suitable for small- and medium-sized breeds of dogs but would be inadequate for large breeds of dog (catheter too short to reach cervix and the cuff too small of a diameter to seal and distend the vagina).

Foley catheter
These catheters are flexible with an inflatable cuff near the distal opening and come in a range of sizes. The size is adaptable to different sized dogs, and there is a cuff to distend and seal the vagina. Although the semen is instilled through the lumen and the syringe should be left attached to prevent backflow through the catheter, it is unlikely that the distal opening is able to get close to the cervix because of its flexibility.

Bovine artificial insemination pipette
These catheters are rigid with no cuff. Their rigidity and small diameter allows for passage of the catheter to the level of the cervical os; however, the absence of a cuff results in no vaginal distension or prevention of backflow of semen.

Mavic catheter
These catheters (MOFA Global, Verona, WI) are plastic with a stylet through the center of them (**Fig. 2**). They have an inflatable cuff at the distal end, and the stylet through which the semen is inseminated contains a one-way valve to prevent leakage through the catheter when the syringe containing semen is empty and removed or changed. They come in 3 sizes, meaning they are suitable for all sizes of bitches; the inflatable cuff, like the Osiris catheter, allows for vaginal stimulation and sealing of the vagina to prevent backflow.

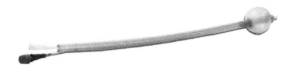

Fig. 1. Osiris catheter for vaginal insemination in the bitch. (*Courtesy of* IMV Technologies, Normandy, France.)

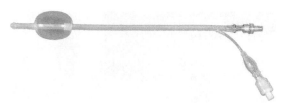

Fig. 2. A 250-mm Mavic catheter for vaginal insemination in the bitch. (*Courtesy of* MOFA Global, Verona, WI.)

Once the chosen catheter is in place and the cuff inflated, the SRF is inseminated slowly, followed by the prostate fluid (or artificial extender if not enough prostate fluid is able to be collected or the prostate fluid shows evidence of disease, namely, blood). The prostate fluid used for insemination is thought to push and help carry the semen through the cervix and into the uterus. With different pH values and viscosities, it is thought best to keep the fractions separate and inseminate them separately, as would occur during the ejaculation process of a tied natural mating to maximize pregnancy rates.[36] Some investigators advocate elevation of the hind quarters of the bitch during and after insemination to aid the flow of semen into the uterus.[27] It is the author's opinion that the use of the Mavic catheter, with massage of the vulva during and after insemination until the Mavic catheter is removed, is of more benefit. Although it is easy to hold up the hindquarters of a small bitch, it is very difficult to do the same in large- and giant-breed bitches; additionally, there is nothing to stimulate uterine contractions during this particular process (hindquarter elevation alone). Vaginal insemination is mostly commonly used for fresh or fresh chilled semen and not recommended for frozen semen (poor published success rates).[19,44] Other than failure to attain pregnancy, rarely other complications of vaginal insemination are perforation of the vagina (observed by the author after breeder performed own insemination) and the introduction of infection through the use of unclean equipment.

Intrauterine Insemination

Laparotomy

Laparotomy intrauterine insemination, or commonly known as surgical AI or surgical implant (SIU), is the insemination of semen into the uterus of the bitch under general anesthesia by laparotomy. In order to perform the procedure, the bitch is anesthetized and placed in dorsal recumbency with the hind end elevated. A midline incision is made approximately 25 mm caudal to the umbilicus extending in a caudal direction. The uterus is exteriorized and inspected for evidence of disease. 22-gauge intravenous (IV) catheters or needles may be used for the insemination. IV catheters are preferred for the procedure, as the uterus can be pierced with the stylet and then the catheter advanced through the uterine lumen (similar to IV placement) to ensure the opening is intraluminal and not intramural. Most operators recommend either 2 catheters (one in each uterine horn, see **Fig. 3**) or one catheter in the uterine body may be used, although the site of insemination has been shown to not affect distribution of semen throughout both uterine horns.[34,45] After placement of the catheter (or needle) the uterus is occluded above the cervix with the index finger and thumb of one hand, while the syringe containing semen is attached to the catheter (or needle) with the other hand and inseminated slowly to fill the uterus. After the semen is inseminated, the uterus should be massaged to enhanced passage of semen to the uterine tube, as there is no uterine motility under anesthesia. The catheter (or needle) is removed from the uterus and the needle hole occluded for a short while to stem

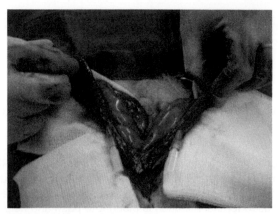

Fig. 3. Laparotomy frozen semen insemination in a bitch. Two catheters have been placed, one in each horn ready for insemination of semen. (*Courtesy of* Dr Stuart Mason, Monash Veterinary Clinic, Oakleigh East, Victoria, Australia.)

any bleeding. The abdomen Is then closed routinely.[26,46] The use of pain relief post-operatively remains controversial, with nonsteroidal antiinflammatory drugs (NSAIDs) advocated by many; however, it is known prostaglandins are required for fertilization, and there is no published work on the effects of NSAIDs and fertilization/pregnancy in the bitch.

SIU is advocated by many; however, there is very little published work as to its true success relative to pregnancy, with most publications consisting of small sample sizes and only one with clinical data.[32] This procedure is illegal in some countries (Norway, Sweden), as it is seen as unethical and unnecessary when there are other methods of intrauterine insemination that are much less invasive,[27,28] whereas in the United Kingdom special permission must be sought to perform the procedure.[47]

Many operators advocate the use of SIU to evaluate the uterus and to pop cysts of the uterus.[48] Although this is commonly believed, there is currently no published evidence to support the procedure of rupturing uterine cysts to improve pregnancy rates to the author's knowledge. It is important to understand that serosal cysts of the uterus are not pathogenic; cystic endometrial hyperplasia (CEH) is often not visible grossly unless severe, in which case it is not recommended to inseminate the affected bitch. CEH is detectable by ultrasound by an experienced clinician and can be managed without surgery with the aim to breed on the subsequent season and avoid an unnecessary surgery.

There is little published evidence to support SIU that is not purely descriptive in nature,[46] confounded by a mixture of fresh, fresh chilled and frozen semen results collated together,[32] experimental with small numbers of selected research breeding bitches,[49,50] or driven largely by opinion.[48]

Laparoscopic insemination

Insemination by laparoscopy has been described; however, it has never become a common procedure in clinical practice because of the high setup costs, steep learning curve, and lack of advantages over SIU and is not discussed here. The procedure is more difficult than SIU and still requires general anesthesia to perform the technique.[51]

Transcervical insemination

Norwegian catheter The Norwegian catheter was the first developed nonsurgical intrauterine device in 1975[38] (**Fig. 4**). It consists of an outer nylon sheath with an inner

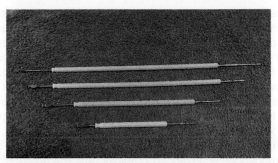

Fig. 4. A complete set of Norwegian catheters for blind transcervical insemination. (*Courtesy of* Jan T. Basberg, Gartnerservice, Haslum, Norway.)

metal stylet with a blunted, rounded distal tip. The procedure is performed in any size of bitch without the need of any anesthesia. With the bitch standing, restrained on a table, the operator will transabdominally palpate the cervix of the bitch while passing the catheter into the vagina of the bitch with the opposing hand. While holding the cervix steady with the thumb and index finger, the stylet is passed into the cervical os and through the cervix of the bitch. The semen is then inseminated through the stylet into the uterine lumen.[27,28]

The procedure is quick, simple, and cheap to perform; however, the learning curve is steep and the procedure difficult on large-breed bitches. Unlike SIU, the procedure may be performed more than once if required, as there is no anesthesia or surgery required.[28] Stimulation of the vestibule during this procedure is likely to stimulate uterine contractions resulting in an insemination process more like a natural mating than that obtained by SIU.[52] The Norwegian catheter may be used for fresh, fresh chilled, or frozen semen. Most published reports on the use of frozen semen in the bitch pertain to the use of the Norwegian catheter.[19,20,28–31]

Endoscopic-assisted transcervical insemination EIU, or commonly known as transcervical insemination (TCI), was first described in 1993 with the use of a cystoscope.[53] EIU is simple to learn with persistence and care; however, it is a technique wherein all steps must be monitored closely to maximize results.[25,26] Nowadays most operators use a uterorenoscope (**Fig. 5**), as this endoscope is longer and thinner (in

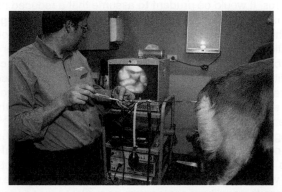

Fig. 5. Performing an EIU in a bitch. The cervix can be seen clearly catheterized by the TCI catheter on the monitor. (*Courtesy of* Dr Stuart Mason, Monash Veterinary Clinic, Oakleigh East, Victoria, Australia.)

diameter) than the cystoscope, allowing it to be used more adequately in all bitches from toys to giant breeds.[25,26] The cystoscope was often too large in diameter for toy bitches and too short to reach the cervix of large bitches. The procedure is performed with the bitch standing, restrained on a table. Using a uterorenoscope, cold xenon, halogen, or LCD light source and a camera with images projected onto a monitor, the operator is able to pass the endoscope to the level of the cervical os. The endoscope is initially passed into the vagina, and at this point air is instilled into the vagina via a rectal insufflation pump attached to the endoscope (30,200 rectal insufflation bulb Welch Allyn, Skaneateles, NY, USA). The use of a vaginal shunt (MOFA Global, Verona, WI, USA) may aid in sealing the vagina to maintain vaginal distension. The endoscope is advanced cranially past the dorsomedian folds to the cervix. The cervical os is visualized on the ventral aspect of the cervix in most cases. A CH-5 (or CH-4) TCI catheter (MOFA Global) is advanced through the endoscope and through the cervical os. Once the catheter is within the cervix, the stylet is removed and the catheter only advanced into the body of the uterus. The TCI catheter has marks at increments of 1 cm to aid in positioning the opening to the catheter within the body of the uterus. The semen is then inseminated through the catheter, slowly, watching for leakage at the cervical os[25,26,53,54] and massaging of the vulva to aid in uterine contractions. The semen is inseminated first, followed by prostate fluid (fresh semen, if prostate fluid is not diseased) or additional extender (fresh chilled, frozen semen) until the uterus is deemed full (appearance of fluid at the cervical os).[25,26] Slow insemination will allow for the insemination of large volumes.[25]

EIU is suitable for fresh, fresh chilled, and frozen semen. EIU has been shown to be more successful than SIU when performed appropriately,[26] and EIU has been shown to be more successful than vaginal insemination with fresh semen.[55,56] Unlike with the Norwegian catheter, with EIU the cervix is visualized so it is guaranteed the catheter is intrauterine 100% of the time.[25,26,53,54]

COMPARISONS OF DIFFERENT ARTIFICIAL INSEMINATION TECHNIQUES

Comparative studies of vaginal insemination of fresh semen with EIU show an approximately 33% to 35% improved pregnancy rate with EIU.[55,56] This improved rate is likely because with vaginal insemination the semen may not actually be placed at the level of the cervical os; additionally, intravaginal insemination requires the sperm to traverse the cervix into the uterus, compared with EIU wherein the sperm is placed directly in the uterus. It would be prudent to assume that a reduced number of sperm traverse the cervix into the uterus than the number placed in the vagina. This loss of sperm entering the uterus is counteracted by the recommendation of more than one vaginal insemination; however, the pregnancy results are still inferior to EIU.[55,56]

Although transcervical insemination by EIU or Norwegian catheter can be repeated, there is no benefit to more than one insemination unless timing of insemination is not optimal.[29,31] In the case of frozen semen, many advocates of SIU have discounted EIU as wasting more semen by doing the procedure twice (compared with one SIU); however, the pregnancy rate of one EIU is widely published[19,25,26,53,54,57] and, more recently, the pregnancy rate of EIU compared with SIU.[26] The author recommends only performing one intrauterine insemination with optimal timing of insemination.[25] The publications describing 2 inseminations by Norwegian catheter or EIU were only in situations when the timing was poor (to cover a larger possible window of fertilization)[29,31] or when the quality of semen was poor.[26]

If the timing of insemination is poor, and the intrauterine insemination occurs in diestrus, there is both a reduced expected pregnancy rate[13,20,33] and an increased probability of inducing CEH and/or pyometra whether it be by laparotomy, EIU, or Norwegian catheter. This point has been illustrated by Nomura and colleagues'[21-24] experiments of introducing many types of foreign material into the uterus of diestrus and causing endometrial hyperplasia/CEH ± pyometra.

Additionally, SIU continues to be advocated by many, as the semen can be inseminated closer to the oviduct than with EIU or Norwegian catheter. Uterine motility studies have shown that the site of insemination is irrelevant, as long as the semen is inseminated into the uterus.[34,45]

The higher success rate of EIU with frozen semen than SIU is most likely due to the lack of stress of surgery and anesthesia, the presence of uterine contractions during the procedure, and lack of effects of wound healing and inflammation.[25,26,52] Aside from the reduced success rate, the ethical issues of SIU (anesthesia, surgery, healing, risk of death from anesthesia, production of antisperm antibodies via blood sperm contact) lead many to question why the procedure continues to be advocated.

SUMMARY

AI of the bitch is commonly required for several reasons, most commonly the inability to attain a mating, owner request (including for semen assessment for suitability of mating), fresh chilled semen, and frozen semen use. Although vaginal insemination provides adequate results of pregnancy, better pregnancy results are attainable using EIU; EIU has been shown to be more successful than SIU. In order to perform AIs adequately, an understanding of the physiology and anatomy of the bitch is imperative, semen must be collected carefully, timing of the bitches cycle must occur, and the most appropriate route of administration must be used for the type of semen being used. Owners should be counseled on the different procedures available to help them have a clear understanding of what is best for their situation.

REFERENCES

1. Heape W. Artificial insemination of mammals and the subsequent fertilisation or impregnation of their ova. Proc Royal Soc, London 1897;61:52–63.
2. Simpson G, England G, Harvey M, editors. Manual of small animal reproduction and neonatology. Gloucester (England): British Small Animal Veterinary Association; 2004.
3. Johnson SD, Root-Kustritz M, Olson PNS, editors. Canine and feline theriogenology. Philadelphia: Saunders; 2001.
4. England GCW, Burgess CM, Freeman SL, et al. Relationship between the fertile period and sperm transport in the bitch. Theriogenology 2006;66(6–7):1410–8.
5. Tsutsui T. Gamete physiology and timing of ovulation and fertilization in dogs. J Reprod Fertil Suppl 1989;39:269–75.
6. Reynaud K, Fontbonne A, Marseloo N, et al. In vivo meiotic resumption, fertilization and early embryonic development in the bitch. Reproduction 2005;130(2): 193–201.
7. Phemister RD, Holst PA, Spano JS, et al. Time of ovulation in the beagle bitch. Biol Reprod 1973;8(1):74–82.
8. Concannon PW, McCann JP, Temple M. Biology and endocrinology of ovulation, pregnancy and parturition in the dog. J Reprod Fertil Suppl 1989;39:3–25.
9. Root Kustritz MV. Managing the reproductive cycle in the bitch. Vet Clin North Am Small Anim Pract 2012;42(3):423–37, v.
10. Concannon PW. Endocrinologic control of normal canine ovarian function. Reprod Domest Anim 2009;44(Suppl 2):3–15.

11. Concannon PW, Hansel W, Visek WJ. The ovarian cycle of the bitch: plasma estrogen, LH and progesterone. Biol Reprod 1975;13(1):112–21.

12. Silva LD, Onclin K, Verstegen JP. Cervical opening in relation to progesterone and oestradiol during heat in beagle bitches. J Reprod Fertil 1995;104(1):85–90.

13. Verstegen JP, Silva LD, Onclin K. Determination of the role of cervical closure in fertility regulation after mating or artificial insemination in beagle bitches. J Reprod Fertil Suppl 2001;57:31–4.

14. Volkmann DH. The effects of storage time and temperature and anticoagulant on laboratory measurements of canine blood progesterone concentrations. Theriogenology 2006;66(6–7):1583–6.

15. Jeffcoate IA, Lindsay FE. Ovulation detection and timing of insemination based on hormone concentrations, vaginal cytology and the endoscopic appearance of the vagina in domestic bitches. J Reprod Fertil Suppl 1989;39:277–87.

16. Olson PNTM, Wykes PM, Nett TM. Vaginal cytology. Part I. A useful tool for staging the canine oestrous cycle. Compend Contin Educ Pract Vet 1984;6:288–98.

17. Goodman MF. Canine ovulation timing. Probl Vet Med 1992;4(3):433–44.

18. Lindsay FEF. The normal endoscopic appearance of the caudal reproductive-tract of the cyclic and non-cyclic bitch - post-uterine endoscopy. J Small Anim Pract 1983;24(1):1.

19. Linde-Forsberg C, Strom Holst B, Govette G. Comparison of fertility data from vaginal vs intrauterine insemination of frozen-thawed dog semen: a retrospective study. Theriogenology 1999;52(1):11–23.

20. Linde-Forsberg C, Forsberg M. Fertility in dogs in relation to semen quality and the time and site of insemination with fresh and frozen semen. J Reprod Fertil Suppl 1989;39:299–310.

21. Nomura K. Histological evaluation of canine deciduoma induced by silk suture. J Vet Med Sci 1995;57(1):9–16.

22. Nomura K. Induction of a deciduoma in the dog. J Vet Med Sci 1994;56(2):365–9.

23. Nomura K, Funahashi H. Histological characteristics of canine deciduoma induced by intrauterine inoculation of E. coli suspension. J Vet Med Sci 1999; 61(4):433–8.

24. Nomura K, Nishida A. Histological variations of canine deciduoma induced in non pregnant horn at different stages of unilateral pregnancy. J Vet Med Sci 1998; 60(5):623–6.

25. Mason SJ. A retrospective clinical study of endoscopic-assisted transcervical insemination in the bitch with frozen-thawed dog semen. Reprod Domest Anim 2017;52(Suppl 2):275–80.

26. Mason SJ, Rous NR. Comparison of endoscopic-assisted transcervical and laparotomy insemination with frozen-thawed dog semen: a retrospective clinical study. Theriogenology 2014;82(6):844–50.

27. Linde-Forsberg C. Artificial insemination. Paper presented at: ESAVS-EVSSAR-ENVN reproduction in companion, exotic and laboratory animal 2005. Nantes.

28. Linde-Forsberg C. Achieving canine pregnancy by using frozen or chilled extended semen. Vet Clin North Am Small Anim Pract 1991;21(3):467–85.

29. Thomassen R, Farstad W, Krogenaes A, et al. Artificial insemination with frozen semen in dogs: a retrospective study. J Reprod Fertil Suppl 2001;57:341–6.

30. Linde-Forsberg C, Forsberg M. Results of 527 controlled artificial inseminations in dogs. J Reprod Fertil Suppl 1993;47:313–23.

31. Thomassen R, Sanson G, Krogenaes A, et al. Artificial insemination with frozen semen in dogs: a retrospective study of 10 years using a non-surgical approach Theriogenology 2006;66(6–7):1645–50.

32. Burgess DM, Mitchell KE, Thomas PG. Coeliotomy-assisted intrauterine insemination in dogs: a study of 238 inseminations. Aust Vet J 2012;90(8):283–90.
33. Tsutsui T, Takahashi F, Hori T, et al. Prolonged duration of fertility of dog ova. Reprod Domest Anim 2009;44(Suppl 2):230–3.
34. Tsutsui T, Shimizu T, Ohara N, et al. Relationship between the number of sperms and the rate of implantation in bitches inseminated into unilateral uterine horn. Nihon Juigaku Zasshi 1989;51(2):257–63.
35. Grandage J. The erect dog penis: a paradox of flexible rigidity. Vet Rec 1972; 91(6):141–7.
36. England GCW, Allen WE. Factors affecting the viability of canine spermatozoa .1. Potential influences during processing for artificial-insemination. Theriogenology 1992;37(2):363–71.
37. Oettle EE. Sperm morphology and fertility in the dog. J Reprod Fertil Suppl 1993; 47:257–60.
38. Andersen K. Insemination with frozen dog semen based on a new insemination technique. Zuchthygiene 1975;10(1):1–4.
39. Phillips TC, Dhaliwal GK, Verstegen-Onclin KM, et al. Efficacy of four density gradient separation media to remove erythrocytes and nonviable sperm from canine semen. Theriogenology 2012;77(1):39–45.
40. Dorado J, Alcaraz L, Galvez MJ, et al. Single-layer centrifugation through PureSperm(R) 80 selects improved quality spermatozoa from frozen-thawed dog semen. Anim Reprod Sci 2013;140(3–4):232–40.
41. Dorado J, Galvez MJ, Demyda-Peyras S, et al. Differences in preservation of canine chilled semen using simple sperm washing, single-layer centrifugation and modified swim-up preparation techniques. Reprod Fertil Dev 2016;28(10): 1545–52.
42. Dorado J, Galvez MJ, Morrell JM, et al. Use of single-layer centrifugation with Androcoll-C to enhance sperm quality in frozen-thawed dog semen. Theriogenology 2013;80(8):955–62.
43. Urbano M, Dorado J, Ortiz I, et al. Effect of cryopreservation and single layer centrifugation on canine sperm DNA fragmentation assessed by the sperm chromatin dispersion test. Anim Reprod Sci 2013;143(1–4):118–25.
44. Fontbonne A, Badinand F. Canine artificial insemination with frozen semen: comparison of intravaginal and intrauterine deposition of semen. J Reprod Fertil Suppl 1993;47:325–7.
45. Fukushima FB, Malm C, Henry M, et al. Site of intrauterine artificial insemination in the bitch does not affect sperm distribution within the uterus. Reprod Domest Anim 2010;45(6):1059–64.
46. Hutchison R. Vaginal & surgical intra-uterine deposition of semen. Paper presented at: Canine theriogenology short course; August, 1993.
47. England GC, Millar KM. The ethics and role of AI with fresh and frozen semen in dogs. Reprod Domest Anim 2008;43(Suppl 2):165–71.
48. Goodman MF. Just because I can, doesn't mean I should: the application of evidence-based medicine to small animal theriogenology. Clin Theriogenology 2015;7(3):147–52.
49. Anderson K. Fertility of frozen dog semen. Acta Vet Scand 1972;13(1):128–30.
50. Ferguson JM, Renton JP, Farstad W, et al. Insemination of beagle bitches with frozen semen. J Reprod Fertil Suppl 1989;39:293–8.
51. Silva LD, Onclin K, Snaps F, et al. Laparoscopic intrauterine insemination in the bitch. Theriogenology 1995;43(3):615–23.

52. England GC, Moxon R, Freeman SL. Stimulation of mating-induced uterine contractions in the bitch and their modification and enhancement of fertility by prostatic fluid. Reprod Domest Anim 2012;47(Suppl 6):1–5.
53. Wilson MS. Non-surgical intrauterine artificial insemination in bitches using frozen semen. J Reprod Fertil Suppl 1993;47:307–11.
54. Wilson MS. Transcervical insemination techniques in the bitch. Vet Clin North Am Small Anim Pract 2001;31(2):291–304.
55. Eilts B. Fertility in a canine breeding colony using vaginal artificial insemination or transcervical insemination of fresh semen. Paper presented at: ANZCVS Science Week, July 5, 2013; Gold Coast, Queensland, Australia.
56. Daskin A, Tekin N, Akcay E. The effect of transcervical intrauterine and intravaginal insemination methods on fertility in dogs. Turk J Vet Anim Sci 2003;27(1):235–9.
57. Pretzer SD, Lillich RK, Althouse GC. Single, transcervical insemination using frozen-thawed semen in the Greyhound: a case series study. Theriogenology 2006;65(6):1029–36.

Estrous Cycle Manipulation in Dogs

Michelle Anne Kutzler, DVM, PhD

KEYWORDS

- Dopamine agonist • Estrus induction
- Gonadotropin releasing hormone (GnRH) agonist

KEY POINTS

- Although many methods of estrus induction exist for both canids and felids, success rates vary between and within various protocols.
- Long-acting preparations are convenient for the owner and less stressful for the patient, but are associated with premature luteal failure and subsequent reduced birthing rates.
- Knowledge of the strengths and weakness of each regimen will assist the veterinarian in making a selection that will be best suited for the patient and client.

INTRODUCTION

Canine reproductive physiology has unique characteristics that make extrapolation from farm animals (horses, cows, sheep, goats, pigs) unsuccessful in this species. Domestic bitches are nonseasonally monoestrous. Bitches ovulate only once or twice per year with few exceptions.[1] The period from the onset of proestrus to the onset of the next proestrus is referred to as the interestrous interval (IEI). Unique to dogs, the IEI includes proestrus, estrus, diestrus, and anestrus. During anestrus, neither the ovary nor the pituitary are quiescent. The IEI averages 31 weeks[2,3] with a typical range of 16 to 56 weeks.[2] However, the IEI may be more or less frequent depending on the duration of anestrus, which varies between and within individual bitches.[4] Estrous cycle manipulation in dogs is used for both shortening and lengthening the IEI, depending on the desired outcome. This review focuses on shortening the IEI for purposes of estrus induction.

In the bitch, progression from early to late anestrus is characterized by a higher amplitude and a greater number of hypothalamic gonadotropin-releasing hormone (GnRH) pulses.[5] The GnRH pulse frequency is significantly increased during late anestrus.[5] The sensitivity of the pituitary to GnRH and the indirect response of the ovary to

Disclosure Statement: The author has nothing to disclose.
Department of Animal and Rangeland Sciences, Oregon State University, 112 Withycombe Hall, Corvallis, OR 97331, USA
E-mail address: michelle.kutzler@oregonstate.edu

Vet Clin Small Anim 48 (2018) 581–594
https://doi.org/10.1016/j.cvsm.2018.02.006
0195-5616/18/© 2018 Elsevier Inc. All rights reserved.
vetsmall.theclinics.com

GnRH also changes from early to late anestrus, with both a significant increase in pituitary sensitivity to GnRH (as expressed by circulating luteinizing hormone [LH] concentrations)[6] and an increase in ovarian responsiveness to LH and follicle-stimulating hormone (FSH).[6,7] Serum FSH concentrations are increased throughout much of canine anestrus, but are significantly higher during late anestrus compared with during mid and early anestrus.[8] Conversely, LH concentrations are low except near the end of anestrus.[9] An increase in plasma FSH concentration is critical for the initiation of folliculogenesis and, consequently, for the termination of anestrus in dogs.[8,10] In most domestic mammals, FSH is regarded as the most important factor in the early stages of follicular development, whereas LH is regarded as the primary regulatory factor in the more mature follicles.[11,12] It has been suggested that, for canine anestrus to end, an increasing plasma FSH concentration must exceed some threshold level of enough sensitive antral follicles to result in the progression of these follicles to the pre-ovulatory stage.[13] FSH induces expression of LH receptors in the ovarian granulosa cells.[4] After initial follicle recruitment, LH is progressively able to replace FSH in the support of follicular maturation.[12] In fact, supraphysiologic doses of LH alone administered to bitches in anestrus will induce follicle growth and proestrus.[9,14]

PATIENT EVALUATION OVERVIEW

Methods for inducing estrus in bitches need to be safe and reliable. Methods for estrus induction in bitches include the use of dopamine agonists (bromocriptine, cabergoline, metergoline), GnRH agonists (lutrelin, buserelin, fertirelin, deslorelin, and leuprolide), and exogenous gonadotropins (LH, FSH, human chorionic gonadotropin [hCG], equine chorionic gonadotropin [eCG], and human menopausal gonadotropin). These methods vary greatly in their efficacy of inducing estrus as well as in the pregnancy rates after the induced estrus. In addition, the applicability of some of these methods for clinical practice is questionable. Indications for inducing estrus include management of prolonged anestrus (prologed IEI) in conjunction with routine breeding management when breeding opportunities are missed or after conception failure, or if a particular mating must be timed around the availability of the stud dog or whelping around a certain time of the year (eg, before hunting season). Estrus induction is most successful in fertile females that are at least 120 days from the onset of their last proestrus.[15] Although several studies have demonstrated that ovulation can be induced after diestrus termination, bitches rarely become pregnant from this approach.[16–18] In the dog, histologic changes similar to endometrial involution are not complete until 135 days after the last proestrus, regardless of whether the bitch was pregnant or not.[19]

PHARMACOLOGIC OPTIONS FOR ESTRUS INDUCTION
Dopamine Agonists

Dopamine agonists are ergot derivatives that inhibit prolactin secretion by directly stimulating dopamine receptors.[20] In species other than the dog, dopamine agonists inhibit gonadotrophin secretion during anestrus and dopamine antagonists induce reproductive activity. In the bitch, however, dopamine agonists induce the onset of estrus. It was previously believed that prolactin inhibition was necessary for canine estrus induction to occur. However, Beijerink and colleagues[21] (2003) demonstrated that bromocriptine shortens the IEI in the bitch, even when the dose is so low that it does not lower the plasma prolactin concentration. In addition, bitches treated with low doses of a serotonin receptor antagonist (metergoline) had reduced prolactin concentrations, but did not go into estrus.[22–24] These observations suggested that dopamine agonists induce estrus with another mechanism other than via lowering plasma prolactin concentration. Kooistra and coworkers[25] (1999) reported that follicle development and resulting estrus induction with bromocriptine was associated with an increase in plasma FSH concentration without a concomitant increase in plasma LH concentration. The dopamine agonist–induced increase in the basal plasma FSH concentration was similar to what is observed during physiologic late anestrus.[4] In the mare, dopamine receptors are present in the ovary[26] and, in rats, dopamine agonists and antagonists directly affect ovarian steroidogenesis.[27] It is not known if there is a direct gonadal effect of dopamine agonists in the dog. However, it should be noted that prolonged cabergoline administration during proestrus and estrus does not affect follicular development.[28]

The pregnancy rate after estrus induction using dopamine agonists varies depending on dose,[21] treatment duration, and stage of anestrus.[29] Several estrus induction protocols using dopamine agonists have been reported (**Table 1**). Within the United States, the most common dopamine agonist treatment used is cabergoline at a

Table 1
Protocols using dopamine agonists for estrus manipulation in the bitch

Reference	n	Estrus Induction Protocols	Pregnancy Rate (%)
Zoldag et al,[36] 2001	48	Bromocriptine 0.3 mg/bitch for 3 d, then 0.6–2.5 mg/bitch PO SID for 3–6 d after onset of estrus	83
Verstegen et al,[29] 1999	5	Cabergoline 0.005 mg/kg PO SID until 3–8 d after onset of proestrus or 40 d	60
Verstegen et al,[29] 1999	5	Cabergoline 0.005 mg/kg PO SID until 3–8 d after onset of proestrus or 40 d	100
Verstegen et al,[29] 1999	5	Cabergoline 0.005 mg/kg PO SID until 3–8 d after onset of proestrus or 40 d	80
Gobello et al,[86] 2002	5	Cabergoline 0.005 mg/kg SID PO until second d of proestrus	100
Rota et al,[87] 2003	12	Cabergoline 0.005 mg/kg PO SID until progression of proestrus to estrus	83
Gunay et al,[38] 2004	13	Cabergoline 6 mg/kg[c] SID PO until onset of estrus or up to 14 d	84.6
Cirit et al,[31] 2007	28	Cabergoline 0.005 mg/kg PO SID for 7–10 d	93.3
Cirit et al,[31] 2007	10	Cabergoline 0.005 mg/kg PO SID until second d of proestrus or d 42 of treatment	60
Cirit et al,[31] 2007	19	Cabergoline 0.0006 mg/kg PO SID until second d of proestrus or d 42 of treatment	57.9
Cirit et al,[31] 2007	8	Cabergoline 0.0006 mg/kg PO SID until second d of proestrus or d 42 of treatment[a]	75
Nak et al,[88] 2012	20	Cabergoline 0.005 mg/kg SID PO until second d of proestrus or d 42 of treatment	80
Kusuma & Tainturier,[39] 1993	10	Metergoline 0.56–1.2 mg/kg IM every third d until proestrus of d 40 of treatment	90
Kusuma & Tainturier,[39] 1993	10	Metergoline 0.56–1.2 mg/kg IM every third d until proestrus of d 40 of treatment[b]	40

Abbreviations: IM, intramuscularly; PO, per os; ISD, once per day.
[a] Human chorionic gonadotropin 500 IU administered IM in late proestrus to induce ovulation.
[b] Human chorionic gonadotropin 500 IU administered IM on the first and third days of estrus to induce ovulation.
[c] Dose appears to be 1000X but reported three times in reference at this amount.

dosage of 0.005 mg/kg administered once daily orally until 1 to 2 days after the onset of induced proestrus. Cabergoline (available as Dostinex [Pfizer] and in generic forms) is a human product containing 0.5 mg of cabergoline per tablet and sold at about $10 per tablet. Aside from the cost, cabergoline can be difficult to dose accurately, especially in small animals.[30] For accurate dosing in dogs, tablets can either be compounded into the appropriate-strength capsules or a portion of the tablet can be crushed and diluted with fluid just before dosing.[30] Cirit and coworkers[31] (2007) observed that a 0.5 mg Dostinex tablet completely dissolves in 50 mL of distilled water at room temperature, producing a solution that is 0.01 mg of cabergoline/mL. It was reported by Persiani and colleagues[32] (1994) that the relative bioavailability of tablets versus an aqueous solution of cabergoline was 99% and the pharmacodynamics and relative bioavailability was not influenced by formulation (tablet vs solution). However, cabergoline is inactivated over time in aqueous solutions containing water, such that the cabergoline solutions should be prepared fresh daily and used within 15 minutes of preparation.[31] McLean and coworkers[30] reported that cabergoline could be stable for 28 days if compounded in acidic fluids (1% acetic acid solution).

There are 2 prominent side effects with dopamine agonists: coat color changes and vomiting. Approximately 25% of bitches that received cabergoline for 14 to 45 days developed coat color changes beginning the second week of administration and lasting until the next coat shedding.[33] Of these, fawn-colored bitches developed a yellowish coat color whereas Argentine boarhounds became black spotted, mainly on their extremities.[33] In previous untreated estrous periods, these bitches had shown no coat color changes.[33] These authors postulated that a color shift in certain hair coats of particular breeds could be mediated through inhibition of melanocyte-stimulating hormone secretion.[33] Transient coat color changes should be considered a possible side effect when planning long-term treatment with dopamine agonists in dogs.[33]

Vomiting was a frequent side effect (3%–25% of cases) with bromocriptine or cabergoline occurring within 1 hour after the first treatment.[6,20,29,34–36] Vomiting tends to be a less common side effect after cabergoline when compared with bromocriptine,[20] probably because cabergoline binds more specifically to dopamine type-2 receptors in the hypothalamus and pituitary gland.[37] It is important to note that Gunay and colleagues[38] did not observe any side effects of vomiting when they administered cabergoline to German Shepherds using a much higher dose of cabergoline (6 mg/kg) than the optimal effective dose (0.005 mg/kg) as determined by dose response.[20] Beginning with lower doses of bromocriptine initially can result in habituation, which will almost completely eliminate emesis as a side effect of treatment.[34] It should be noted that even very high doses of metergoline do not induce vomiting in bitches.[39]

Gonadotropin-Releasing Hormone and Gonadotropin-Releasing Hormone Agonists

GnRH is a hypothalamic decapeptide that mediates the synthesis and release of pituitary LH and FSH. In the bitch, progression from early to late anestrus is characterized by a higher amplitude and a greater number of GnRH pulses,[5] and an increase in pituitary sensitivity to GnRH.[7,40] Different approaches have been investigated to directly stimulate the activity of the pituitary with GnRH and GnRH agonists to induce estrus (**Table 2**). Pulsatile administration of GnRH at doses of 0.0002 to 0.0004 mg/kg at 90-minute intervals is sufficient to obtain increases in LH similar to the endogenous pulses that normally occur at the end of proestrus.[9] By making molecular changes to native GnRH, more than 700 GnRH agonists have been synthesized that have an increased receptor affinity and enhanced stability.[41] High rates of fertile estrus induction were reported with less than 0.0024 mg/kg/d of lutrelin for more than 8 days.[42]

Table 2
Protocols using GnRH and GnRH agonists for estrus manipulation in the bitch

Reference	N	Estrus Induction Protocols	Pregnancy Rate (%)
Vanderlip et al,[89] 1987	8	GnRH 0.000040–0.000430 mg/kg IV every 87 min for 9 d	37.5
Cain et al,[90] 1988	8	GnRH 0.000096–0.000139 mg/kg IV every 90 min for 11–13 d	87.5
Concannon et al,[91] 1997	36	GnRH 0.000015–0.000500 mg/kg IV every 90 min for 7–9 d	33
Rota et al,[87] 2003	10	Buserelin 0.0015 mg/kg SQ TID for 11 d and 0.00075 mg/kg SQ TID for 3 d	20
Inaba et al,[44] 1998	18	Leuprolide 0.10 mg/kg SQ once[a]	78
Hatoya et al,[45] 2006	7	Leuprolide 0.0036 mg intranasal spray once daily until onset of proestrus up to 14 d	42.9
Concannon,[43] 1989	24	Lutrelin 0.0017–0.0025 mg/kg/d SQ for 12–14 d via osmotic mini pump	37.5[b]
Concannon et al,[42] 2006	6	Lutrelin 0.0024 mg/kg/d SQ for 12–14 d via osmotic mini pump	33.3
Concannon et al,[42] 2006	20	Lutrelin 0.0018 mg/kg/d for SQ 12–14 d via osmotic mini pump	35
Concannon et al,[42] 2006	6	Lutrelin 0.0012 mg/kg/d for SQ 12–14 d via osmotic mini pump	33.3
Concannon et al,[42] 2006	18	Lutrelin 0.0006–0.0024 mg/kg/d SQ for 12–14 d via osmotic mini pump	88.9
Concannon et al,[42] 2006	7	Lutrelin 0.0002 mg/kg/d SQ for 12–14 d via osmotic mini pump	57.1
Concannon et al,[42] 2006	24	Lutrelin 0.0006–0.0024 mg/kg/d SQ for 7–8 d via osmotic mini pump	16.7
Concannon et al,[42] 2006	6	Lutrelin 0.048 mg/kg/d SQ for 12–14 d via osmotic mini pump	0
Kutzler et al,[51,52] 2001	7	Deslorelin 2.1 mg SQ once over the shoulder blades	43[b]
Kutzler et al,[56] 2002	6	Deslorelin 2.1 mg vestibular submucosa once	67
Kutzler et al,[56] 2002	5	Deslorelin 2.1 mg vestibular submucosa once	40
Volkmann et al,[57] 2006	3	Deslorelin 2.1 mg vestibular submucosa once	67
Volkmann et al,[57] 2006	10	Deslorelin 1.05 mg vestibular submucosa once	70
Kutzler et al,[56] 2002	5	Deslorelin 1.5 mg IM once	60
Walter et al,[92] 2011	11	Deslorelin 4.7 mg SQ medial side of the leg once	63.6
Fontaine et al,[93] 2011	6	Deslorelin 4.7 mg SQ ventral abdomen close to the umbilicus once[c]	25
Fontaine et al,[93] 2011	23	Deslorelin 4.7 mg SQ ventral abdomen close to the umbilicus once[d]	78.3
Von Heimendahl et al,[94] 2012	16	Deslorelin 4.7 mg SQ ventral abdomen close to the umbilicus once	68.8
Borges et al,[95] 2015	19	Deslorelin 4.7 mg SQ ventral abdomen close to the umbilicus once	36.8
Borges et al,[95] 2015	17	Deslorelin 4.7 mg SQ ventral abdomen close to the umbilicus once	70.6

Abbreviations: IM, intramuscularly; IV, intravenously; SQ, subcutaneously; TID, 3 times per day.
[a] Fertirelin 0.003 mg/kg IM given on the first day of estrus to induce ovulation.
[b] Premature luteal failure.
[c] Administered 80 to 160 days after their previous estrus.
[d] Administered 200 to 590 days after their previous estrus.

However, reduced efficacy occurred at doses of 0.0048 mg/kg/d owing to a failed or insufficient LH surge at the end of proestrus.[42] Concannon and colleagues[42] concluded that the dose of GnRH agonist needed to be sufficiently large enough to stimulate the initial increase in LH and FSH but modest enough to not excessively downregulate the spontaneous preovulatory surge and be administered for at least 10 to 13 days.

Increases in GnRH do not need to be pulsatile to induce estrus.[9] Constant infusion or release of a GnRH agonist (lutrelin, deslorelin, leuprolide) via a subcutaneous osmotic mini pump or implant resulted in similar estrus induction and pregnancy rates as GnRH pulsatile infusion, provided that the GnRH agonist therapy is discontinued.[9,43] According to Concannon and colleagues,[42] GnRH agonist needs to be administered for at least 10 to 13 days, but removed shortly before or at the time when the LH surge typically occurs, to prevent downregulation. A single injection of leuprolide (0.1 mg/kg subcutaneously) induced estrus in prepubertal bitches as well as bitches 120 and 150 days postpartum.[44] An intranasal spray containing a GnRH agonist (Leupron Depot, Takeda Chemical Industries, Osaka, Japan) used to induce estrus produced no negative clinical effects and seemed to cause little stress to the animals.[45] As mentioned, prolonged administration of GnRH agonists results in pituitary overstimulation, downregulation of GnRH receptor transcription in the pituitary,[46] suppression of LH (and in some species FSH) secretion,[47,48] decreased luteal responsiveness to LH, and decreased progesterone secretion.[41,49,50] Premature luteal failure resulting in a shortened diestrus with subsequent pregnancy loss has been reported with GnRH agonist therapy for estrus induction.[43,46–52]

The GnRH agonist that has been most widely studied in canine estrus manipulation is deslorelin. Deslorelin is a D-Trp[6]-Pro[9]-des-Gly[10]GnRH agonist with 2 amino acid substitutions. Veterinary clinical applications of deslorelin in bitches were first introduced by Trigg and colleagues[53] (2000) during an investigation for a novel contraceptive (Suprelorin), which is now commercially available in Europe, Australia, and New Zealand. Preliminary investigations with this product demonstrated that it induced estrus in all anestrous bitches treated initially, which was followed by prolonged estrus suppression.[54,55] Administration of a 2.1-mg deslorelin implant resulted in reliable, rapid, and synchronous estrus when administered to anestrous bitches[50–52,56] or to diestrous bitches after termination of diestrus using prostaglandin F-2α in.[57] Although all of these methods resulted in rapid and dependable estrus induction in bitches, pregnancy rates (fertility) varied from 8% to 100% depending on the stage of estrous cycle in which the induction was initiated and the protocol used. GnRH and GnRH agonists are not approved for use in bitches in the United States. Although readily available, the extralabel use of a GnRH agonist (Suprelorin-F, Virbac Animal Health, Fort Worth, TX) in species other than ferrets is strictly prohibited.

Gonadotropins

Both LH and FSH are follicotropic in the dog; administration of pharmacologic doses of either LH or FSH alone induces estrus (**Table 3**).[9,58] However, an estrus induction protocol established with combined dosages of FSH and LH designed to resemble the gradual increase of endogenous FSH coincidentally with the LH increase during proestrus was not successful.[58] The LH potency within purified or partially purified FSH products used may interfere with endogenous LH release.[59] Bouchard and coworkers[59] (1991) demonstrated that LH cross-reactivity from contamination of porcine-derived FSH lasts 48 hours after administration. In addition, acute allergic reactions have been reported after intravenous administration of LH (5 mg) in 2 bitches.[60]

In addition to exogenous pituitary gonadotropins, eCG (formerly known as pregnancy mare serum gonadotropin) and human menopausal gonadotropin have been

Table 3
Protocols using gonadotropins for estrus manipulation in the bitch

Reference	N	Estrus Induction Protocol	Pregnancy Rate
Verstegen et al,[14] 1997	16	LH 0.1 IU/kg TID for 7 d	37.5
Shille et al,[58] 1984	5	FSH 0.77–1.1 mg IM once	40
Shille et al,[58] 1984	4	FSH 0.077–0.11 mg to 1.23–1.78 mg IM SID for 10 d, doubling dose of FSH every 2 d	50
Nickson et al,[66] 1992	18	eCG 187 MU[a] IM once[b]	50
Hancock & Rowlands,[96] 1949	9	eCG 200–300 IU SQ once or 100 IU SQ every 4 d for a total of 200–300 IU	11.1
Thun et al,[97] 1977	6	eCG 15.6–35.7 IU/kg SID SQ for 10 d[c]	50
Thun et al,[97] 1977	7	eCG 15.6–35/7 IU/kg SID SQ for 10 d[c]	57
Thun et al,[97] 1977	12	eCG 1.25–2.8 IU/kg SID SQ for 10 d[c]	58
Archbald et al,[98] 1980	8	eCG 44 IU/kg SID IM for 9 d[c]	60
Archbald et al,[98] 1980	5	eCG 44 IU/kg SID SQ for 9 d[d]	60
Allen,[99] 1982	4	eCG 21.2–26.9 IU SQ every 48 h for a total of 5 injections (1250 IU total)	25
Renton et al,[100] 1984	3	eCG 500 IU SID SQ until onset of proestrus or up to 10 d	0[e]
Chaffaux et al,[101] 1984	5	eCG 27.8–41.6 IU/kg SID IM for 10 d[f]	0
Chaffaux et al,[101] 1984	15	eCG 27.8–41.6 IU/kg SID IM for 10 d[c]	20
Nakao et al,[73] 1985	11	eCG 44 IU/kg SID IM for 9 d[c]	13[e]
Arnold et al,[102] 1989	17	eCG 20 IU/kg SID IM for 10 d[c]	0
Arnold et al,[102] 1989	6	eCG 20 IU/kg SID IM for 5 d[g]	50
Kusuma & Tainturier,[39] 1993	10	eCG 33.3–71.4 IU/kg SID IM until proestrus or up to 9 d	0
Weilenmann et al,[74] 1993	14	eCG 20 IU/kg SID IM for 5 d[g]	43[e]
Wanke et al,[103] 1997	10	hMG 1.7 U/kg SID IM for 9 d	40
Nak et al,[88] 2012	19	eCG 20 IU/kg SID IM for 5 d[g]	0
Stornelli et al,[62] 2012	15	eCG 50 IU/kg IM once[h]	80

Abbreviations: eCG, equine chorionic gonadotropin; FSH, follicle-stimulating hormone; hMG, human menopausal gonadotropin; IM, intramuscularly; IV, intravenously; LH, luteinizing hormone; SQ, subcutaneously; SID, once per day; TID, 3 times per day.
[a] Mouse units.
[b] Human chorionic gonadotropin 50 MU IM at time of eCG injection.
[c] Human chorionic gonadotropin 500 IU IM or SQ on the 10th day of treatment.
[d] Human chorionic gonadotropin 500 IU IM on the second day of estrus.
[e] Premature luteal failure.
[f] Gonadoliberin 0.05 mg IM on the 10th day of treatment.
[g] Human chorionic gonadotropin 500 IU IM on the fifth day of treatment.
[h] Human chorionic gonadotropin 500 IU IM on the seventh day of treatment.

used for estrus induction in bitches (see **Table 3**). The most widely studied gonadotropin for estrus induction in the dog is eCG, with protocols ranging from daily to weekly injections using either subcutaneous or intramuscular routes of administration. Studies using eCG have generally been more successful for estrus induction in bitches than those using FSH. Bitches treated with eCG at a dose of 20 IU/kg subcutaneously for 5 consecutive days with an additional 500 IU subcutaneously per bitch of hCG on the last day of treatment had similar estrus induction and ovulation rates to cabergoline treated bitches.[61]

A protocol using 50 IU/kg (intramuscularly once) of eCG combined 7 days later with 500 IU (intramuscularly once) of hCG induced normal and fertile estrus (the mean interval from treatment to estrus was 4.0 ± 0.4 days) with an 80% pregnancy rate (12/15) and no reported side effects.[62] Although eCG induces follicular development and in some bitches allows spontaneous ovulation, not all animals will ovulate spontaneously with a single eCG dose.[62] Hence, the use of hCG after eCG treatment is often recommended. However, the administration of hCG for the induction of ovulation is controversial and several groups have reported no benefit or serious side effects. The administration of hCG has no positive effects on ovulation rates, pregnancy rates, or number of offspring per pregnancy when administered at the onset of or during estrus.[31] In fact, treatment with hCG on the first and third days of estrus significantly prolongs behavioral estrus and lowers serum progesterone concentration of day 5 of estrus.[31] Volkmann and coworkers[63] found similar results when hCG was administered to bitches after day 40 of gestation, in that after an initial increase in serum progesterone concentrations, hCG dramatically suppressed progesterone secretion. In addition to a reduction in ovulation and pregnancy rates, Kusuma and Tainturier[39] (1993) reported both prolonged proestrus and shortened proestrus (with concomitant shortened estrus) in bitches treated with hCG in late proestrus. Nevertheless, Wright[64,65] (1972) reported that ovulation in the bitch occurs 26 to 30 hours after the administration of hCG and that eCG-induced bitches treated with hCG at the onset of estrus had better ovulatory responses than those only treated with eCG.[64]

Although widely available around the world under the brand name of Folligon (Intervet, Osaka, Japan), eCG is not commercially available in the United States except in combination with hCG (PG600; Intervet). This product contains 80 IU eCG and 40 IU hCG per milliliter. Nickson and associates[66] (1992) demonstrated that a single 5-mL injection of PG600 was highly effective at inducing proestrus in bitches (17 of 19). Unfortunately, the ovulation rate was poor (8 of 19); superovulation may have occurred and pregnancy rates were not reported.[66] However, others have reported 50% to 84% whelping rates when eCG and HCG are given in combination to induce estrus in bitches.[67,68]

Numerous side effects have been reported with eCG, from immune-mediated reactions[69] to sudden death.[70] The most frequent problems encountered with eCG arise from the unpredictability of an individual bitch's response both in the number of follicles that develop and in the potential for premature luteal failure. Premature luteal failure with subsequent shortening of diestrus and pregnancy loss is a frustrating sequela of eCG use in canids.[71–74] In 1 study, treatment with eCG was followed by a progressive decline in progesterone concentrations to less than 1 ng/mL between 38 and 40 days after estrus.[71] Histologically, luteal cells from corpora lutea formed in bitches after eCG treatment have reticulated and vacuolated cytoplasm compared with luteal cells from corpora lutea of normal, nonfertile estrous cycles that have compact and granulated cytoplasm.[75] Premature luteolysis of induced corpora lutea have also been reported in ewes,[76] beef cows,[77] and dairy cows.[78] In ruminants, pretreatment with a progestin before ovulation induction increases luteal weight[79] and secretion of progesterone.[80–83] However, bitches pretreated with megestrol acetate (2.2 mg/kg orally once daily for 8 days) before undergoing an estrus induction with eCG (44 IU/kg intramuscularly once daily for 9 days) were not prevented from undergoing premature luteolysis as progesterone values were less than 1 ng/mL by 50 days after estrus in all eCG-treated bitches.[84] It is of interest to note that such premature luteal regression seems to be independent of the presence or absence of the uterus. This was demonstrated after hysterectomy of normal, nonpregnant bitches on day 4 of estrus during a noninduced cycle. Hysterectomy resulted in premature regression of the corpora lutea.[85] The authors speculated that a luteotrophic factor of uterine origin, which may be active in the normal cycle of the bitch at 24 days of diestrus, may be involved in luteal maintenance.[85]

SUMMARY

Although many methods of estrus induction exist for both canids and felids, success (induction of estrus, ovulation, pregnancy, and delivery of offspring) rates vary between and within various protocols. Knowledge of the strengths and weakness of each regimen will assist the veterinarian in making a selection that will be best suited for the patient and client. Long-acting preparations (eCG, GnRH agonist implants) are convenient for the owner and less stressful for the patient, but are associated with premature luteal failure and subsequent reduced pregnancy rates. For these reasons, practitioners should use of dopamine agonists when needing to induce estrus in the bitch.

REFERENCES

1. Fuller JL. Photoperioidic control of estrus in the Basenji. J Hered 1956;47: 179–80.
2. Christie DW, Bell ET. Some observations on the seasonal incidence and frequency of oestrus in breeding bitches in Britain. J Small Anim Pract 1971;12: 159–67.
3. Rowlands IW. Some observations on the breeding of dogs. J Hered 1950;47: 40–55.
4. Okkens AC, Kooistra HS. Anoestrus in the dog: a fascinating story. Reprod Domest Anim 2006;41:291–6.
5. Tani H, Inaba T, Tamada H, et al. Increasing gonadotropin-releasing hormone release by perfused hypothalamus from early to late anestrus in the beagle bitch. Neurosci Lett 1996;207:1–4.
6. Van Haaften B, Dieleman SJ, Okkens AC, et al. Induction of estrus and ovulation in dogs by treatment with PMSG and/or bromocriptine. J Reprod Fertil Suppl 1989;39:330–1 [abstract].
7. Jeffcoate IA. Endocrinology of anestrous bitches. J Reprod Fertil Suppl 1993;47: 69–76.
8. Kooistra HS, Okkens AC, Bevers MM, et al. Concurrent pulsatile secretion of luteinizing hormone and follicle-stimulating hormone during different phases of the estrous cycle and anestrus in beagle bitches. Biol Reprod 1999;60: 65–71.
9. Concannon PW. Biology of gonadotropin secretion in adult and prepubertal female dogs. J Reprod Fertil Suppl 1993;47:3–27.
10. Onclin K, Lauwers F, Verstegen JP. FSH secretion patterns during pregnant and nonpregnant luteal periods and 24h secretion patterns in male and female dogs. J Reprod Fertil Suppl 2001;57:15–21.
11. Moyle WR, Campbell RK. Gonadotropins. In: Adashi EY, Rock JA, Rosenwaks Z, editors. Reproductive endocrinology, surgery and technology. Philadelphia: Lippincott-Raven; 1995. p. 683–724.
12. Monniaux D, Huet C, Besnard N, et al. Follicular growth and ovarian dynamics in mammals. J Reprod Fertil Suppl 1997;51:3–23.
13. de Gier J, Beijerink NJ, Kooistra HS, et al. Physiology of the canine anoestrus and methods for manipulation of its length. Reprod Domest Anim 2008; 43(Suppl 2):157–64.

14. Verstegen J, Onclin K, Silva L, et al. Termination of obligate anestrus and induction of fertile ovarian cycles by administration of purified pig LH. J Reprod Fertil 1997;111:35–40.

15. Chakraborty PK, Wildt DE, Seager SWJ. Induction of estrus and ovulation in the cat and dog. Vet Clin North Am Small Anim Pract 1982;12:85–91.

16. Jeukenne P, Verstegen J. Termination of diestrus and induction of estrus in diestrous non pregnant bitches by the prolactin antagonist cabergoline. J Reprod Fertil Suppl 1997;51:59–66.

17. Leyva-Ocariz H. Effect of hyperadrenocorticism and diabetes mellitus on serum progesterone concentrations during early metoestrus of pregnant and non-pregnant cycles induced by pregnant mares' serum gonadotrophin in domestic dogs. J Reprod Fertil Suppl 1993;47:371–7.

18. Ohmura M, Torii R, Hatoya S, et al. Induction of fertile oestrus in dioestrous bitches using prostaglandin F2α and a GnRH agonist. Vet Rec 2011;168:669.

19. Anderson AC, Simpson ME. The ovary and reproductive cycle of the dog (Beagle). Los Altos (CA): Geron-X Inc; 1973.

20. Jöchle W, Arbeiter K, Post K, et al. Effects on pseudopregnancy, pregnancy and interoestrous intervals of pharmacological suppression of prolactin secretion in female dogs and cats. J Reprod Fertil Suppl 1989;39:199–207.

21. Beijerink NJ, Dieleman SJ, Kooistra HS, et al. Low doses of bromocriptine shorten the interestrous interval in the bitch without lowering plasma prolactin concentration. Theriogenology 2003;60:1379–86.

22. Krulich L, McCann SM, Mayfield MA. On the mode of the prolactin release-inhibiting action of the serotonin receptor blockers metergoline, methysergide and cyproheptadine. Endocrinology 1981;108:1115–24.

23. Müller EE, Locatelli V, Cella S, et al. Prolactin-lowering and –releasing drugs. Mechanisms of action and therapeutic applications. Drugs 1983;25:399–432.

24. Okkens AC, Kooistra HS, Dieleman SJ, et al. Dopamine agonistic effects as opposed to prolactin concentrations in plasma as the influencing factor on the duration of anestrus in bitches. J Reprod Fertil 1997;51(Suppl):55–8.

25. Kooistra HS, Okkens AC, Bevers MM, et al. Bromocriptine-induced premature oestrus is associated with changes in the pulsatile secretion pattern of follicle-stimulating hormone in beagle bitches. J Reprod Fertil 1999;117:387–93.

26. King SS, Campbell AG, Dille EA, et al. Dopamine receptors in equine ovarian tissues. Domest Anim Endocrinol 2005;28:405–25.

27. Mori H, Arakawa S, Ohkawa T, et al. The involvement of dopamine in regulation of steroidogenesis in rat ovarian cells. Horm Res 1994;41:36–40.

28. De Rensis F, Spattini G, Ballabio R, et al. The effect of administering a dopamine agonist (cabergoline) on follicular and luteal development during proestrus and estrus in the female greyhound. Theriogenology 2006;66:887–95.

29. Verstegen JP, Onclin K, Silva L, et al. Effect of stage of anestrus on the induction of estrus by the dopamine agonist cabergoline in dogs. Theriogenology 1999; 51:597–611.

30. McLean S, Brandon S, Kirkwood R. Stability of cabergoline in fox baits in laboratory and field conditions. Wildl Res 2007;34:239–46.

31. Cirit Ü, Bacinoglu S, Cangul IT, et al. The effects of a low dose of cabergoline on induction of estrus and pregnancy rates in anestrous bitches. Anim Reprod Sc 2007;101:134–44.

32. Persiani S, Sassolas G, Piscitelli G, et al. Pharmacodynamics and relative bioavailability of cabergoline tablets vs. solution in healthy volunteers J Pharm Sci 1994;83(10):1421–4.

33. Gobello C, Castex G, Broglia G, et al. Coat colour changes associated with cabergoline administration in bitches. J Small Anim Pract 2003;44(8):352–4.
34. Arbeiter K, Barsch E. Possibilities of oestrus induction in the bitch with an ergoline derivate. J Vet Med 1988;35:111–7.
35. Janssens LAA. Treatment of pseudopregnancy with bromocriptine, an ergot alkaloid. Vet Rec 1986;119:172–4.
36. Zoldag L, Fekete S, Csaky I, et al. Fertile estrus induced in bitches by bromocriptine, a dopamine agonist: a clinical trial. Theriogenology 2001;55:1657–66.
37. Rains CP, Bryson HM, Fitton A. Cabergoline: a review of its pharmacological properties and therapeutic potential in the treatment of hyperprolactinaemia and inhibition of lactation. Drugs 1995;49(2):255–79.
38. Gunay A, Gunay U, Soylu MK. Cabergoline applications in early and late anoestrus periods on German Shepherd dogs. Revue Méd Vét 2004;155(11):557–60.
39. Kusuma PS, Tainturier D. Comparison of induction of oestrus in dogs using metergoline, metergoline plus human chorionic gonadotrophin, or pregnant mares' serum gonadotrophin. J Reprod Fertil Suppl 1993;47:363–70.
40. Hull ME, Kenigsberg DJ. Gonadotropin releasing hormone: function and clinical use. Lab Management 1987;25:51–8.
41. Jacobi GH, Wenderoth UK. Gonadotropin-releasing hormone analogues for prostate cancer: untoward side effects of high-dose regimens acquire a therapeutical dimension. Eur Urol 1982;8:129–34.
42. Concannon PW, Temple M, Montanez A, et al. Effects of dose and duration of continuous GnRH-agonist treatment on induction of estrus in beagle dogs: competing and concurrent up-regulation and down-regulation of LH release. Theriogenology 2006;66:1488–96.
43. Concannon PW. Induction of fertile oestrus in aneostrus dogs by constant infusion of GnRH agonist. J Reprod Fertil Suppl 1989;39:149–60.
44. Inaba T, Tani H, Gonda M, et al. Induction of fertile estrus in bitches using a sustained-release formulation of a GnRH agonist (leuprolide acetate). Theriogenology 1998;49:975–82.
45. Hatoya S, Torii R, Wijewardana V, et al. Induction of fertile oestrus in bitches by an intranasal spray of gonadotrophin-releasing hormone agonist. Vet Rec 2006; 158:378–9.
46. Cheng KW, Ngan ESW, Kang SK, et al. Transcriptional down-regulation of human gonadotropin-releasing hormone (GnRH) receptor gene by GnRH: role of protein kinase C and activating protein 1. Endocrinology 2000;141:3611–22.
47. Garrel G, Lerrant Y, Siriostits C, et al. Evidence that gonadotropin-releasing hormone stimulates gene expression and levels of active nitric oxide synthase type I in pituitary gonadotrophs, a process altered by desensitization and, indirectly, by gonadal steroids. Endocrinology 1998;139:2163–70.
48. Maclellan LJ, Bergfeld EG, Earl CR, et al. Influence of the luteinizing hormone-releasing hormone agonist, deslorelin, on patterns of estradiol-17β and luteinizing hormone secretion, ovarian follicular responses to superstimulation with follicle-stimulating hormone, and recovery and in vitro development of oocytes in heifer calves. Biol Reprod 1997;56:878–84.
49. McRae GI, Roberts BB, Worden AC, et al. Long-term reversible suppression of oestrus in bitches with nafarelin acetate, a potent LHRH agonist. J Reprod Fertil 1985;74:389–97.
50. D'Occhio MJ, Aspden WJ. Endocrine and reproductive responses of male and female cattle to agonists of gonadotrophin-releasing hormone. J Reprod Fertil Suppl 1999;54:101–14.

51. Kutzler MA, Wheeler R, Volkmann DH. Serum deslorelin concentrations in bitches after Ovuplant® administration. Proc Ann Meet Soc Theriogenology. Vancouver, 2001. p. 13. [abstract].

52. Kutzler MA, Wheeler R, Volkmann DH. Canine estrus induction using the GnRH agonist, deslorelin. Proc Ann Meet Eur Vet Soc Small Anim Reprod. Milan, March 1, 2001. p. 147–8.[abstract].

53. Trigg TE, Wright PJ, Armour AF, et al. Long term reversible desexing of male dogs and oestrus postponement of bitches, using a GnRH analogue implant. J Reprod Fertil Suppl 2001;57:255–61.

54. Trigg TE, Wright PJ, Armour AF, et al. Use of a GnRH analogue implant to produce reversible long-term suppression of reproductive function in male and female domestic dogs. J Reprod Fertil Suppl 2001;57:255–61.

55. Wright PJ, Verstegen JP, Onclin K, et al. Suppression of the oestrous responses of bitches to the GnRH analogue deslorelin by progestin. J Reprod Fertil Suppl 2001;57:263–8.

56. Kutzler MA, Wheeler R, Lamb S, et al. Deslorelin implant administration beneath the vulvar mucosa for the induction of synchronous estrus in bitches. Proc Ann Meet Eur Vet Soc Small Anim Reprod. Liege, May 11, 2002. [abstract].

57. Volkmann DH, Kutzler MA, Wheeler R, et al. The use of deslorelin implants for the synchronization of estrous in diestrous bitches. Theriogenology 2006;66: 1497–501.

58. Shille VM, Thatcher MJ, Simmons KJ. Efforts to induce estrus in the bitch, using pituitary gonadotropins. J Am Vet Med Assoc 1984;184:1469–73.

59. Bouchard G, Youngquist RS, Clark B, et al. Estrus induction in the bitch using a combination diethylstilbestrol and FSH-P. Theriogenology 1991;36(1): 51–65.

60. Bardens JW. Hormonal therapy for ovarian and testicular dysfunction in the dog. J Am Vet Med Assoc 1971;159:1405.

61. Jurczak A, Domosławska A, Bukowska B, et al. Equine chorionic gonadotropin and human chorionic gonadotropin stimulation increase the number of luteinized follicles and the progesterone level compared with cabergoline stimulation in anoestrus bitches. Reprod Domest Anim 2016;51(4):562–8.

62. Stornelli MC, Garcıa Mitacek MC, Gimenez F, et al. Pharmacokinetics of eCG and induction of fertile estrus in bitches using eCG followed by hCG. Theriogenology 2012;78:1056–64.

63. Volkmann DH, Kutzler MA, Wheeler R, et al. Failure of hCG to support luteal function in bitches after estrus induction using deslorelin implants. Theriogenology 2006;66:1502–6.

64. Wright PJ. A study of the response of the ovaries of bitches to pregnant mare serum (PMS) and human chorionic gonadotrophin (hCG). Proc 7th International Congress Anim Reprod held at Munich (Germany), June 6–9, 1972, vol. 2. p. 1075–9.

65. Wright PJ. The induction of oestrus and ovulation in the bitch using pregnant mare serum gonadotrophin and human chorionic gonadotrophin. Aust Vet J 1980;56(3):137–40.

66. Nickson D, Renton JP, Harvey MJA, et al. Oestrus induction in the bitch. Proc 12th International Congress Anim Reprod held at The Hague (The Netherlands), August 23–27, 1992, vol. 4. p. 1799–801.

67. Scrogie NJ. The treatment of sterility in the bitch by use of gonadotrophic hormones. Vet Rec 1939;51:265–8.

68. Takeishi M, Kodoma Y, Mikami T, et al. Studies on reproduction in the dog. XI. Induction of estrus by hormonal treatment and results of the following insemination. Jap J Anim Reprod 1976;22(2):71–5.
69. Carter JG. Hormone treatment for nonproductive bitches. Can Vet J 1980;21: 185.
70. Greenblatt RB, Pund ER. The gonadotrophins: a clinical and experimental study. South Med J 1941;36:730–42.
71. Barta M, Archibald LF, Godke RA. Luteal function of induced corpora lutea in the bitch. Theriogenology 1982;18:541–9.
72. Ishihara M, Kita I, Honjo H, et al. Clinical studies on the artificial estrus of bitches. Res Bull Fac Agr Gifu Univ 1982;46:249–56.
73. Nakao T, Yukiyo A, Fukushima S, et al. Induction of estrus in bitches with exogenous gonadotropins, and pregnancy rate and blood progesterone profiles. Nihon Juigaku Zasshi 1985;47:17–24.
74. Weilenmann R, Arnold S, Dobeli M, et al. Estrus induction in bitches by the administration of PMSG and hCG. Schweiz Arch Tierheilkd 1993;135:236–41 [in German].
75. Jones GE, Boyns AR, Bell ET, et al. Immunoreactive luteinizing hormone and progesterone during pregnancy and following gonadotropin administration in beagle bitches. Acta Endocrinol 1973;72:573–81.
76. Haresign W, Foster JP, Haynes NB, et al. Progesterone levels following treatment of seasonally anestrous ewes with synthetic LH-releasing hormone. J Reprod Fertil 1975;43:269–79.
77. Kessler DJ, Weston PG, Pimentel CA, et al. Diminution of the in vitro response to luteinizing hormone by corpora lutea induced by gonadotropin releasing hormone treatment of postpartum suckled beef cows. J Anim Sci 1981;53:749–54.
78. Morrow DA, Roberts SJ, McEntee K, et al. Postpartum ovarian activity and uterine involution in dairy cattle. J Am Vet Med Assoc 1966;149:1596–609.
79. Woody CO, Ginther OJ, Pope AL. Effects of exogenous progesterone on corpora lutea induced in anestrous ewes. J Anim Sci 1967;26:1113–5.
80. Williams GL, Petersen BJ, Tilton JE. Pituitary and ovarian responses of postpartum dairy cows to progesterone priming and single or double injections of gonadotropin-releasing hormone. Theriogenology 1982;18:561–72.
81. Scheffel CE, Pratt BR, Inskeep EK. Induced corpora lutea in the postpartum beef cow. II. Effects of treatment with progesterone and gonadotropins. J Anim Sci 1982;54:830–6.
82. Ramirez-Godinez JA, Kiracofe GH, McKee RM, et al. Reducing the incidence of short estrous cycles in beef cows with Norgestomet. Theriogenology 1981;15: 613–23.
83. Pratt BR, Berardinelli JG, Stevens LP, et al. Induced corpora lutea in the postpartum beef cow. I. Comparison of gonadotropin releasing hormone and human chorionic gonadotropin and effects of progestagen and estrogen. J Anim Sci 1982;54:822–9.
84. Archbald LF, Ingraham RH, Godke RA. Inability of progestogen pretreatment to prevent premature luteolysis of induced corpora lutea in the anestrus bitch. Theriogenology 1984;21:419–26.
85. Hadley JC. The effect of serial uterine biopsies and hysterectomy on peripheral blood levels of total unconjugated oestrogen and progesterone in the bitch. J Reprod Fertil 1975;45:389–93.
86. Gobello C, Castex G, Corrada Y. Use of cabergoline to treat primary and secondary anestrus in dogs. J Am Vet Med Assoc 2002;220(11):1653–4.

87. Rota A, Mollo A, Marinelli L, et al. Evaluation of cabergoline and buserelin efficacy for oestrous induction in the bitch. Reprod Domest Anim 2003;38:440–3.
88. Nak D, Nak Y, Simsek G. Comparison of the use of cabergoline and gonadotrophin to treat primary and secondary anoestrus in bitches. Aust Vet J 2012;90: 194–6.
89. Vanderlip SL, Wing AE, Felt P, et al. Ovulation induction in anestrous bitches by pulsatile administration of GnRH. Lab Anim Sci 1987;27:459–68.
90. Cain JL, Cain GR, Feldman EC, et al. Use of pulsatile intravenous administration of gonadotropin-releasing hormone to induce fertile estrus in bitches. Am J Vet Res 1988;49:1993–6.
91. Concannon P, Lasley B, Vanderlip S. LH release, induction of oestrus and fertile ovulations in response to pulsatile administration of GnRH to anoestrous dogs. J Reprod Fertil Suppl 1997;51:1–54.
92. Walter B, Otzdorff C, Brugger N, et al. Estrus induction in beagle bitches with the GnRH-agonist implant containing 4.7 mg deslorelin. Theriogenology 2011; 75:1125–9.
93. Fontaine E, Mir F, Vannier F, et al. Induction of fertile oestrus in the bitch using deslorelin, a GnRH agonist. Theriogenology 2011;76(8):1561–6.
94. Von Heimendahl A, Miller C. Clinical evaluation of deslorelin to induce oestrus, ovulation and pregnancy in the bitch. Reprod Domest Anim 2012;47(Suppl 6): 398–9.
95. Borges P, Fontaine E, Maenhoudt C, et al. Fertility in adult bitches previously treated with a 4.7 mg subcutaneous deslorelin implant. Reprod Domest Anim 2015;50(6):965–71.
96. Hancock JL, Rowlands IW. The physiology of reproduction in the dog. Vet Rec 1949;61:771.
97. Thun R, Watson P, Jackson GL. Induction of estrus and ovulation in the bitch, using exogenous gonadotropins. Am J Vet Res 1977;38:483–6.
98. Archbald LF, Baker BA, Clooney LL, et al. A surgical method for collecting canine embryos after induction of estrus and ovulation with exogenous gonadotropins. Vet Med Small Anim Clin 1980;75:228–38.
99. Allen WE. Attempted oestrus induction in four bitches using pregnant mare serum gonadotrophin. J Small Anim Pract 1982;23:223–31.
100. Renton JP, Harvey MJA, Eckersall PD. Apparent pregnancy failure following mating of the bitches at PMSG induced oestrus. Vet Rec 1984;115:383–4.
101. Chaffaux S, Locci D, Pontois M, et al. Induction of ovarian activity in anoestrous beagle bitches. Br Vet J 1984;140:191–5.
102. Arnold S, Arnold P, Concannon PW, et al. Effects of duration of PMSG treatment on induction of estrus, pregnancy rates and the complications of hyperestrogenism in dogs. J Reprod Fertil Suppl 1989;39:115–22.
103. Wanke M, Farina J, Loza M, et al. Induction of oestrus in bitches with normal and persistent anestrus using human menopausal gonadotropin (hMG). Theriogenology 1997;47:935–42.

Estrus Suppression in Dogs

Michelle Anne Kutzler, DVM, PhD

KEYWORDS

- Agonist • Androgen • Antagonist • GnRH • Hormonal downregulation
- Progestogen

KEY POINTS

- Although progestogen administration is the most commonly used method of estrus suppression in dogs, there has not been and it is unlikely there will be a universally safe or effective progestogen in dogs.
- Continuous treatment with androgens for up to 5 years has been demonstrated, but it is generally not recommended to treat continuously for more than 24 months.
- Following an initial flare-up in gonadotropin concentrations, sustained exposure to gonadotropin-releasing hormone (GnRH) agonists reduces gonadotropin secretion through GnRH receptor downregulation, internalization, signal uncoupling, and a decrease in GnRH receptor expression.
- GnRH antagonists directly block pituitary GnRH receptors resulting in immediate suppression of gonadotropin release without a flare-up, but currently available products are too short-lived to be clinically beneficial.

INTRODUCTION

Within the United States, suppression of the canine estrous cycle is predominately attained by surgically removing the ovaries (ovariectomy) with or without the uterus (ovariohysterectomy). However, not all owners have their pets surgically sterilized. For purpose-bred bitches, the safest and most effective and least expensive method to prevent unwanted pregnancy is indoor confinement and segregation from intact males. For those bitches not intended for breeding, pet owners may still be reluctant to consider traditional surgical sterilization given recent (albeit confounding) evidence of long-term health problems associated with gonad removal, including obesity,

Disclosure Statement: The author has no relationship with any commercial company that has a direct financial interest in this subject matter or the materials discussed within this article or with a company making a competing product. However, the author is a scientific advisor for the Alliance for Contraception in Cats and Dogs (ACCD). The mission of the ACCD is to advance nonsurgical fertility control so as to effectively and humanely reduce the number of unwanted cats and dogs.
Department of Animal and Rangeland Sciences, Oregon State University, 112 Withycombe Hall, Corvallis, OR 97331, USA
E-mail address: michelle.kutzler@oregonstate.edu

Vet Clin Small Anim 48 (2018) 595–603
https://doi.org/10.1016/j.cvsm.2018.04.001
0195-5616/18/© 2018 Elsevier Inc. All rights reserved.

urinary incontinence, endocrine disorders (eg, hypothyroidism, diabetes), musculo-skeletal disorders (eg, cranial cruciate ligament rupture, hip dysplasia), behavioral disorders (eg, aggression, fear) and cognitive dysfunction, and neoplasia (eg, osteosarcoma, hemangiosarcoma, mastocytoma, lymphoma).

There are numerous nonsurgical methods for estrus suppression that have been used previously and that are currently being used. Pharmacologic methods of estrus suppression must be safe, reliable, and reversible. Hormonal treatments using reproductive steroid hormones (progestogens or androgens) or gonadotropin-releasing hormone (GnRH) analogues result in negative feedback, effectively shutting down the hypothalamic-pituitary-gonadal axis.

PATIENT EVALUATION OVERVIEW

Indications for suppressing estrus for bitches intended for future breeding include inconvenient timing of estrus for owner (American Kennel Club [AKC] performance classes prohibit exhibition of bitches in season) and long-term medical management of pyometra. For bitches not intended for breeding and when surgical sterilization is not an option, estrus suppression is important for prevention of pregnancy. Commercially available options in the United States for estrus suppression in dogs have declined over the last 3 decades, although most are still available through veterinary compounding pharmacies. Estrus-suppression protocols mediate their action by inhibiting pituitary gonadotropin secretion and release, mainly that of luteinizing hormone (LH). These protocols include the use of progestogens, androgens, GnRH agonists, or GnRH antagonists. Because LH is luteotropic in the dog, administration of estrus-suppression drugs to pregnant dogs may result in abortion and/or fetal urogenital malformations (eg, hypospadias in males, masculinization in females). Practitioners should first confirm that patients are not pregnant or that their owners know about and are ready to accept the consequences.

PHARMACOLOGIC TREATMENT OPTIONS FOR ESTRUS SUPPRESSION
Progestogens

Canine estrus suppression using progestogens has been practiced for many decades with the first report by Murray and Eden[1] in 1952. The mechanism of the estrus suppressive activity of progestogens in dogs is still unclear. In many species, there is evidence that progestogens reduce serum concentrations of gonadotropins. However, high doses of medroxyprogesterone acetate (MPA) or megestrol acetate (MA) administered to ovariectomized beagle bitches for several months did not reduce the increased circulating concentrations of LH nor did it lower LH concentrations in intact bitches.[2,3] On the contrary, basal plasma follicle-stimulating hormone (FSH) and LH concentrations increase during the first months of MPA treatment,[4] which may be due to a direct inhibitory effect of MPA at the ovarian level, resulting in suppression of the ovarian secretion of estradiol or inhibin.[5,6]

MPA (Depo-Provera) is a long-acting injectable progestin that was labeled for estrus suppression in the bitch (Promone).[7] MPA may be administered as a single subcutaneous injection (2 mg/kg; maximum 60 mg per animal)[8] or orally (5 mg once daily [10 mg for large dogs during the first 5 days]) for a maximum of 21 days.[9] Delmadinone acetate is similar to MPA and is used to postpone estrus.[10] MA has been used extensively for temporary estrus suppression in the bitch and is rapidly metabolized when given orally.[11] When given at a daily dose of 2.2 mg/kg body weight orally for 8 days beginning in early proestrus, estrus was suppressed in 92% of cases.[12] Two- to 4-week administration of MA during anestrus alternating with an untreated period of 3 to 4 months is also effective. Chlormadinone acetate 2 mg orally once a week[13] or (0.5 mg/kg, n = 2) orally for 8 days is equally effective as MA.[14] Proligestone is commercially manufactured in Europe (Delvosteron) and is labeled for estrus suppression (10–30 mg/kg subcutaneously repeated at 3 and 7 months following the initial injection).[15]

All of these drugs should be administered during anestrus approximately 1 month before the expected onset of the next estrous cycle. The first estrus after the use of proligestone can be expected in most bitches within 9 to 12 months but may take up to 2 to 3 years. With respect to MPA, the return to estrus may vary from 2 to 9 months.[9] It is important to note the subcutaneous contraceptive implants labeled for human use containing levonorgestrel (Norplant) do not suppress estrus in dogs.[16]

Although progestogen administration is the most commonly used method of estrus suppression in dogs,[17] there has not been and it is unlikely there will be a universally safe or effective progestogen in dogs. Reported adverse effects depend on the type of progestogen administered, dose, treatment duration, and age of the animal.[18,19] The most commonly reported adverse effect is increased appetite leading to weight gain, lethargy, or restlessness.[4,11–13,20] Progestogens have a moderate affinity for the glucocorticoid receptor[21] and can result in clinical signs consistent with adrenocortical suppression (eg, alopecia, hair discoloration, thinning of the skin).[22] Progestogens can also cause acromegaliclike symptoms, including hypertrophy of skin and other soft tissues and overgrowth of some bone and cartilage, occurring in response to progesterone-induced hypersecretion of growth hormone by mammary tissue as well as the pituitary, and resulting in increased serum concentrations of insulinlike growth factor 1.[23] Elevations in serum progesterone can also cause diabetic insulin resistance, acting either directly or via increased growth hormone production.[24–27] This hypersecretion of growth hormone as a result of progestogen administration can be successfully treated by the progesterone receptor blocker aglepristone.[28]

The next most significant adverse effect reported are uterine pathologic conditions, with the prevalence of cystic endometrial hyperplasia-endometritis as high as 45%.[29–31] Pyometra developed in 0.8% of bitches treated with progestogens.[12] It is important to note that the canine mammary gland produces pathologic changes following progestogen administration in a way that is not seen in other species.[32,33] Apparently a significant level of constitutive expression of progesterone receptors occurs in canine mammary tissues.[23] Unlike laboratory animals, progestogen administration induces progesterone receptor synthesis in the canine mammary gland.[34] In addition, the dog seems to have a unique sensitivity to the mammary tumor-promoting effect of progestogens via progestin-induced growth hormone induction.[35] Progestogen-induced neoplastic transformation of mammary tissue starts with the proliferation of undifferentiated terminal ductal structures,[36] leading to hyperplasia, adenomatous changes, and eventually adenocarcinoma.[23,26,27,31,37]

Androgens

Androgens have also been used for canine estrus suppression. Mibolerone is a synthetic androgen that was commercially manufactured (formerly sold under the name of Cheque Drops) and labeled for estrus suppression in dogs.[17,38,39] The dose for mibolerone varies in bitches depending on body weight and breed.[11] For bitches up to 12 kg, the mibolerone dosage is 30 μg/d. For bitches 12 to 23 kg, the mibolerone dosage is 60 μg/d. For bitches 23 to 45 kg, the mibolerone dosage is 120 μg/d. For bitches more than 45 kg, the mibolerone dosage is 180 μg/d. Any German shepherd dog or any Alsatian-derived mixed breed should receive the maximum daily dosage 180 μg/d). The reason for the higher dosage requirement within Alsatian lineage is unknown.[40] If treatment is initiated at least 30 days before the onset of proestrus, estrus can be postponed for up to 2 years. Following cessation of the treatment, return to estrus will occur within 70 days on average (1–7 months).[38] Continuous treatment up to 5 years has been demonstrated without data on reversal rates to normal fertility following cessation of long-term treatment. The original manufacturer recommended to not treat continuously for more than 24 months. Testosterone (weekly intramuscular injections of testosterone propionate 110 mg or oral administration of 25–50 mg of methyltestosterone twice weekly) also suppresses estrus in bitches.[41]

The most common side effects reported with androgen use in bitches is clitoral hypertrophy and vaginitis.[39,42] Other side effects include increased body odor, urinary incontinence and spraying, mounting behavior, cervical dermis thickening, and epiphora.[11,38,42] It is important to note that androgens are contraindicated for use in Bedlington terriers because of an increased risk of hepatic dysfunction and in patients with androgen-responsive neoplasias.

Gonadotropin-Releasing Hormone Agonists

GnRH acts as the master reproductive hormone through regulation of the release of LH and FSH from the pituitary. In females, both LH and FSH are required to stimulate the ovarian changes leading to ovulation. However, sustained exposure to GnRH reduces GnRH-stimulated gonadotropin secretion through GnRH receptor downregulation, internalization, signal uncoupling, and a decrease of receptor expression.[43] Within the past 2 decades, long-acting GnRH agonists have been developed for canine estrus suppression.[44,45] GnRH agonists mimic GnRH by initially stimulating LH and FSH secretion (flare-up effect), which is generally regarded as an inherent disadvantage because it will induce estrus and delays the effects of estrus suppression by 7 to 14 days.[46] The induced estrus is associated with normal estrous signs (eg, vulvar edema, sanguineous vaginal discharge, estrous behavior).[47–49] The duration of the induced estrus is shorter compared with a natural estrus,[50] but the fertility in the induced estrus was high (ovulation rate, pregnancy rate, litter size) and not significantly different from untreated cycles.[50,51]

Biocompatible subcutaneous implants containing 4.7 mg or 9.4 mg of deslorelin acetate (Suprelorin) are commercially available in Europe, Australia, and New Zealand and labeled contraception of male dogs with a 98% efficacy for at least 6 months.[52] Although an extralabel application, when Suprelorin was administered to anestrous bitches, an ovulatory estrus was induced 4 to 8 days after implantation because of the initial flare-up effect, which was followed by estrus suppression up to 27 months.[53] When a subcutaneous deslorelin implant was administered to prepubertal female dogs, estrus was suppressed for 23 months.[54]

A subcutaneously administered goserelin acetate implant (Zoladex) containing 3.6 mg of goserelin suppressed estrous cyclicity for 12 months.[55] In addition, several buserelin acetate implants labeled for human reproductive purposes are commercially available (eg, Suprefact). Male dogs treated with a single buserelin implant containing 3.3 mg had testosterone suppression and suppression of spermatogenesis for 6 to 12 months. Recent data in female dogs show that buserelin implants will result in estrus suppression following an initial flare-up similar to what has been reported for deslorelin.[56]

The predominant complication of GnRH agonist administration for estrus suppression is the initial flare-up. When administered to some diestrous bitches (serum progesterone concentrations >5 ng/mL), the initial flare-up was suppressed.[53,57,58] However, several other investigators reported estrous signs after administering deslorelin implants to diestrous bitches.[47,59,60] Administration of MA concurrently with a deslorelin implant has also been widely investigated. Treatment with MA (2 mg/kg) for 14 or 21 days beginning 1 week before deslorelin implant administration prevented the estrous response, but a lower dose (1 mg/kg) of MA would not.[57] Corrada and colleagues[61] (2006) reported that administration of MA (2.2 mg/kg) for 8 days with the deslorelin implant administered on the fourth day was more effective at preventing the initial flare-up than when deslorelin was administered on the first day.

Another limitation to this method of estrus suppression is that the duration efficacy seems to be dose related, and even at the same dose, varies greatly between individuals.[53] However, research in males has shown that multiple serial implant administration did not cause adverse effects or diminished efficacy. Dogs that have been reimplanted for 4 consecutive doses at 6-month intervals with the 4.7 mg deslorelin implant returned to normal steroidogenesis after cessation of treatment.[62] Serial studies similar to this have not been reported for females; however, females that have received implants have had normal fertility at subsequent estrous cycles.

Side effects reported following deslorelin implant administration include persistent estrus (including ovarian cysts, 15%), induced lactation (11%), some behavioral changes (6%) and miscellaneous problems (cystitis, vomiting, allergic reactions; 2%),[60] and pyometra (1 case reported).[63] For this reason, GnRH agonist implants should be subcutaneously administered cranial to the umbilicus in case removal becomes necessary.[64]

Gonadotropin-Releasing Hormone Antagonists

Both GnRH agonists and antagonists suppress gonadotropins and gonadal steroids, but administration of agonists is accompanied by an initial gonadotropin and gonadal hormone surge that will induce estrus in anestrous bitches. GnRH antagonists directly block pituitary GnRH receptors resulting in immediate suppression of gonadotropin release.[45,65] This suppression leads to an immediate dose-related arrest of gonadotropin secretion without the initial flare effect.[46,65] The degree and duration of LH and FSH suppression depends on the amount of GnRH antagonist administered.[66]

In general, GnRH antagonists require high doses to competitively inhibit responses to endogenous GnRH.[45] Subcutaneous administration of acycline (0.11–0.33 mg/kg) to bitches in early proestrus (<3 days) suppressed estrus for 3 weeks without any side effects observed.[67] If acyline is administered to anestrous bitches within the first 48 hours after administration of a long-acting deslorelin acetate implant, the initial ovarian stimulation and ovulation are not prevented,[68,69] suggesting that GnRH agonist stimulation overrode the effects of the GnRH antagonist.[70]

Other GnRH antagonists have been used in humans (degarelix for prostate cancer,[71,72] cetrorelix for infertility,[73] sufugolix for postmenopausal women,[74] relugolix for uterine fibroids,[75] elagolix for endometriosis).[76,77] However, a common problem with all GnRH antagonists is that they must be administered by injection.[78]

SUMMARY

In summary, surgical sterilization will likely remain the procedure of choice for permanent estrus suppression within the United States. However, practitioners have several options for short-term, reversible estrus suppression in dogs. Reproductive and nonreproductive side effects (eg, progestogens, androgens) and product availability (eg, mibolerone, deslorelin) continue to be significant limiting factors to greater adoption of these methods in veterinary practice. There is great hope for continued improvement in GnRH antagonists increasing their applicability for use in canine estrus suppression.

REFERENCES

1. Murray GH, Eden EL. Progesterone to delay estrum in bitches. Vet Med 1952;47: 467–8.
2. McCann JP, Altszuler N, Hampshire J, et al. Growth hormone, insulin, glucose, cortisol, luteinizing hormone, and diabetes in beagle bitches treated with medroxyprogesterone acetate. Acta Endocrinol 1987;116:73–80.
3. Colon J, Kimball M, Hansen B, et al. Effects of contraceptive doses of the progestagen megestrol acetate on luteinizing hormone and follicle-stimulating hormone secretion in female dogs. J Reprod Fertil Suppl 1993;47:519–21.
4. Beijerink NJ, Bhatti SF, Okkens AC, et al. Adenohypophyseal function in bitches treated with medroxyprogesterone acetate. Domest Anim Endocrinol 2007;32: 63–78.
5. Mann GE, Campbell BK, McNeilly AS, et al. The role of inhibin and oestradiol in the control of FSH secretion in the sheep. J Endocrinol 1992;133:381–91.
6. Shupnik MA. Gonadal hormone feedback on pituitary gonadotropin genes. Trends Endocrinol Metab 1996;7:272–6.
7. Jackson EKM. Contraception in the dog and cat. Br Vet J 1984;140:132–7.
8. Schaefers-Okkens AC, Kooistra HS. Use of progestogens. Tijdschr Diergeneeskd 1996;121:335–7 [in Dutch].
9. Max A, Jurka P, Dobrzynski A, et al. Non-surgical contraception in female dogs and cats. Acta Sci Pol Zootechnica 2014;13(1):3–18.
10. Romagnoli S, Sontas H. BSAVA manual of canine and feline reproduction and neonatology. Gloucester (United Kingdom): British Small Animal Veterinary Association; 2010. p. 23–33.
11. Plumb DC. Veterinary drug handbook. 4th edition. Ames (IA): Iowa State University Press; 2002.
12. Burke TJ, Reynolds HA Jr. Megestrol acetate for estrus postponement in the bitch. J Am Vet Med Assoc 1975;167:285–7.
13. Sawada T, Tamada H, Inaba T, et al. Prevention of estrus in the bitch with chlormadinone acetate administered orally. J Vet Med Sci 1992;54:595–6.
14. Wanke MM, Loza ME, Rebuelto M. Progestin treatment for infertility in bitches with short interestrus interval. Theriogenology 2006;66:1579–82.
15. Evans JM, Sutton DJ. The use of hormones, especially progestagens, to control oestrus in bitches. J Reprod Fertil 1989;39:163–73.
16. Baldwin CJ, Peter AT, Bosu WT, et al. The contraceptive effects of levonorgestrel in the domestic cat. Lab Anim Sci 1994;44:261–4.
17. Wiebe VJ, Howard JP. Pharmacologic advances in canine and feline reproduction. Top Companion Anim Med 2009;24:71–99.
18. Jochle W. Pet population control in Europe. J Am Vet Med Assoc 1991;198: 1225–30.
19. Misdorf W. Progestagens and mammary tumors in dogs and cats. Acta Endocrinol (Copenh) 1991;125:27–31.
20. Sahara K, Tsutsui S, Naitoh Y, et al. Prevention of estrus in bitches by subcutaneous implantation of chlormadinone acetate. J Vet Med Sci 1993;55:431–4.
21. Selman PJ, Wolfswinkel J, Mol JA. Binding specificity of medroxyprogesterone acetate and proligestone for the progesterone and glucocorticoid receptor in the dog. Steroids 1996;61:133–7.
22. Nelson M. After-effect of injection. Vet Rec 1977;100:78.
23. Concannon PW. Reproductive cycles of the domestic bitch. Anim Reprod Sci 2011;124:200–10.

24. Yu EN, Winnick JJ, Edgerton DS, et al. Hepatic and whole-body insulin metabolism during proestrus and estrus in mongrel dogs. Comp Med 2016;66:235–40.
25. Selman PJ, Mol JA, Rutteman GR, et al. Effects of progestin administration on the hypothalamic-pituitary-adrenal axis and glucose-homeostasis in dogs. J Reprod Fertil Suppl 1997;51:345–54.
26. Weikel JH Jr, Nelson LW. Problems in evaluating chronic toxicity of contraceptive steroids in dogs. J Toxicol Environ Health 1977;3:167–77.
27. Beck P. Effect of progestins on glucose and lipid metabolism. Ann N Y Acad Sci 1977;286:434–45.
28. Bhatti SFM, Duchateau L, Okkens AC, et al. Treatment of growth hormone excess in dogs with the progesterone receptor antagonist aglepristone. Theriogenology 2006;66:797–803.
29. Von Berky AG, Townsend WL. The relationship between the prevalence of uterine lesions and the use of medroxyprogesterone acetate for canine population control. Aust Vet J 1993;70:249–50.
30. Sokolowski JH, Zimbelman RG. Canine reproduction effects of multiple treatments of medroxyprogesterone acetate on reproductive organs of the bitch. Am J Vet Res 1974;35:1285–7.
31. Nelson LW, Kelly WA. Progesterone-related gross and microscopic changes in female beagles. Vet Pathol 1976;13:143–56.
32. Owen LN, Briggs MH. Contraceptive steroid toxicology in the beagle dog and its relevance to human carcinogenicity. Curr Med Res Opin 1976;4:309–29.
33. McKenzie BE. Guidelines and requirements for the evaluation of contraceptive steroids. Toxicol Pathol 1989;17:377–84.
34. Briggs MH. Progestogens and mammary tumours in the beagle bitch. Res Vet Sci 1980;28:199–202.
35. Rutteman GR. Contraceptive steroids and the mammary gland: is there a hazard?–Insights from animal studies. Breast Cancer Res Treat 1992;23:29–41.
36. Russo IH, Russo J. Progestagens and mammary gland development: differentiation versus carcinogenesis. Acta Endocrinol 1991;125(Suppl. 1):7–12.
37. Van Os JL, Van Laar PH, Oldenkamp EP, et al. Oestrus control and the incidence of mammary nodules in bitches, a clinical study with two progestogens. Vet Q 1981;3:46–56.
38. Johnston SD, Root Kustritz MV, Olson PNS. Canine and feline theriogenology. Philadelphia: W.B. Saunders Co; 2001.
39. Burke TJ, Reynolds HA, Sokolowski JH. A 280-day tolerance-efficacy study with mibolerone for suppression of estrus in the cat. Am J Vet Res 1977;38:469–77.
40. Sokolowski JH. The evaluation of efficacy of mibolerone for estrus prevention in the bitch. Proceedings of the Symposium on Cheque® for Canine Estrus Prevention. Augusta (MI), March 13–15, 1978.
41. Blythe LL, Gannon JR, Craig AM, et al. Endocrine glands, hormones and the reproductive system. In: Care of the Racing and Retired Greyhound. Topeka, Kansas: Hall Commercial Printing; 2007. p. 161–73.
42. Burke TJ. Pharmacologic control of estrus in the bitch and queen. Vet Clin North Am Small Anim Pract 1982;12:79–84.
43. Vickery BH, Mc Rae GI, Goodpasture JC, et al. Use of potent LHRH analogues for chronic contraception and pregnancy termination. J Reprod Fertil 1989;39:175–87.
44. Nestor JJ. Development of agonistic LHRH analogs. In: Vickery BH, Nestor JJ, Hafez ESE, editors. LHRH and its analogues: contraceptive and therapeutics applications. Lancaster (PA): MTP Press; 1984. p. 3–10.

45. Vickery BH. Comparisons of the potential utility of LHRH agonists and antagonists for fertility control. J Steroid Biochem 1985;23:779–91.

46. Herbst KL. Gonadotropin-releasing hormone antagonists. Curr Opin Pharmacol 2003;3:1–7.

47. Körber H, Wehrend A, Hoffmann B, et al. The use of Suprelorin® for estrus suppression in the bitch. Reprod Biol 2013;13(Suppl 2):30–1 (abstract).

48. Rubion S, Desmoulins PO, Riviere-Godet E, et al. Treatment with a subcutaneous GnRH agonist prevents puberty in bitches. Proc 5th International Symposium on Canine and Feline Reproduction. Sao Paulo, Brazil, August 4–6, 2004. p. 56–8. [abstract].

49. McRae GI, Roberts BB, Worden AC, et al. Long-term reversible suppression of oestrus in bitches with nafarelin acetate, a potent LHRH agonist. J Reprod Fertil 1985;74:389–97.

50. Fontaine E, Mir F, Vannier F, et al. Induction of fertile oestrus in the bitch using deslorelin, a GnRH agonist. Theriogenology 2011;76:1561–6.

51. Borges P, Fontaine E, Maenhoudt C, et al. Fertility in adult bitches previously treated with a 4.7 mg subcutaneous deslorelin implant. Reprod Domest Anim 2015;50:965–71.

52. Herbert CA, Trigg TE. Applications of GnRH in the control and management of fertility in female animals. Anim Reprod Sci 2005;88:141–53.

53. Trigg TE, Wright PJ, Armour AF, et al. Use of a GnRH analogue implant to produce reversible long-term suppression of reproductive function in male and female domestic dogs. J Reprod Fertil Suppl 2001;57:255–61.

54. Lacoste D, Dube D, Trudel C, et al. Normal gonadal functions and fertility after 23 months of treatment to prepubertal male and female dogs with the GnRH agonist [D-Trp-6, des-Gly-NH2-10] GnRH ethylamide. J Androl 1989;10:456–65.

55. Lombardi P, Florio S, Paganini U, et al. Ovarian function suppression with a GnRH analogue (goserelin) in hormone-dependent canine mammary cancer. J Vet Pharmacol Ther 1999;22:56–61.

56. Piepenbrink A, Failing K, Riesenbeck A, et al. Downregulation of LH in the bitch after application of the GnRH-agonist buserelin as a slow-release implant. Tierarztl Prax Ausg K Kleintiere Heimtiere 2017;45(3):147–52 [in German].

57. Wright PJ, Verstegen JP, Onclin K, et al. Suppression of the oestrous responses of bitches to the GnRH analogue deslorelin by progestin. J Reprod Fertil Suppl 2001;57:263–8.

58. Sung M, Armour A, Wright P. The influence of exogenous progestin on the occurrence of proestrous or estrous signs, plasma concentrations of luteinizing hormone and estradiol in deslorelin (GnRH agonist) treated anestrous bitches. Theriogenology 2006;66:1513–7.

59. Maenhoudt C, Santos NR, Fontbonne A. Suppression of fertility in adult dogs. Reprod Domest Anim 2014;49(Suppl 2):58–63.

60. Fontaine E, Fontbonne A. Use of deslorelin to control fertility in the bitch. In: Symposium deslorelin: deslorelin in practice, 7th EVSSAR Congress. Louvain la Neuve, Belgium, May 14–15, 2010. p. 15–7.

61. Corrada Y, Hermo G, Johnson CA, et al. Short-term progestin treatments prevent estrous induction by a GnRH agonist implant in anestrous bitches. Theriogenology 2006;65(2):366–73.

62. Trigg TE, Doyle AG, Walsh JD, et al. Advances in the use of the GnRH agonist deslorelin in control of reproduction. Proc 5th International Symposium on Canine and Feline Reproduction. Sao Paulo, Brazil, August 4–6, 2004. p. 49–51 [abstract].

63. Arlt SP, Spankowsky S, Heuwieser W. Follicular cysts and prolonged oestrus in a female dog after administration of a deslorelin implant. New Zealand Vet J 2011; 59:87–91.
64. Schafer-Somi S, Kaya D, Gultiken N, et al. Suppression of fertility in pre-pubertal dogs and cats. Reprod Dom Anim 2014;49(Suppl 2):21–7.
65. Heber D, Dobson R, Swerdloff RS, et al. Pituitary receptor site blockade by a gonadotrophin-releasing antagonist in vivo: mechanism of action. Science 1982;216:420–1.
66. Fraser HM. LHRH analogues: their clinical physiology and delivery systems. Baillieres Clin Obstet Gynaecol 1988;2:639–58.
67. Valiente C, Garcia Romero G, Corrada Y, et al. Estrous cycle interruption with a low and a high dose of the GnRH antagonist, acyline, in bitches. Theriogenology 2009;79:408–11.
68. Valiente C, Diaz J, Rosa D, et al. Effect of a GnRH antagonist on GnRH agonist-implanted anoestrous bitches. Theriogenology 2009;72:926–9.
69. Hermo G, Corrada Y, Arias D, et al. Failure of a single GnRH antagonist administration to prevent estrous induction by a GnRH agonist implant in anestrous bitches. In: Proceedings of the World Small Animal Association (WSAVA). Prague, Czech Republic, October 11–14, 2006. [abstract].
70. Sharma OP, Weinbauer GF, Behre HM, et al. The gonadotropin releasing hormone (GnRH) agonist induced initial rise of bioactive LH and testosterone can be blunted in a dose dependent manner by GnRH antagonist in the non-human primate. Urol Res 1992;20:317–21.
71. Sonesson A, Koechling W, Stalewski J, et al. Gonadotropin-releasing hormone receptor antagonist, in rat, dog, and monkey. Drug Metab Dispos 2011;39(10): 1895–903.
72. Doehn C, Sommerauer M, Jocham D. Degarelix for prostate cancer. Expert Opin Investig Drugs 2009;18:851–60.
73. Merviel P, Najas S, Campy H, et al. Use of GNRH antagonists in reproductive medicine. Minerva Ginecol 2005;57:29–43.
74. Boyce M, Clark E, Johnston A, et al. Effects of single and repeated oral doses of TAK-013, a new nonpeptide gonadotropin-releasing hormone (GnRH) antagonist, in healthy post-menopausal women. Fertil Steril 2002;78(3):S281.
75. Takeda. A placebo-controlled, phase 3 study of TAK-385 40 mg in the treatment of pain symptoms associated with uterine fibroids. In: ClinicalTrials.gov. Bethesda (MD): National Library of Medicine (US). Available at: https://clinicaltrials.gov/ct2/show/study/NCT02655224. Accessed July 20, 2016.
76. Chen C, Wu D, Guo Z, et al. Discovery of sodium R-(+)-4-{2-[5-(2-fluoro-3-methoxyphenyl)-3-(2-fluoro-6-[trifluoromethyl]benzyl)-4-methy l-2, 6-dioxo-3, 6-dihyro-2H-pyrimidin-1-yl]-1-phenylethylamino}butyrate (elagolix), a potent and orally available nonpeptide antagonist of the human gonadotropin-releasing hormone receptor. J Med Chem 2008;51:7478–85.
77. AbbVie. A global phase 3 study to evaluate the safety and efficacy of elagolix in subjects with moderate to severe endometriosis-associated pain. In: ClinicalTrials.gov. Bethesda (MD): National Library of Medicine (US). Available at: https://clinicaltrials.gov/ct2/show/study/NCT01931670. Accessed March 10, 2018.
78. García Romero G, Valiente C, Aquilano D, et al. Endocrine effects of the GnRH antagonist, acyline, in domestic dogs. Theriogenology 2009;71:1234–7.

Mismating Diagnosis and Protocols

Natalie S. Fraser, DVM, MS

KEYWORDS

- Mismating • Misalliance • Prostaglandin F2α • Aglepristone • Prolactin inhibitors

KEY POINTS

- Animals unwanted for future breeding can undergo ovariohysterectomy at any time.
- Ascertain, if possible, if the bitch or queen has been mated and determine pregnancy status before initiating therapy.
- There is no US Food and Drug Administration–approved mismating treatment in the United States and Canada; aglepristone is available in Mexico.
- Combination therapy with prostaglandins and prolactin inhibitors is highly effective, and reduced dosages when used in combination reduce adverse effects.

INTRODUCTION

Mismating, or termination of pregnancy, may be requested for a variety of reasons in the bitch and queen, most commonly to eliminate an unwanted pregnancy. There is currently no US Food and Drug Administration (FDA)-approved medication for mismating in the United States. However, there are several medical protocols that can be used for this purpose in an off-label manner. The ideal mismating treatment would be effective during any stage of estrus or pregnancy, would be free from side effects, would be aesthetically pleasing to the owner (ie, no vaginal discharge or fetal remnants passed from the vulva), would have no negative effects on future fertility, and would be inexpensive and readily available. At this time, no such drug exists, and thus, clinicians must weigh the various benefits of each protocol to select the one that best suits the individual patient and owner's needs. Alternately, ovariohysterectomy offers a surgical treatment option that both eliminates the unwanted pregnancy and prevents future occurrences.

PATIENT EVALUATION OVERVIEW

Practitioners presented with bitches or queens for mismating must first ascertain if mating has occurred or has likely occurred. In studies performed on bitches

Theriogenology, School of Veterinary Science, The University of Queensland, 8114, Gatton, Queensland 4343, Australia
E-mail address: natalie.fraser@uq.edu.au

Vet Clin Small Anim **48** (2018) 605–615
https://doi.org/10.1016/j.cvsm.2018.02.007
0195-5616/18/© 2018 Elsevier Inc. All rights reserved.

presented for mismating, only 62% to 70% accidentally bred once during behavioral estrus were actually pregnant.[1,2] Thus, pregnancy termination may not be necessary in a large percentage of bitches presented for accidental mating. Owners of estrus females may present the animal for mismating without having actually witnessed breeding; the bitch or queen may have gone missing for a period of time long enough for copulation to have occurred. Bitches should be evaluated using behavioral assessment (tail flagging), vaginal cytology, measurement of blood serum progesterone, and/or vaginoscopy to determine the stage of the estrus cycle and proximity to ovulation. Canine sperm can survive in the female reproductive tract for prolonged periods of time[3]; thus, bitches bred before the window of peak fertility may still become pregnant. The presence of spermatozoa on a vaginal cytology is indicative that mating has occurred.[4] However, practitioners should not assume that the absence of spermatozoa indicates that the bitch was not mated; thus, positive evidence of mating is only of diagnostic use when selecting a mismating treatment option that can be used during estrus. Sensitivity of vaginal cytology assessment can be improved by leaving a saline-moistened cotton swab in the vaginal vault (as for vaginal cytology) for 1 minute to absorb fluid and then extracting the vaginal fluid by placing the swab in a centrifuge tube containing 0.4 mL saline for 10 minutes. After agitating the swab in the fluid and squeezing it out against the side of the tube, the sample is centrifuged at 2000 rpm for 10 minutes and the sediment is examined after staining with Diff-Quick stain. When using this technique, it has been reported that 100% of bitches mated in the preceding 24 hours had spermatozoa in the sample and that 75% of bitches mated in the preceding 48 hours had spermatozoa in the sample.[4]

In contrast, queens are reflex ovulators; estrus is exhibited for 5 to 7 days on average every 2 to 3 weeks.[5] Cats in estrus display characteristic behaviors, such as excessive vocalization, rolling, facial scent marking, raising of the hindquarters, rhythmic treading of the hind limbs, and excessive grooming; vaginal cytology can also be used to assess for the presence of keratinized epithelial cells in the vaginal mucosa. Queens may also have excoriations around the scapulae from the tom biting the scruff of the queen during mating. The likelihood of ovulation increases with multiple copulations in queens.[5]

Definitive pregnancy diagnosis can be performed in mid gestation by abdominal palpation or transabdominal ultrasound in bitches and queens. Ultrasound is preferred by the author because it is highly sensitive and specific; with experience, gestational sacs can be identified as early as 20 days after the luteinizing hormone (LH) surge using this technique, but by 30 days of gestation, pregnancy diagnosis via ultrasound is straightforward.[6] An additional benefit to ultrasound diagnosis of pregnancy is the ability to determine the approximate gestational age, allowing the practitioner to anticipate whether the fetal fluids and tissues are likely to be resorbed or passed from the vulva after mismating. Alternatively, serum relaxin can be used in bitches to determine pregnancy status as early as 20 days post-LH surge because this is the only specific pregnancy-associated protein identified in the dog.[7] In queens, elevated progesterone levels indicate that ovulation has occurred and thus are suggestive that mating has taken place but cannot be used for definitive diagnosis of pregnancy. Abdominal radiographs can be used for pregnancy diagnosis later in gestation (>43 days after LH peak), but before skeletal mineralization, other causes of uterine enlargement cannot be ruled out radiographically. Thus, radiographs are not the diagnostic method of choice for early pregnancy diagnosis so that mismating treatments can be performed in a timely fashion, during a period where resorption, as opposed to expulsion of fetuses, is more likely to occur.

PHARMACOLOGIC TREATMENT OPTIONS

Several classes of drugs can be used for mismating and are discussed in detail.

Estrogens

Estrogens inhibit oocyte movement and implantation of embryos; thus, this is the only treatment option that can be used while the bitch is still in estrus. Administration of this regimen is viewed by some veterinarians as malpractice because other alternatives for mismating have arisen. Many resources cite the use of estrogens as unsafe, but few published data are available to substantiate these statements.[8] In order to be effective, the injection must be given after ovulation while the bitch is still in cytologic estrus because administration to bitches in diestrus may result in pyometra.[9] Given the mechanism of action of estrogens, administration during diestrus will not be effective if the embryos have already migrated into the uterus. Other potential adverse effects include bone marrow toxicity, including aplastic anemia, thrombocytopenia, and leukopenia. Estradiol cypionate is the classic "mismate shot" requested by bitch owners; this drug is administered at a dose rate of 44 μg/kg once during estrus. Diethylstilbestrol (75 mcg/kg, orally for 7 days) appeared to have little effect on pregnancy, with 11 out of 12 treated bitches confirmed pregnant on day 25 of diestrus.[9] Estradiol benzoate, administered once 2 days after mating (5 days after ovulation), resulted in 0/10 bitches diagnosed as pregnant at a dose of 0.2 mg/kg, compared with 5/5 control bitches pregnant. The investigators reported no side effects with this dosing regimen.[10] However, given the severe nature of the potential adverse effects associated with administration, estrogens are generally not recommended for mismating. Consideration of adverse effects is particularly prudent when considering that the bitch presented for mismating may in fact not be pregnant, and that other safer alternatives are available. Estrogen mismate protocols do have distinct advantages in that they can be administered once and are inexpensive. If estrogens are used, the client should be advised of their potential adverse effects before administration.

Tamoxifen citrate has antiestrogen activity in humans, but in canines, it has estrogenic activity. When administered at a dose of 1.0 mg/kg every 12 hours orally, for 10 days, and if initiated before day 15 of diestrus, tamoxifen was 100% successful at preventing pregnancy.[11] When initiated after day 15 of diestrus, it was not effective, with 2/4 bitches carrying normal fetuses to term. When initiated after day 30 of diestrus, 4/4 bitches produced clinically normal pups. In addition, reported side effects included ovarian cysts, pyometra, and endometritis. Considering the side effects and poor efficacy, this drug is generally not used for mismating in the bitch.

Prostaglandin F2α and Analogues

Both dinaprost (Lutalyse), naturally occurring prostaglandin, and cloprostenol (Estrumate), a synthetic prostaglandin, can be used for mismating in small animals, although neither drug is labeled for this purpose. Other synthetic prostaglandins commercially available include fluprostenol and alfaprostol. Synthetic prostaglandins have a higher receptor affinity and half-life than natural prostaglandin. The mechanism of action for mismating is to induce luteolysis,[12–14] and the corpus luteum (CL) of the bitch is more resistant to the effects of prostaglandins earlier in gestation. It is recommended that pregnancy be confirmed at approximately 30 days' gestation before instituting a prostaglandin-based protocol to ensure the CL is likely to respond. A single dose of prostaglandin will not induce luteolysis in bitches, and multiple doses are required for abortion to occur.

Side effects include nausea, ptyalism, vomiting, abdominal pain, malaise, and profound hypotension and circulatory collapse with high doses. Side effects are secondary to nonspecific smooth muscle contraction. Adverse effects typically lessen with administration of subsequent doses. Some practitioners prefer to admit bitches to the hospital for the duration of treatment because of the side effects of prostaglandins; animals treated on an outpatient basis should be monitored for 20 to 60 minutes after injection to ensure no significant side effects occur before discharge from the hospital. Although circulatory collapse is rare, some practitioners prefer to place an intravenous catheter preemptively if fluid therapy is needed. The author has also personally observed severe respiratory distress in a brachycephalic dog after administration of prostaglandins that resolved with supportive care within 30 minutes. Side effects from synthetic prostaglandins are typically less than those seen with treatment using natural prostaglandin.

Reported treatment protocols for dinoprost are 0.1 to 0.25 mg/kg subcutaneously every 8 to 12 hours; to reduce side effects, treatment can be initiated at the lower end of the dose range and increased after 48 hours of treatment.[1] Cloprostenol has been used at a dose of 1.0 to 2.5 μg/kg subcutaneously every 24 hours for 4 to 5 days; 100% of bitches aborted after a 4- to 7-day treatment regimen.[8] Anecdotally, some practitioners have reported success with mismating using cloprostenol at a further reduced frequency of 1.0 to 2.5 μg/kg every 48 hours; the vast majority of bitches tolerate this protocol with minimal or no side effects. Cloprostenol administration for mismating has also been evaluated in queens at a dose rate of 5 μg/kg subcutaneously daily for 3 days,[15] with poor efficacy whereby only 10% of queens aborted after 3 days of treatment[15] and no queens aborted after 2 days of treatment.[16] Treatment failure may be due to therapy being discontinued prematurely.

One of the major drawbacks to prostaglandin therapy for mismating is the need for extended treatment periods. It is vitally important that bitches and queens continue treatment until pregnancy termination is complete and progesterone has dropped to less than 2 ng/mL. Progression of pregnancy termination can be easily monitored via ultrasonography to ensure all fetuses have been resorbed or expelled. Bitches have lost a portion of a litter and carried remaining fetuses to term after incomplete treatment with prostaglandins.[17] Personnel handing these medications should be aware of the risk to pregnant women and asthmatics. Owners should be advised that bitches treated with prostaglandins may exhibit an early return to estrus because of the shortening of diestrus.

Dopamine Agonists

Prolactin is luteotropic in bitches and required to maintain luteal function in the second half of gestation,[18] and thus drugs that inhibit prolactin can be used alone or in conjunction with prostaglandins for mismating. Dopamine agonists act by binding directly to dopamine receptors in lieu of dopamine and thus cause dopamine-like effects; this includes the antagonism of prolactin production.[19] The subsequent lowering of prolactin results in regression of the CL and ultimately pregnancy termination. Drugs in this category include bromocriptine, cabergoline, and metergoline.

Treatment with bromocriptine for mismating has been studied using both injectable and oral formulations; only the oral tablets are available in the United States. Bitches treated with bromocriptine at a dose of 0.1 mg/kg intramuscularly once daily for 6 days resulted in pregnancy termination in all bitches (n = 3) after 42 days' gestation, but termination did not occur in early pregnant bitches (<23 days' gestation).[20] The investigators did not specify whether resorption or abortion occurred. Gastrointestinal side effects and listlessness were noted after treatment. Bromocriptine administered at a dose of 62.5 μg/kg twice daily by mouth to bitches at 43 to 45 days' gestation resulted in only 50% of bitches aborting.[21] Bromocriptine tablets are commercially available as 2.5-mg tablets; this can make appropriate dosing problematic for smaller patients, necessitating procurement of a compounded product. Because the use of bromocriptine alone has variable effects as an abortifacient in bitches, it is more common to combine bromocriptine with prostaglandins for mismating. Combining medications allows the dosage of both medications to be reduced, resulting in a reduction in adverse effects, and is discussed further under the section Combination therapy.

Cabergoline has also been evaluated as an abortifacient in bitches and queens. Bitches were treated with 1.65 μg/kg subcutaneously once daily for 5 days at 25 to 40 days after mating.[22] All bitches that were greater than 40 days' gestation resulted in pregnancy termination (n = 5), but only half of the bitches treated before day 40 of gestation showed termination of pregnancy. Fetal resorption occurred in 75% of cases. Side effects were reported as minimal. In another study, cabergoline was administered at 5 μg/kg orally once daily as an abortifacient.[23] This dose was partially luteolytic in the first half of gestation and fully luteolytic in the second half of gestation, resulting in pregnancy termination in the second half of gestation. In queens, cabergoline administered 15 μg/kg by mouth daily induced abortion in 100% of queens treated from days 34 to 42 after mating, but 2 queens failed to abort when treated after day 45 postmating.[24] Cabergoline is commercially available in the United States as a 0.5-mg tablet, often necessitating the procurement of a compounded formulation for treatment.

Metergoline, similar to other prolactin inhibitors, causes complete luteolysis and can be used reliably to terminate pregnancy. An earlier study showed that at a dose of 0.4 to 0.5 mg/kg orally for 5 days from days 18 to 20 of gestation did not terminate pregnancy but resulted in a reduction in serum progesterone levels.[25] In a more recent study, metergoline administered at a dose of 0.6 mg/kg orally twice daily, starting on day 28 after the onset of cytologic diestrus, terminated pregnancy in 8 of 9 treated bitches.[26] There were no side effects associated with metergoline administration, but some bitches required a prolonged period of treatment, with a mean 12.5 days of treatment (range 3–23 days).

Dexamethasone

Oral administration of dexamethasone has been evaluated for termination of pregnancy in bitches from 30 to 50 days' gestation.[27,28] Reported dosing regimens include a 9.5-day course of treatment as follows: 0.2 mg/kg every 12 hours for 7 days, 0.16 mg/kg the morning of the eighth day, 0.12 mg/kg in the evening of the eighth day, 0.08 mg/kg in the morning of the ninth day, 0.04 mg/kg in the evening of the ninth day, and 0.02 mg/kg the morning of the 10th day. Compared with a 7.5-day dosing regimen, the 9.5-day course of treatment was more effective. Another investigator reported success with administration of 0.2 mg/kg orally every 12 hours for 10 days with no tapering of the dose with minimal side effects.[8]

Fetal death after treatment with dexamethasone began 5 to 9 days after starting therapy, but live fetuses were identified up to 12 days after treatment was initiated.[27,28] Early pregnancies (<40 days) had few to no clinical signs of pregnancy loss excluding mild vaginal discharge in approximately one-third of cases. The main side effects of treatment included polyuria, polydipsia, and anorexia.

The mechanism of action of corticosteroids in termination of pregnancy is unknown. However, treatment with dexamethasone has many advantages, namely that the drug is readily available, inexpensive, easy to administer, and generally safe. However, dexamethasone treatment requires prolonged periods of treatment; depending on the stage of gestation when pregnancy termination is initiated, the length of treatment may result in abortion of fetuses rather than resorption.

Competitive Progesterone Receptor Blockers

RU-486, or mifepristone, is available in the United States for termination of pregnancy in women. It is highly regulated and difficult to obtain for other uses, but has been reported as an abortifacient drug in bitches.[29] Restricted access makes it impractical for use in veterinary patients.

Aglepristone (RU 46534) is a competitive progesterone antagonist that is used for the treatment of various progesterone-dependent conditions, including termination of pregnancy in bitches and queens. Aglepristone is not currently approved by the FDA, but is registered for use in Europe and Australia. The product is labeled for use at any stage of gestation and is administered as 2 injections 24 hours apart at a dose rate of 10 mg/kg. It is highly efficacious at all stages of gestation whereby a CL is present. Bitches treated with aglepristone approximately 30 days after ovulation aborted 4 to 7 days after the start of treatment, and the drug was well tolerated with the only side effect reported being slight vaginal discharge.[30] Efficacy in mid gestation has been reported to be as high as 95% with few and transient side effects.[31] There has been one report of fetal retention following aglepristone treatment in a bitch.[32] The bitch failed to respond to an initial course of therapy with aglepristone and was re-treated 15 days later; 5 weeks after aborting, uterine wall distention and a retained fetal skull was identified. The manufacturer recommends in the package insert that bitches should not be administered aglepristone for mismating until the end of estrus to assure maximal effectiveness of the drug.[33] Given the relative expense of this medication, it may be beneficial to determine pregnancy status, particularly in large-breed bitches where treatment may cost several hundred dollars. Although this drug is considered highly efficacious, bitches should still have follow-up ultrasonography performed to ensure pregnancy loss is complete.

Although aglepristone is not labeled for use in cats, there are several studies highlighting its efficacy in early,[15] mid,[34,35] and late gestation.[36] Efficacy was reported at 100% in early gestation, and 88.5% in mid gestation; queens exhibited brief periods of anorexia and depression before fetal expulsion. In late gestation, only 67% of queens aborted. Aglepristone treatment does not appear to affect fertility in subsequent estrous cycles. Similar to recommendations for bitches, queens should undergo ultrasonography to determine that abortion is complete, particularly considering the apparent reduction in efficacy later in gestation.

Monitoring Response to Therapy

Bitches and queens should be serially monitored via ultrasound and/or serum progesterone measurement to confirm that pregnancy termination is complete. Treatment options that rely on destruction of the CL (prostaglandins, prolactin inhibitors) should be continued until serum progesterone levels are less than 2 ng/mL. Treatment with aglepristone may result in a transient increase in serum progesterone levels. Fetal distress (bradycardia) is not consistently identified on ultrasound before fetal death. Depending on gestational age of the pregnancy, the dam may have vaginal discharge and/or pass obvious fetal and placental remnants. Bitches should be observed and fetal tissues removed to prevent consumption of these tissues and subsequent gastrointestinal upset in the dam. Treatment should be continued until abortion is complete, as evidenced by expulsion or resorption of all fetuses from the uterus.

COMBINATION THERAPIES

Prostaglandins and dopamine agonists are commonly combined to increase the efficacy of treatment and reduce adverse effects by a reduction in dose of each drug used. Bromocriptine has been investigated in combination with both dinoprost and cloprostenol from day 25 after mating. Bitches either received bromocriptine at 15 to 30 μg/kg by mouth twice daily and dinoprost at 0.1 to 0.2 mg/kg subcutaneously once daily, or the same dose of bromocriptine with cloprostenol at 1 μg/kg subcutaneously every 48 hours.[37] Treatment success was 100% in both groups, and there was no difference in days of treatment required for pregnancy termination. Pregnancy termination was accompanied by a mucoid sanguineous vaginal discharge for 3 to 10 days after treatment.

Combined treatment of mismating in bitches and queens with cabergoline and cloprostenol has also been evaluated.[38,39] Bitches were treated between 35 and 45 days from the first mating with 5 μg/kg cabergoline by mouth once daily and 1 μg/kg cloprostenol subcutaneously on days 1 and 3 (every 48 hours). If pregnancy was not terminated by day 8, cabergoline was continued until day 12. In 12 of the 13 treated bitches, pregnancy termination was confirmed within 2 to 9 days after the initiation of treatment; one bitch did not respond to treatment. Reported side effects were mild and included nausea, vomiting, and panting; side effects were observed after injection of cloprostenol and resolved within 20 minutes. The results of this study further indicate the need to confirm that pregnancy is completely terminated before discontinuing therapy. It is the author's preference to use a modification of this protocol whereby cloprostenol injections are continued at 48-hour intervals until the pregnancy is completely terminated, with periodic ultrasound monitoring to determine that all fetuses are either resorbed or expelled. In queens, cabergoline was administered orally at 5 μg/kg daily with cloprostenol 5 μg/kg subcutaneously every 48 hours administered 30 days after the first mating.[39] All treated animals aborted in 9 ± 1 days and did not exhibit any adverse effects other than mild hemorrhagic vulvar discharge.

Aglepristone has been evaluated in conjunction with concurrent administration of misoprostol.[40,41] Misoprostol is a synthetic prostaglandin E1 analogue and plays a role in cervical ripening. Bitches were treated between day 25 and 35 of gestation with either of the following: aglepristone at the labeled dose of 10 mg/kg subcutaneously every 24 hours for 2 doses; aglepristone as described with 200 to 400 μg misoprostol administered intravaginally; or aglepristone as described with 400 to 800 mg misoprostol administered orally. Misoprostol was administered daily until abortion was complete. No differences were noted between groups concerning the duration until termination of pregnancy, and in all groups, pregnancies were terminated 2 to 14 days after the first administration of aglepristone. No side effects were seen in any treatment group.

Aglepristone was also evaluated alone and in combination with cloprostenol for its effects on pregnancy termination in bitches.[41] Fourteen pregnant bitches between day 25 and 32 of gestation were used in the study. Two treatment groups were assessed; aglepristone was administered solely at 10 mg/kg, subcutaneously, once daily on 2 consecutive days in the first group and aglepristone as previously described with cloprostenol at 1 μg/kg in the second group. All pregnancies were successfully terminated in both groups; the addition of cloprostenol did not improve the success of treatment.

SURGICAL TREATMENT OPTIONS

Bitches and queens can undergo ovariohysterectomy at any point in gestation, but the procedure is technically easier during early to mid gestation. If presented with a bitch in estrus, it may be preferable to delay ovariohysterectomy until early diestrus because blood flow to the uterus is reduced at this time relative to estrus, but this carries the risk that the owner may not present the bitch or queen for surgery in a timely fashion. If further reproduction is not desired from the animal in question, ovariohysterectomy provides a permanent solution and eliminates any subsequent estrus. Because this is a commonly performed procedure, the surgical technique is not described here further.

In late gestation, the fetuses may still be viable. Current American Veterinary Medical Association guidelines regarding the euthanasia of fetuses in utero recommend that the fetus or fetuses are left in situ for 1 hour or longer and allowed to die of hypoxia[42]; fetuses that are removed from the uterus can be euthanized with barbiturates administered intraperitoneally.

TREATMENT RESISTANCE/COMPLICATIONS

No single therapeutic agent, excluding ovariohysterectomy, is 100% effective in terminating pregnancy at all stages of gestation. In the event of treatment failure, several options exist. First, treatment can be continued until pregnancy termination is complete (ie, continued prostaglandin or prolactin inhibitor therapy). Alternately, a different treatment protocol can be selected, or treatment can be repeated (ie, repeat dosing of aglepristone). The earlier in gestation that treatment is initiated, the more aesthetic the outcome for the owner regarding the passage of fluids and fetal tissues from the vulva. As gestation progresses into late term, mismating protocols may result in the birth of live but nonviable puppies, which may be upsetting to the bitch or queen owner.

EVALUATION OF OUTCOME AND LONG-TERM RECOMMENDATIONS

Bitches and queens not intended for future breeding are good candidates for surgical treatment via ovariohysterectomy because this eliminates the risk of future unwanted pregnancies. Owners of bitches/queens that are treated medically should be educated on strategies for preventing unwanted pregnancies in the future, including understanding of basic estrus cycle physiology and options for confinement of dogs and bitches in the household. Owners should also be made aware that the next anticipated estrus cycle may occur earlier than expected with certain treatment options, such as prostaglandins or aglepristone. Treatment with prostaglandins, dopamine agonists, and aglepristone appears to have no adverse effects on future fertility. Other medical therapies have not been specifically evaluated for effects on future fertility, but anecdotally, animals are often seen for repeated mismating. Protocols that carry the risk of pyometra, particularly estrogens, may result in a reduction in future fertility secondary to cystic endometrial hyperplasia-pyometra complex.

SUMMARY

The most appropriate mismating protocol will vary on a case-by-case basis, dependent on the owner's desire to preserve fertility, drug availability, adverse effects, and gestational age of the pregnancy. Owners must be advised of the extra-label use and any possible side effects from the selected treatment protocol. Although not currently FDA approved, it may be possible to acquire this drug under a special use permit; the feasibility of acquiring aglepristone in North America may be limited by drug cost and the relative infrequency of its use. Combinations of prostaglandins and dopamine agonists offer a good alternative with high efficacy and a low risk of adverse effects when used at low doses.

REFERENCES

1. Feldman EC, Davidson AP, Nelson RW, et al. Prostaglandin induction of abortion in pregnant bitches after misalliance. J Am Vet Med Assoc 1993;202(11):1855–8.
2. Fieni F, Fuhrer M, Tainturier D, et al. Use of cloprostenol for pregnancy termination in dogs. J Reprod Fertil 1989;39:332–3.
3. Doak RL, Hall A, Dale HE. Longevity of spermatozoa in the reproductive tract of the bitch. J Reprod Fertil 1967;13(1):51–8.
4. Whitacre MD, Yates DJ, VanCamp SD, et al. Detection of intravaginal spermatozoa after natural mating in the bitch. Vet Clin Pathol 1992;21(3):85–7.
5. Tsutsui T, Stabenfeldt GH. Biology of ovarian cycles, pregnancy and pseudopregnancy in the domestic cat. J Reprod Fertil Suppl 1993;47:29–35.
6. Davidson AP, Baker TW. Reproductive ultrasound of the bitch and queen. Top companion Anim Med 2009;24(2):55–63.
7. Verstegen-Onclin K, Verstegen J. Endocrinology of pregnancy in the dog: a review. Theriogenology 2008;70(3):291–9.
8. Eilts BE. Pregnancy termination in the bitch and queen. Clin Tech Small Anim Pract 2002;17(3):116–23.
9. Bowen RA, Olson PN, Behrendt MD, et al. Efficacy and toxicity of estrogens commonly used to terminate canine pregnancy. J Am Vet Med Assoc 1985;186(8):783–8.
10. Tsutsui T, Mizutani W, Hori T, et al. Estradiol benzoate for preventing pregnancy in mismated dogs. Theriogenology 2006;66(6–7):1568–72.
11. Bowen RA, Olson PN, Young S, et al. Efficacy and toxicity of tamoxifen citrate for prevention and termination of pregnancy in bitches. Am J Vet Res 1988;49(1):27–31.
12. Concannon PW, Hansel W. Prostaglandin F2alpha induced luteolysis, hypothermia, and abortions in beagle bitches. Prostaglandins 1977;13(3):533–42.
13. Romagnoli SE, Cela M, Camillo F. Use of prostaglandin F2 alpha for early pregnancy termination in the mismated bitch. Vet Clin North Am Small Anim Pract 1991;21(3):487–99.
14. Romagnoli SE, Camillo F, Novellini S, et al. Luteolytic effects of prostaglandin F2alpha on day 8 to 19 corpora lutea in the bitch. Theriogenology 1996;45(2):397–403.
15. Garcia Mitacek MC, Bonaura MC, Praderio RG, et al. Progesterone and ultrasonographic changes during aglepristone or cloprosternol treatment in queens at 21 to 22 or 35 to 38 days of pregnancy. Theriogenology 2017;88:106–17.
16. Garcia Mitacek MC, Stornelli MC, Praderio R, et al. Efficacy of cloprostenol or aglepristone at 21-22 and 35-38 days of gestation for pregnancy termination in queens. Reprod Domest Anim 2012;47(Suppl 6):200–3.
17. Feldman E, Nelson R. Canine and feline endocrinology and reproduction. 3rd edition. St. Louis (MO): Saunders Elsevier; 2004.
18. Okkens AC, Bevers MM, Dieleman SJ, et al. Evidence for prolactin as the main luteotrophic factor in the cyclic dog. Vet Q 1990;12(4):193–201.
19. Beijerink NJ, Kooistra HS, Dieleman SJ, et al. Serotonin antagonist-induced lowering of prolactin secretion does not affect the pattern of pulsatile secretion of follicle-stimulating hormone and luteinizing hormone in the bitch. Reproduction 2004;128(2):181–8.
20. Concannon PW, Weinstein P, Whaley S, et al. Suppression of luteal function in dogs by luteinizing hormone antiserum and by bromocriptine. J Reprod Fertil 1987;81(1):175–80.

21. Wichtel JJ, Whitacre MD, Yates DJ, et al. Comparison of the effects of PGF(2) alpha and bromocryptine in pregnant beagle bitches. Theriogenology 1990; 33(4):829–36.
22. Onclin K, Silva LD, Donnay I, et al. Luteotrophic action of prolactin in dogs and the effects of a dopamine agonist, cabergoline. J Reprod Fertil Suppl 1993;47: 403–9.
23. Jochle W, Arbeiter K, Post K, et al. Effects on pseudopregnancy, pregnancy and interoestrous intervals of pharmacological suppression of prolactin secretion in female dogs and cats. J Reprod Fertil Suppl 1989;39:199–207.
24. Erünal-Maral N, Aslan S, Findik M, et al. Induction of abortion in queens by administration of cabergoline (Galastop™) solely or in combination with the PGF2α analogue Alfaprostol (Gabbrostim™). Theriogenology 2004;61(7):1471–5.
25. Gerstenberg C, Nothling JO. The effects of metergoline combined with PGF2alpha treatment on luteal function and gestation in pregnant bitches. Theriogenology 1995;44(5):649–59.
26. Nothling JO, Gerber D, Gerstenberg C, et al. Abortifacient and endocrine effects of metergoline in beagle bitches during the second half of gestation. Theriogenology 2003;59(9):1929–40.
27. Wanke M, Loza ME, Monachesi N, et al. Clinical use of dexamethasone for termination of unwanted pregnancy in dogs. J Reprod Fertil Suppl 1997;51:233–8.
28. Zone M, Wanke M, Rebuelto M, et al. Termination of pregnancy in dogs by oral administration of dexamethasone. Theriogenology 1995;43(2):487–94.
29. Concannon PW, Yeager A, Frank D, et al. Termination of pregnancy and induction of premature luteolysis by the antiprogestagen, mifepristone, in dogs. J Reprod Fertil 1990;88(1):99–104.
30. Galac S, Kooistra HS, Butinar J, et al. Termination of mid-gestation pregnancy in bitches with aglepristone, a progesterone receptor antagonist. Theriogenology 2000;53(4):941–50.
31. Pettersson CH, Tidholm A. Safety and efficacy of mid-term pregnancy termination using aglepristone in dogs. J small Anim Pract 2009;50(3):120–3.
32. Rigau T, Rodriguez-Gil JE, Garcia F, et al. Partial foetal retention following aglepristone treatment in a bitch. Reprod Domest Anim 2011;46(4):738–41.
33. Alizin Anti Progesterone Injection (aglepristone) [package insert]. Milperra, Australia: Virbac (Australia) Pty Limited; 2017.
34. Fieni F, Martal J, Marnet PG, et al. Clinical, biological and hormonal study of mid-pregnancy termination in cats with aglepristone. Theriogenology 2006;66(6–7): 1721–8.
35. Georgiev P, Wehrend A. Mid-gestation pregnancy termination by the progesterone antagonist aglepristone in queens. Theriogenology 2006;65(7):1401–6.
36. Georgiev P, Bostedt H, Goericke-Pesch S, et al. Induction of abortion with aglepristone in cats on day 45 and 46 after mating. Reprod Domest Anim 2010;45(5): e161–7.
37. Gobello C, Castex G, Corrada Y, et al. Use of prostaglandins and bromocriptine mesylate for pregnancy termination in bitches. J Am Vet Med Assoc 2002;220(7) 1017–9.
38. Corrada Y, Rodriguez R, Tortora M, et al. A combination of oral cabergoline and double cloprostenol injections to produce third-quarter gestation termination in the bitch. J Am Anim Hosp Assoc 2006;42(5):366–70.
39. Onclin K, Verstegen J. Termination of pregnancy in cats using a combination of cabergoline, a new dopamine agonist, and a synthetic PGF2 alpha, cloprostenol J Reprod Fertil Suppl 1997;51:259–63.

40. Agaoglu AR, Aslan S, Emre B, et al. Clinical evaluation of different applications of misoprostol and aglepristone for induction of abortion in bitches. Theriogenology 2014;81(7):947–51.
41. Kaya D, Kucukaslan I, Agaoglu AR, et al. The effects of aglepristone alone and in combination with cloprostenol on hormonal values during termination of mid-term pregnancy in bitches. Anim Reprod Sci 2014;146(3–4):210–7.
42. AVMA. AVMA guidelines for the euthanasia of animals: 2013 edition. Schaumburg (IL): American Veterinary Medical Association; 2013.

Gestational Aging and Determination of Parturition Date in the Bitch and Queen Using Ultrasonography and Radiography

Cheryl Lopate, MS, DVM*

KEYWORDS

- Gestational aging • Canine • Feline • Fetal maturation • Pregnancy length
- Ultrasound

KEY POINTS

- Radiography can be used to diagnose pregnancy and confirm fetal numbers but is less accurate in the determination of fetal age and readiness for birth than ultrasound.
- Ultrasound imaging can be used to determine gestational age via measurement of fetal and extrafetal structures in bitches and queens.
- There is no substitute for accurate ovulation timing at the onset of the estrous cycle to determine gestational age.

INTRODUCTION

Pregnancy in the bitch and queen is a relatively short process, compared with other domestic species, lasting only 65 days from the luteinizing hormone (LH) surge. This short duration of pregnancy means that fetuses are born in an immature state and the final development of most organ systems occurs in the weeks to months after birth. Considerable development of major fetal organ systems occurs during the last days of gestation, in preparation for survival outside the uterus. Failure of the fetuses to complete the maturation process results in failure to survive. Additionally, owing to the nature of the zonary placenta, once a fetus exceeds its due date by more than 2 days, it will demand more nutritional support than the placenta is able to provide, resulting in intrauterine fetal death. Thus, it is critical to ensure that each fetus has attained, but not exceeded, its maximal gestational age before delivery.

Disclosure Statement: The author has nothing to disclose.
Reproductive Revolutions and Wilsonville Veterinary Clinic, 9275 SW Barber Street, Wilsonville, OR 97070, USA
* 18858 Case Road Northeast, Aurora, OR 97002.
E-mail address: lopatec1@gmail.com

There are several situations when the determination of gestational age and fetal maturation are necessary. Most of these situations arise when there is either inadequate or no ovulation timing to allow determination of an accurate due date.

- Patients that will be allowed to deliver naturally but may require veterinary care during parturition. This measure allows the breeder and veterinarian to be prepared and available for the onset of labor.
- Patients that will undergo an elective cesarean delivery for a variety of reasons, such as high-risk breed (brachycephalic dog and cats); large or giant breeds bitches with singleton or small litters that may not initiate labor on their own; bitches with large litters where development of uterine inertia is a concern; and patients with a prior history of dystocia or primary uterine inertia.
- Patients with high-risk pregnancies including gestational diabetes mellitus or pregnancy toxemia. In these cases, the dam is often supported as far into the pregnancy as possible to try to get the fetuses to term. In some cases, it may not be possible to continue owing to the failing health status of the dam and in these cases the fetuses may not survive if they must be delivered preterm.
- Patients requiring tocolytic support during pregnancy. This may include dams that require progesterone supplementation owing to luteal failure as a result of chronic endometritis, stress, partial abortion, or idiopathic luteal insufficiency. It also includes dams that enter preterm labor owing to abnormalities or defects in the myometrium from nutritional, parasitic, environmental, traumatic, or inflammatory causes. Determination of the due date is imperative in these cases to either know when to withdraw the tocolytic agents or to know when to perform a cesarean delivery before fetal demise.

Gestational duration is most accurately determined by using either the LH surge or progesterone concentrations.[1–3] Parturition occurs 65 ± 2 days after the LH surge, and ovulation begins 48 hours after the LH surge.[1–6] Owing to the extreme variability of the duration of the bitch's estrous cycle and receptive behavior, and the amount of time sperm may survive in the bitch's reproductive tract, the use of breeding dates is not an accurate method of estimating gestational age.[1,2,7] Parturition may occur any time from 58 to 71 days after a given breeding date.[1,2,7,8] In contrast, in the queen, knowledge of breeding dates is an accurate method of determining due date because they have induced ovulation, but in some cases breeding dates may not be known.

This article reviews the use of radiography and ultrasound imaging in the determination of gestational age and the assessment of fetal maturation in the bitch and queen. All estimations and calculations of gestational age and fetal maturation in this article are expressed in days after the LH surge unless otherwise noted.

METHODS TO ASSESS FETAL MATURATION
Radiographs

Factors affecting radiographic quality
Proper radiographic technique and adequate patient restraint are critical for accurate assessment.[8,9] A single lateral radiograph of the abdomen is usually sufficient to allow for pregnancy diagnosis and fetal counting. Radiographs are the best method to obtain an accurate fetal count, but must be done in late pregnancy (days 57–65) to ensure mineralization is complete and reduce the chances that fetuses will be missed during evaluation.[4,8,9] A ventrodorsal radiograph allows measurements to be taken to assess the size of the pelvic canal in relation to fetal head size.[8,9] It is necessary to increase the kVP to between 4 and 10 to obtain adequate visualization of the fetal

skeletons. Varying degrees of fetal mineralization are present depending on the day of pregnancy the radiographs are obtained, which may make certain skeletal structures difficult to observe.[8,9] Giant breed bitches may be difficult to get adequate penetration owing to the width of the pregnant abdomen. Sometimes, high fetal numbers prevent accurate visualization of the entire litter. Localization of multiple fetuses overlying each other may make it difficult to evaluate all skeletal components of each individual fetus.[8,9] Abdominal contents (food and gas) may also obscure visualization of the fetus(es).[8,9]

Gestational aging with radiography

Canine Spherical uterine swellings are visible between days 31 and 38 days (average of 35).[1,2,4,7–9] These swellings turn ovoid between days 38 and 44 (average of 41 days). Mineralization of the fetal skull is first evident around between 43 and 46 days (average of 45 days). The scapula, humerus, and femur are visible between 46 and 51 days (average of 48 days). The radius, ulna, and tibia are visible between 50 and 53 days (average of 52 days). The pelvis and all 13 ribs are visible between 53 and 59 days (average of 54 days; **Fig. 1**). The coccygeal vertebrae, fibula, calcaneus, and distal extremities are visible between 55 and 64 days (average of 61 days). Teeth are visible between 58 and 63 days (average of 61 days; **Fig. 2**).

Feline Spherical swellings are visible in all queens by day 21 of pregnancy, but may be seen as early as day 17 after mating in some patients.[4,10,11] The first general mineralization can be seen on average 39 ± 1 days (range, 36–40 days), the vertebral column on 41 ± 1 days (range, 38–43 days), skull 43 ± 1 days (range, 38–44 days), ribs 43 ± 2 days (range, 40–45 days), femur 44 ± 1 days (range, 42–46 days), scapula 45 ± 2 days (range, 41–48 days), humerus 45 ± 1 days (range, 41–45 days), radius 46 ± 2 days (range, 43–50 days), tibia 46 ± 1 days (range, 44–50 days), pelvis 46 ± 1 days (range, 45–57 days), ulna 48 ± 2 days (range, 44–6 days), coccygeal vertebrae 50 ± 2 days (range, 49–57 days), fibula 52 ± 3 days (range, 48–65 days), metacarpals/tarsals 57 ± 3 days (range, 51–62 days), phalanges 59 ± 3 days (range, 54–65 days), calcaneus 59 ± 3 days (range, 55–65 days), and teeth 63 ± 1 days (range, 59–64 days).[4,11,12] Litter size does not affect the predicted parturition date.[12]

Radiographs can help to provide a rough estimate of gestational age, but are not adequate alone to determine fetal readiness for birth because there is some overlap of radiographic detail between dams and among breeds.[1,2,7–9] The fetus may be

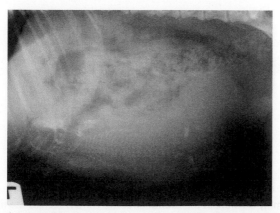

Fig. 1. The fetal pelvis is visible in this radiograph with the fetus in a frontal plane.

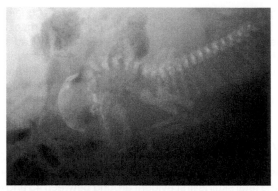

Fig. 2. The fetal teeth are visible as a radiodense straight line running through the middle of the mouth. The fetal extremities of the front feet are also visible.

completely mineralized by as early as 58 days after the LH surge, and at this stage they would not survive ex utero.[1,2,7–9] Furthermore, with the advent of digital radiography, the fetal skeletal components may be visualized even sooner in some cases, making gestational aging by radiography less accurate.

Fetal death
Failure of the uterus to continue to enlarge or a rapid decrease in uterine diameter is indicative of abortion, resorption, or fetal death.[8,13] Fetal death can be identified if the bones of the skull begin to override each other or become otherwise deformed, if there is gas accumulation within the uterus or in or around the fetus (within the blood vessels, heart, body cavities), or if there is abnormal flexion of the fetus (balling) or hyperextension of the hind limbs[8,13] (**Figs. 3** and **4**). When gas is suspected within the uterus, it should be confirmed with a second radiographic view.

Ultrasound Imaging
There are 3 major limitations of ultrasound imaging: (1) the quality of the machine, (2) the experience of the operator, and (3) patient factors (amount of hair, use of quality ultrasound gel, relaxation of the patient, respiratory rate, and patient size). As ultrasound technology continues to evolve and improve, the timing of first visualization of fetal structures becomes earlier and earlier in pregnancy.[14] Ultrasound imaging

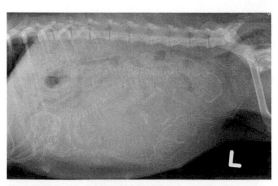

Fig. 3. A fetal mummy is visible in the caudal abdomen and is seen as the much smaller fetus in a balled up in posture.

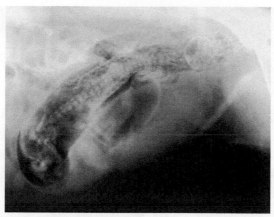

Fig. 4. Emphysema is seen around this dead fetus.

can be used estimate gestational age through the use of gestational sac and/or fetal measurements and through evaluation of the progression of organ development. It may also be used to ascertain fetal viability and to determine if fetal stress is present.

Gestational aging via fetal and extrafetal measurements

Canine Pregnancy may be diagnosed as early as 19 to 21 days of gestation, at which time the conceptuses are approximately 1 cm in diameter.[3,4,7,15–17] Measurement to determine gestational age is more accurate when the bitch is less than 37 days' gestation.[4,15,18–22] Between days 19 and 37 of gestation, measurement of gestational sac diameter (inner chorionic cavity [ICC]) or the crown–rump length of the fetus can easily be obtained.[3,4,15,16,18,19,21–25] If the bitch is more than 37 days' gestation, fetal measurements of the biparietal diameter (BPD), body diameter (BD), and deep portion of the fetal diencephalo-telencephalic vesicle (DPTV) are obtained from 1 or more fetuses.

When measuring the gestational sacs, 2 transverse plane measurements should be taken at 90° angles to each other and these values averaged before using the formulas provided[4,20,22,24,25] (**Fig. 5**). The crown–rump length is measured in a sagittal plane from the most rostral part of the head to the base of the tail (**Fig. 6**). For BPD, the image should be in a midsagittal plane and the markers placed at the parietal bones symmetrically on either side of the fetal skull[4,15,18,19,21,22,24] (**Fig. 7**). Measurement of BD should be taken at the widest portion of the fetal abdomen (level of the stomach and liver; **Fig. 8**).[4,15,18,19,21,22,24] Two transverse plane measurements should be obtained at 90° angles to each other and these measurements are averaged before using with the formulas provided in **Boxes 1** and **2**.[22,25,26] When taking measurements of fetal or extrafetal structures, at least 2 (or more) distinct fetuses or gestational sacs should be measured whenever possible, and the measurements averaged before applying them to formulas.[4,20,22,24,25,27] In cases of singletons, this is of course impossible and measurement of multiple structures (ie, ICC, crown–rump length, BPD, or BD) may be taken to increase the accuracy of any 1 measurement alone[4,22,24,25] (see **Fig. 8**).

The DPTV can be visualized from day 35 of gestation until day 58 of gestation as a symmetric anechoic area viewed on sagittal midline in the fetal skull and has been used to determine gestational age[28,29] (**Fig. 9**). The DPTV represents the fetal thalamus and the primordial basal nuclei.[28,29] The size of the DPTV depends on the size of the bitch

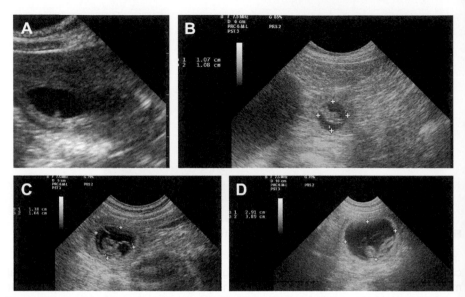

Fig. 5. (*A*) Day 21 embryo is visible protruding from the wall of the gestational sac. (*B*) Day 26 embryo is seen centrally in the gestational sac with membranes attached to the embryo proper on both sides. (*C*) Day 29 embryo is seen with the yolk sac above the embryo. (*D*) Day 40 fetus with the regressing yolk sac seen to the right side of the fetus.

and formulas for gestational aging have been determined for small (<10 kg), medium (11–25 kg), and large breed (26–40 kg) bitches (see **Box 2** below).[28,29]

Other rules of thumb regarding gestational aging are that the BD exceeds head diameter by more than 2 mm between 38 and 42 days gestational age and the fetal crown–rump length first exceeds placental length between 40 and 42 days.[7,15,18,19]

Some factors that may affect the interpretation and accuracy of these measurements are differences in size among breeds (toys vs giants), litter size (singletons vs very large litters), and head shape (brachycephalic vs dolicocephalic). These factors should be taken into consideration when using fetal measurements to predict due dates. Some studies show no effect of litter size on gestation length,[20,22] whereas others show that smaller litter size (either <7 puppies or <3 puppies) is associated

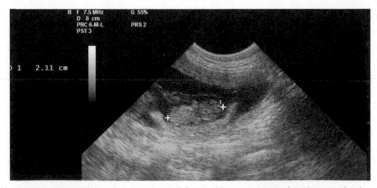

Fig. 6. The crown–rump length is measured from the most rostral point on the head to the base of the tail.

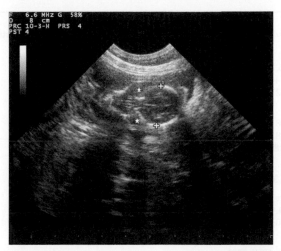

Fig. 7. Biparietal diameter measurement. The markers are placed at the widest portion of the parietal bone with both orbits (*asterisks*) visible to ensure that the image is symmetric.

with longer gestational duration.[21,30–32] There may also be some breed variation with gestation duration, with German Shepherd dogs and Hound dogs having shorter gestations and West Highland White Terriers having longer gestations.[30,31,33] In the author's experience, Cavalier King Charles Spaniels also have a shorter gestation. In another study using Drever bitches, it was shown that, once the litter size exceeds the average for the breed, each additional puppy will reduce gestation length by 0.25 days.[32] Conversely, when litter size is less than average, 0.25 days should be added to the due date for each puppy below breed average.[32]

Ultrasound imaging is less accurate in the determination of litter size compared with radiographs, but can be used at a much earlier stage of pregnancy to estimate litter size, which can then be used to help manage the nutritional demands of pregnancy.[4,34]

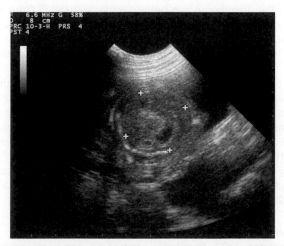

Fig. 8. Body diameter measurement. Markers are placed at 90° angles at the widest part of the fetus, which is the level the stomach and liver. The stomach is seen as an anechoic structure with the uniformly hyperechoic liver adjacent to it.

Box 1
Formulas for calculation of gestational age in the bitches using extrafetal structures

ICC (medium size)
  GA $= 19.66 + 6.27 \times$ (cm)[19] or
  GA $= (6 \times$ cm$) + 20$[15] or
  DBP $= ($mm $- 82.13)/1.8$[24]

ICC (small size)
  DBP $= ($mm $- 68.88)/1.53$[24]
  DBP $= 63.2 - (18.58 + 0.71 \times$ mm) Maltese[25]
  DBP $= 63.4 - (18.92 + 0.65 \times$ mm) Yorkshire[25]

ICC (large breed)
  DBP $= 44.76-(4.34 \times$ ICC) GSD[27]

OUD (medium size)
  GA $= 17.39 + 4.98 \times$ cm[19]
  DBP $= ($mm $- 80.78)/1.57$[24]

OUD (small size)
  DBP $= ($mm $- 85.17)/1.83$[24]

Placental thickness
  GA $= ($mm $+ 0.314)/0.021$[44]

Abbreviations: DBP, days before parturition is calculated based on a 65 ± 2 d gestation length; GA, gestational age is calculated based on days past the luteinizing hormone surge ± 2 d; ICC, inner chorionic cavity; OUD, outer uterine diameter.

Litter size is best evaluated between days 25 and 30 of pregnancy when there is minimal overlapping of fetuses and the horns can be followed along both sides of the body more easily.[34] Scanning should be done from the bladder cranial to each ovary to reduce the likelihood of counting an individual fetus more than once.[34]

Feline Measurement of the ICC and exterior chorionic cavity can be used from day 10 to 25 of pregnancy when the gestational sac maintains a round appearance.[4,35–37] The gestational sacs are spherical until day 20 when they take on a slightly oblong shape with the edges of the gestational sac being slightly tapered.[35] Care should be taken not to deform the gestational sac with pressure and 2 transverse views through the middle of the gestational sac should be obtained on 1 or more sacs and the measurements averaged.[4,35] Formulas for gestational aging using extrafetal structures are presented in **Box 3**.

After 30 days of gestational age, the BPD, BD, and stomach diameter can all be used to determine gestational age.[4,38,39] Stomach diameter is measured at the widest diameter of the stomach in a transverse view.[38,39] The BPD is taken at the widest point on the skull in a frontal or dorsal view, at the central location of the echogenic line produced by the falx cerebri. BD taking 2 transverse measurements at the widest point of the abdomen, which occurs at the level of the stomach and liver.[4,38,39] The crown–rump length may be used from day 38 to term. Formulas for gestational aging via crown–rump length measurement or measurement of fetal structures are presented in **Tables 1** and **2**.

Accuracy of results

In early to midpregnancy (<37–40 days) the use of ICC has been shown to be between 64% and 91% accurate (± 1 days) in both small and medium breeds and between 85% and 88% accurate in large breeds (± 2 days) at predicting the day of

---

Box 2
Formulas for calculation of gestation age in small, medium and large breed bitches using fetal structures

CRL (medium size)
  GA = (3 × CRL) + 27[15]
  GA = 24.64 + 4.54 × cm – 0.24 × cm²[19]

BPD (medium size)
  GA = (15 × HD) + 20[15]
  GA = 21.08 + 14.88 × cm – 0.11 × cm²[19]
  DBP = (mm – 29.18)/0.7[24]

BPD (small size)
  DBP = 63.2 – (24.7 + 1.54 × mm) Maltese[25]
  DBP = 63.4 – (23.89 + 1.63 × mm Yorkshire[25]
  DBP = (mm – 25.11)/0.61[24]

BPD (large breed)
  DPB = 38.65 – (12.86 × BPD) GSD[27]

BD (medium size)
  GA = (7 × BD) + 29[15]
  GA = 22.89 + 12.75 × cm – 1.17 × cm²[19]

BD + BPD
  GA = (6 × BPD) + (3 × BD) + 30[15]
  DBP = 34.27 to 5.89 × BPD (cm) – 2.77 × BD (cm)[18]

DPTV (small size)
  DBP = (mm – 10.11)/0.24[28,29]

DPTV (medium size)
  DBP = (mm – 14.15)/0.4[28,29]

DPTV (large size)
  DBP = (mm – 10.27)/0.24[28,29]

Abbreviations: BD, body diameter; BPD, biparietal diameter; CRL, crown–rump length; DBP, days before parturition is calculated based on a 65 ± 2 day gestation duration; DPTV, deep portion of the diencephalo-telencephalic vesicle; GA, gestational age is calculated based on days past the luteinizing hormone surge ± 2 days; GSD, German Shepherd dogs.

---

parturition.[21,22,24–26] The use of the outer uterine diameter is less accurate because it is more prone to errors in the placement of the markers. Use of the length of the zonary placenta and placental thickness have been proposed for measurement, but have not proven to be accurate in estimating gestational age and should not be used.[22,24,25]

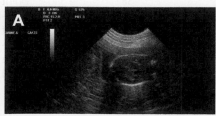 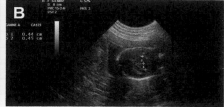

Fig. 9. Deep portion of the diencephalo-telencephalic vesicle (DPTV). (*A*) The DPTVs are visible in the center of the skull on sagittal midline as 2 symmetrically located round to slightly pyriform shaped structures. (*B*) Markers are placed to outline the 2 vesicles. The combined width of the 2 vesicles is used for formula measurement.

> **Box 3**
> **Formulas for calculation of GA (days) in the queen using extrafetal structures before day 40**
>
> GA = 2.0087x − 31.43 where x = embryo/fetus length in mm[a]
>
> GA = 1.602x − 12.13 where x = outer uterine diameter in mm
>
> GA = 1.368x − 11.566 where x = inner chorionic circumference in mm
>
> *Abbreviation:* GA, gestational age.
> [a] Embryo/fetal length is measured from the rostral most point of the skull to the base of the tail on days 17–30.
> *Data from* Zambelli D, Caneppele B, Bassi S, et al. Ultrasound aspects of fetal and extrafetal structures in pregnant cats. J Feline Med Surg 2002:4(2):95–106.

Use of the crown–rump length is accurate in early pregnancy, but is also prone to errors in placement of the markers and, once the fetus reaches approximately 40 days of gestation, it begins to flex significantly making the use of this measure inaccurate.[20,22,25]

In later pregnancy (>40 days of gestation) the use of BPD is the most accurate measurement tool.[20,22,25,26] BPD is more accurate than BD in the bitch after day 37.[20–22,24,25] Combining the use of BD and BPD increases the accuracy from using BD alone. Accuracy with the use of BPD measurements within 1 day of actual parturition was 64% to 75% in small breeds and 65% in medium breeds; and within 2 days this increased to 85% to 88% and 81% to 86%, respectively.[21,22,25,26] In cases of singletons or very small litters, BPD may be less accurate than in bitches with normal size litters.[21] Formulas for determining gestational age are presented in **Boxes 1** and **2**.

A study by Socha and Janowski[40] using the ICC and BPD in a bitches of various breeds and sizes (from <10 kg to >40 kg), revealed similar accuracy to those found with breed-specific research. The ICC was more accurate than the BPD for all sizes of bitches. The ICC predicted parturition date within 1 day 60.00% to 78.95% of the time and within 2 days 80.00% to 92.31% of the time. The BPD predicted parturition within 1 day, 42.31% to 63.04% of the time and within 2 days 64.29% to 91.30% of the time.[40]

Groppetti and colleagues[27] looked at breed specific measurements of ICC and BPD in German Shepherd dogs. They found the ICC to be 94.5% accurate at predicting

Table 1
Use of crown–rump length to determine gestational age (days) in the queen

Days from Coitus	Crown–Rump Length (mm)
38	58
41	75
44	84
47	94
50	106
53	114
56	121
58	130
60	136
65 (day of parturition)	145

Data from Refs.[35,37,42]

Table 2
Formulas for calculation of GA (days) in the queen using fetal structures

BPD (after 40 d)[15,34]	$GA = 25 \times BPD + 3$ Where DBP $= 61 - GA$
BD (after 40 d)[15,34]	$GA = 11 \times BD + 21$ Where DBP $= 61 - GA$
BPD[42]	$DPB = BPD \, (mm) - 23.39/0.47 \, d$
DPTV[28]	$BPD = DPTV \, (mm) - 10.74/0.22 \, d$
BD[38]	$BD \, (mm) = 0.405565e^{0.0372141*t}$ $t = \dfrac{\log(BD/0.405565)}{0.0372141}$
BPD[38]	$BPD \, (mm) = 0.483873e^{0.02756*t}$ $t = \dfrac{\log(BPD/0.483873)}{0.02756}$
GD[38]	$GD \, (mm) = 0.115113e^{0.0388901*t}$ $t = \dfrac{\log(GD/0.115113)}{0.0388901}$

Abbreviations: BD, body diameter; BPD, biparietal diameter; DBP, days before parturition; DPTV, diencephalo-telencephalic vesicle; GA, gestational age; GD, gastric diameter; t, gestational age.
  Data from Refs.[15,35,38,42]

parturition within 2 days and 81.8% accurate within 1 day. The BPD was found to be 91.7% at predicting parturition within 2 days and 83.3% within 1 day.[27] Accuracy was higher in litters with more than 3 pups.[27]

Socha and coworkers[5] compared the use of the ICC or BPD with LH surge, progesterone concentrations, and day 1 of cytologic diestrus. They found that the ICC was 66.67% accurate within 1 day and 100% within 2 days of actual parturition, BPD was 83.33% for 1 day and 100% for 2 days, LH surge was 66.67% for 1 day and 100% for 2 days, progesterone was 100% for both 1 and 2 days, and cytologic diestrus was 50% for 1 days and 66.67% for 2 days.[5] This cohort was small (only 6 bitches) and all of medium size. The study indicates what others have also shown in that hormonal analysis is more accurate than fetal biometry, but fetal biometry does provide an accurate means of estimating the due date when hormonal analysis has not been performed.

The accuracy of predicting parturition using DPTV measurements within 1 day of actual parturition was 40%, 50%, and 38% for small, medium, and large breed bitches, respectively, and increased to 62%, 65%, and 60%, respectively, when the estimated due date was extended to within 2 days of actual parturition.[28,29]

The difference in accuracy of parturition prediction for giant or toy breeds compared with the medium breeds has been examined and it was concluded that one could use the measurement formulas for medium sized bitches if one corrected for the extremes in size.[20] To obtain more accurate due dates, the authors recommended subtracting 2 days for giant breed bitches and adding 1 day for small breed bitches after the gestational age is calculated.[20] After adjusting for weight, these authors found an accuracy of 75% and 87% for gestational aging for ±1 day and ±2 days, respectively, for bitches evaluated by day 30 of gestational age.[20] Another study looked at gestational aging in giant breeds and found that their accuracy using previously calculated formulas for medium breed bitches was 76.6% for ICC for ±1 day and 90% for ±2 days; for BPD, it was 54.16% for ±1 days and 79.16 for ±2 days.[24,40] They concluded, as have other researchers, that ICC measured in midpregnancy is more accurate and should be the preferred method and timing of gestational aging when possible.[40] Other formulas have since been provided for small breeds, but none have been proposed for giant breeds.[22,24,25]

A study by Lenard and colleagues[41] comparing the use of midpregnancy fetal organ development (fetal heartbeat, limb development, and brain development) and late pregnancy BPD and BD measurements showed that the use of both methods predicted parturition date within 65 ± 1 days was 74.6% and 65 ± 2 days was 86.1%, whereas the use of midpregnancy fetal organ development alone predicted parturition date within 65 ± 1 days was 74.6% and 65 ± 2 days was 91.9%. Using either method alone, midpregnancy fetal organ development was more accurate at predicting parturition date than was fetal body measurements in late pregnancy.[41] The use of midpregnancy fetal organ development tended to overestimate gestational age, whereas the use of BD measurements in late pregnancy tended to underestimate gestational age.[41] Maternal body weight and litter size had no significant impact on the accuracy of the prediction method.[41] The earlier in pregnancy the bitch is scanned for gestational aging estimation, the more accurate the results.[41] This study also found that litter size could be estimated accurately in early to midpregnancy, but that fetal numbers may change owing to fetal resorption (before day 37), fetal mummification, or by missing some fetuses owing to maternal colonic or intestinal gas, poor patient compliance, or operator experience with the technique.[41]

The combined use of organ developmental changes along with fetal and extrafetal measurements provides a more accurate estimation of gestational aging than the use of either modality alone.[19,26]

In the feline, the use of these measurements predicts parturition within 1 to 2 days. BPD provides the greatest accuracy, with 64.3% queening within 1 day of the predicted due date and 85.7% queening within 2 days of the predicted due date.[42] The DPTV can be identified after day 34 of pregnancy[42]; however, it has poor accuracy in terms of prediction of due date (±1 day 38.5%; ±2 days 61.5%).[42]

Gestational aging via estimation of fetal maturation

Canine The use of a 6.5- to 12.5-mHz probe is ideal for assessing fetal organ development.[7,15,18,19,26] Gestational age may be estimated through the assessment of organ development.[7,15,18,19,26] Serial examinations may provide more accurate information than a single examination and the examination of multiple fetuses is better than 1 or 2.[4,27] The embryo is first noted within the gestational sac by day 25 or 26 after the LH surge.[7,14,15,18,19,26,34] It seems to be oblong and rests adjacent to the wall of the uterus. The heartbeat is first visible at 23 to 26 days of gestation, when the embryonic mass is 1 to 4 mm in length and lying adjacent to the wall of the gestational sac.[4,7,15,17–19,26,34] Fetal heartbeats and movement may be detected as early as day 23 of gestation.[4,7,15,17,18] The heartbeat is typically noted on the first day the embryo proper is visible or the next day.[17] At day 27 to 28, the embryo moves away from the endometrial wall and seems to be suspended by the fetal membranes with the yolk sac being the larger of the 2 cavities.[7,15,18,19,26] The placenta can be seen as early as days 26 to 27 of gestation as a distinct structure lining the uterus; it becomes zonary in appearance by days 29 to 31 of gestation and the edges curl inward by days 32 to 34.[7,14,15,18,19,26] The embryo is located dependently in the chorionic cavity by days 29 to 33 of gestation and the yolk sac takes on a tubular appearance at this time as it shrinks away.[7,15,18,19,26] The bladder is first visible between 35 and 39 days of gestation, the stomach between 36 and 39 days, the kidneys and eyes between 39 and 47 days, and the intestine between 57 and 63 days.[7,14,15,18,19,26] The lungs become more hyperechoic than the liver between 38 and 42 days of gestation and the liver becomes more hyperechoic than the other abdominal organs between 39 and 47 days[7,14,15,18,19,26] (**Fig. 10**).

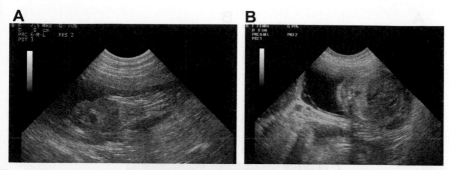

Fig. 10. (*A*) Day 37 fetus in a sagittal view. The lung is hyperechoic to the liver. The bladder is also visible in the caudal abdomen. (*B*) Day 45 fetus in a transverse view with the liver seen as hyperechoic to the other abdominal contents.

The kidneys mature on ultrasound imaging as the pregnancy progresses, initially being hypoechoic compared with other abdominal contents and having prominent anechoic pelves[7,15,19] (**Fig. 11**). The renal cortex is differentiated from the medulla as maturation continues and the pelves are less dilated.[15] The medulla and renal pelvis become increasingly prominent until term.[15] Intestines can be visualized from days 39 to 44 of pregnancy, but visualization of the different layers is not possible until days 48 to 54, and these layers become increasingly prominent until term[7,15,19,43] (**Fig. 12**). In the term fetus, the surface mucosa is hyperechoic; the mucosa, submucosa, and muscle are hypoechoic, and the serosa is hyperechoic.[43] Peristalsis becomes evident between 62 and 64 days of gestation. Panting may make visualization of peristalsis more difficult. Once all layers of the intestine are visible and peristalsis is prominent on serial examinations, fetal survival ex utero should be good.[43] However, the researchers noted that simply the presence of full gut development and peristalsis does not guarantee readiness for birth; in some bitches whelping naturally, 4 days elapsed from the point where peristalsis was prominent and intestinal development considered complete, and another 2 days after that transpired before fetal distress was evidenced by a decrease in the fetal heart rate (FHR).[43]

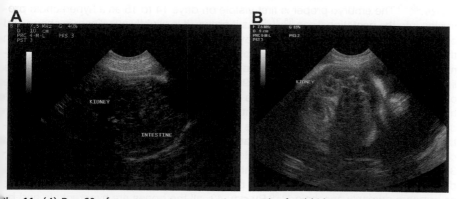

Fig. 11. (*A*) Day 60 of pregnancy transverse image. The fetal kidney is visible in the upper left quadrant of the image and is seen as an elliptically shaped hypoechoic structure with anechoic renal pelves present. (*B*) Day 63 of pregnancy transverse image. The renal cortex and medulla are clearly differentiated and the renal pelves are visible.

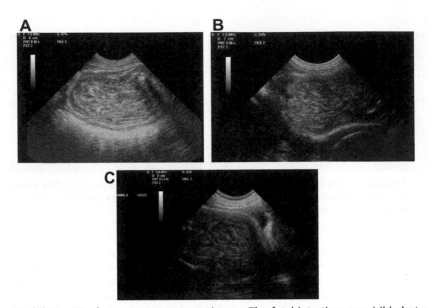

Fig. 12. (*A*) Day 58 of pregnancy transverse image. The fetal intestines are visible but minimal layering is evident. The fetal kidney is also visible in the dorsal central portion of the abdomen. (*B*) Day 62 of pregnancy. Intestinal layering is more evident. (*C*) Day 65 of pregnancy. Intestinal layering is complete and very prominent.

Placental thickness can be used to determine gestational age by measuring the outer layer of the placenta in a longitudinal/transverse view that is perpendicular to the placenta's plane.[44] It is accurate for all size bitches (R^2 = 0.8–0.87). The formula is presented in **Box 1**.[44]

Feline Use of a 7.5- to 12.5-mHz probe is ideal for assessing organ maturation.[35,36,38,45] The gestational sac is first visible on days 10 to 11 of gestation as an anechoic structure, measuring 6.9 mm that is spherical but slightly compressed on both ends.[4,34–37,46] The size of the embryonic vesicle in a single litter may vary slightly in size.[36,46] The embryo proper is first visible on days 14 to 15 as a hyperechoic protrusion into the gestational sac.[35,37,45] As it grows, it is slightly curvilinear in shape and eventually becomes slightly C-shaped by day 18, allowing definition of the head from the trunk.[35–38,45,46] The heartbeat is visible after days 16 to 17.[4,36,37,45,46] The lung parenchyma is hyperechoic to the liver parenchyma at this stage of pregnancy.[45] The limb buds are evident on days 18 to 19.[35,36,45] The neural tube and liver are visible on day 20.[36] The neural tube continues to develop a dorsal sagittal structure with a hyperechoic wall with anechoic content.[35] The bladder and stomach are visible on days 26 to 30 as anechoic structures in the caudal and mid abdomen, respectively.[4,35–37] The crown–rump length can be measured using the most rostral point on the cranium and the base of the tail as landmarks and is useful from days 17 to 30 of pregnancy.[35,36] On day 22, the embryo assumes a figure of 8 shape with a clear demarcation of the head from the body proper.[36] The head is full of fluid at this stage so appears primarily anechoic.[35,36] By day 42, all the bones are hyperechoic and by day 50 the marrow cavity can be seen in the long bones as a hypoechoic central zone.[35] Obvious fetal movements are evident from day 33 to term and swallowing can be identified from day 37 to term.[35,37] The eyes are visible from day 35 to term as 2 anechoic round structures at the lateral aspect of the skull, and the lens of the eye can be identified as a round hyperechoic structure within the globe after day 50.[35] The great vessels can be seen after day 42 as 2 anechoic tubular structures running the full length of the body.[35] The kidneys are visible after day 39 as elliptical structures sitting ventrolateral to the spine and are the same echogenicity as the liver.[4,35,37] After day 50, the renal cortex can be differentiated from the medulla and the architecture of the parenchyma becomes completely defined on day 60.[35,37] The gallbladder is evident on day 54.[35] The heart chambers can be identified after day 50.[35] The small and large intestines are distinguishable on day 40, when they become hypoechoic to the liver in echogenicity.[4,35,37] The mucosa becomes visible as a hypoechoic central area compared with the more hyperechoic muscularis layers after day 54 and this continues to develop until term.[35,37] The author has found that intestinal peristalsis is evident in the last 4 to 5 days of pregnancy.

The yolk sac fills the majority of the gestational sac from days 10 to 18.[35,37] On day 20, the yolk sac and the allantois occupy equal portions of the gestational sac and the yolk sac continues to regress through day 30, when it is barely visible ventral to the fetus.[35,37] The zonary placenta can be identified from day 25 to term.[35,37] The placenta is more hyperechoic at the internal and external surface and slightly hypoechoic centrally.[35,36] The amnion can be seen closely adherent to the fetus after day 45 and the amount of allantoic fluid visible around the fetus decreases significantly from day 45 to term.[35]

Doppler ultrasound imaging of maternal and fetal blood vessels

The relationship between gestational age, fetal size, fetal well-being, and characteristics uterine artery blood flow may help with assessing fetal readiness for birth in the bitch.[47] Color and spectral (Triplex) Doppler imaging may be used to assess blood flow through the uterine artery, umbilical artery (Uma) using the resistive index (RI) and the pulsatility index (PI) and the alterations in the diastolic notch and diastolic flow through these vessels.[47] Five- to 12-MHz range scanners can be used for these studies.[47] It is difficult to measure the same vessel in the same location in the same fetus in canine pregnancies owing the presence of multiple fetuses and repositioning of the uterine horns during the pregnancy, so unless a fetus or feti are identified as abnormal based on fetal development, it may be difficult to follow a single fetus and the subsequent changes in vessel blood flow.[48] The 3 most commonly measured parameters are the:

RI = peak systolic velocity – end-diastolic velocity/peak systolic velocity[47];

PI = peak systolic velocity – end-diastolic velocity/mean velocity[47]; and the

A:B ratio = systolic peak velocity/end-diastolic velocity.[48]

The RI, PI, and A:B ratio decrease as gestational age advances, indicating perfusion in the vessels likely associated with increased nutritional demands from the growing feti.[47,48] The diastolic notch in the Uma disappears at 16 ± 5 days before parturition and Uma diastolic flow appears at 21 ± 1 days before parturition.[47] The absence of Uma diastolic flow along with elevation in RI and PI indicate high blood flow resistance and may indicate intrauterine growth restriction, which can affect fetal well-being.[47] Abnormal placentation and trophoblast invasion may result in abnormal uterine artery and Uma waveforms and increased RI and PI.[47] Concurrent measurements of fetal body dimensions (BPD and BD) along with serial measurements of uterine artery and Uma blood flow may help to assess fetal well-being, may be used to help determine if fetal stress is present, and may impact decision making on the day to perform a cesarean delivery.[47]

Fetal sex determination

Canine Fetal sex determination is possible from day 55 to term.[49] The perineal area is scanned in the longitudinal plane. The best image is obtained with the fetus in a ventral decubitus position with the pelvic limbs flexed and the ileal wings parallel to each other[49] (**Fig. 13**). Female fetuses are identified by the presence of 2 hyperechoic lines that join anteriorly with a triangular shape and a central hyperechoic line (the vulva lips). Male fetuses are identified by a central hyperechoic line caudal to the inguinal area (representing the penis/prepuce).[49] The more fetuses present, the lower the accuracy of determining fetal gender on all fetuses because there is less space in the abdomen and so fetal movement is diminished, making it less likely to get the fetus in the plane needed to visualize the external genitalia.[49]

Feline Fetal sex determination can be performed starting between days 38 and 43 of pregnancy[37,38] (**Fig. 14**). Male fetuses can be identified by the bulging of the scrotum dorsally and the prepuce ventrally, both located under the tail base in a midsagittal view.[37,38] Female fetuses may be identified by the single triangular bulge of the vulvar lips distant to the tail base in the same midsagittal view.[37,38] Beyond 43 days of gestational age, the tail is more closely adherent to the perineum and the amount of fetal fluid near the perineum decreases, so it is more difficult to identify these structures.[37,38]

ASSESSMENT OF FETAL STRESS

Ultrasound imaging is also routinely used to assess the fetus for signs of stress. The FHR is an excellent indicator of fetal stress. Normally, FHRs are 2 to 3 times greater that of the maternal heart rate (MHR) or 220 to 240 bpm[15,50–52] (**Fig. 15**). It is generally accepted that a FHR of greater than 190 is normal and that decelerations, especially when prolonged (more than a few minutes) or sustained, indicate fetal stress.[53] The FHR increases from early pregnancy until 20 days before parturition, when it slowly

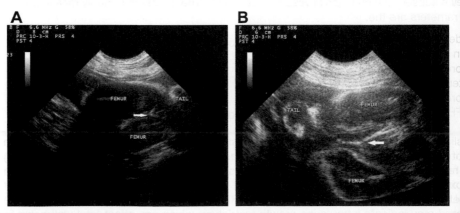

Fig. 13. Canine. (*A*) Female fetus in a ventral decubitus position. The vulva is seen in between the rear legs as a triangular structure with a central hyperechoic line (*arrow*). (*B*) Male fetus in a ventral decubitus position. The hyperechoic line running between the rear legs depicting the penis/prepuce is visible (*arrow*).

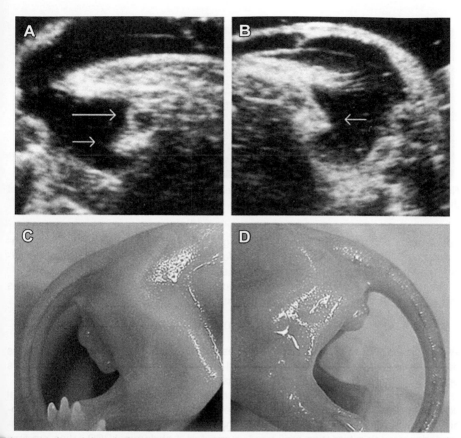

Fig. 14. Feline. (*A*) Male fetus mid-sagittal view – the scrotum is seen bulging dorsally (*short arrow*) and the penis bulging ventrally (*long arrow*) to the tail base. (*B*) Female fetus mid sagittal view – the single triangular bulge of the vulvar lips (*arrow*) distant to the tail base is evident. (*C, D*) gross lateral anatomical view of the external genitalia of 43 day fetuses. (*From* Zambelli D, Prati F. Ultrasonography for pregnancy diagnosis and evaluation in queens. Theriogenology 2006;66:140; with permission.)

decreases until term.[51,54] The FHR is initially under sympathetic control thus resulting in higher heart rate, and then when parasympathetic tone begins to develop in late pregnancy, the FHR starts to decline.[54] In both large and small breeds, the FHR tended to be higher than in medium sized breeds.[54] The MHR increases throughout pregnancy, likely owing to the need to supply the enlarging uterus with more blood.[54] FHR accelerations may be associated with fetal movement.[54]

In 1 study, heart rates between 180 and 220 bpm were considered indicative of slight fetal stress and rates consistently less than 180 bpm were considered indicative of severe fetal distress owing to hypoxia.[52] In other studies, FHRs consistently less than 140 to 180 bpm are considered indicative of sustained fetal stress owing to hypoxia.[15,50,51,53] Intermittent uterine contractions over a fetus can temporarily reduce the fetus' heart rate significantly, but it should return to a normal rate within 1 to 2 minutes and remain within the normal range if there is no fetal stress.[53] These decelerations may be due to pressure on the fetus while in the vaginal canal or from uterine contractions.[53] Signs of FHR deceleration may begin up to 48 to 72 hours before parturition.[53] In general, the FHR declines as parturition approaches.[53] A bitch with fetuses having

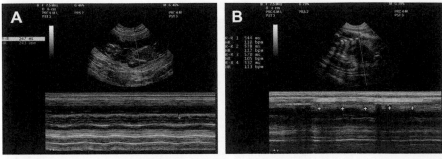

Fig. 15. (A) Normal fetal heart rate (FHR) taken using M-mode ultrasonography. (B) Fetal distress demonstrated by the low FHR.

deceleration and then acceleration, showing signs of delivery (panting, nesting, contractions) that then stops having FHR deceleration and has diminished signs of delivery, may be in uterine inertia and cesarean delivery should be considered.[53]

Evaluation of FHR and the FHR/MHR ratio may be helpful in evaluating fetal stress more than FHR alone.[54] Using the equation:

$$Z = 1.8284 - 0.0137x + 0.00014x + 0.05071y - 0.00099y^2$$

Where z is the FHR:MHR ratio, x is the pregestational dam weight in kilograms, and y is days before parturition. Both the FHR and FHR:MHR increase until 35 to 20 days before parturition and then begin to decrease.[54]

Fetal stress can also be assessed by examining the fetal fluids and fetoplacental units. Increases in the echogenicity of the fetal fluids may indicate passage of meconium or hemorrhage into the fetal fluids owing to premature placental separation.[52] Intrauterine growth retardation may be documented if abdominal:BPD ratios are less than 2 from day 48 of pregnancy until birth.[52] Puppies with low abdominal:BPD ratios tend to weigh less than 20% of the average birth weight for the breed and are at risk for early neonatal loss.[52]

An increase or decrease in the volume of fluid surrounding a fetus may indicate rupture of 1 or both fetal membranes, abnormalities of placental function, or

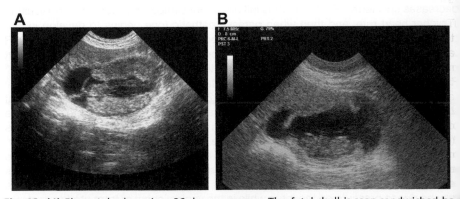

Fig. 16. (A) Placental edema in a 36-day pregnancy. The fetal skull is seen sandwiched between the 2 sides of the placenta. (B) Normal placental thickness in the same age pregnancy for comparison. The placenta is lying between the 2 sides of the placenta.

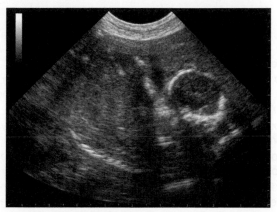

Fig. 17. Fetal death is evident by the lack of definition of the internal organs and abnormal posture of the fetus. The rib cage and skull are still identifiable.

abnormalities of fetal swallowing and waste fluid disposition. It is important to remember that, as the gestation progresses, the amount of fluid surrounding the fetus decreases as the fetus itself enlarges.

Detachment of the placenta may be partial or complete, and fetuses generally do not survive for long after the placenta begins to detach. Edema or thickening of the placenta may indicate abnormalities or alterations in blood flow, a diminished ability of the placenta to drain fetal waste fluids properly, or placentitis (**Fig. 16**). The author's experience is that the normal canine placenta does not exceed 1.2 cm at its centermost point at any stage of pregnancy, regardless of breed.

Fetal death in both the canine and feline species is documented by a lack of heartbeat when it is expected to be present or when littermates are clearly viable.[46] The morphology of the fetal organs becomes less distinct within 12 hours of fetal death and is indiscernible within 24 hours.[46] Fetal mass decreases and condenses into a ball-like structure of uniform density over time.[46] Fetal spine, ribs, and skull can be identified for the longest time in mummified fetuses[46] (**Fig. 17**).

SUMMARY

There is no substitute for accurate ovulation timing at the onset of the estrous cycle to determine gestational age. Determination of the time of the LH surge (81% accuracy at ±1 day) or day of ovulation remain the most accurate methods to determine fetal readiness for birth.[4–6] Although we do have the means to assess gestational age and fetal viability beyond ovulation timing, none of the methods currently available are completely accurate for determining fetal readiness for birth or the bitch's actual due date. If the day of the LH surge is not known, the next most accurate means of predicting parturition date is measurement of extrafetal structures (ICC) by ultrasound imaging before day 37 of pregnancy.[4,26] Additional measurement of fetal structures (BPD, BD, and DPTV) and the assessment of organ development by ultrasound imaging can help to increase the accuracy of due date estimation by increasing the available database of information.[4] Combining the use of fetal biometry with ovulation timing using hormonal analysis, cytology, speculum examination, and behavioral assessment will provide the most accurate assessment gestational age.[6]

REFERENCES

1. Rendano VT, Lein DH, Concannon PW. Radiographic evaluation of prenatal development in the Beagle: correlation with time of breeding, LH release, and parturition. Vet Radiol 1984;132–41.
2. Johnston SD, Kustritz MVR, Olson PS. Canine pregnancy. In: Johnston SD, Kustritz MVR, Olson PS, editors. Canine and feline theriogenology. Philadelphia: Saunders; 2001. p. 66–104.
3. Shille VM, Gontarek J. The use of ultrasonography for pregnancy diagnosis in the bitch. J Am Vet Med Assoc 1985;187:1021–5.
4. Michel E, Sporri M, Ohlerth S, et al. Prediction of parturition date in the bitch and queen. Reprod Domest Anim 2011;46:926–32.
5. Socha P, Rudowska M, Janowski T. Effectiveness of determining the parturition date in bitches using the ultrasonographic fetometry as compared to hormonal and cytological methods. Pol J Vet Sci 2012;15(3):447–53.
6. Kim Y, Travis AJ, Meyers-Wallen VN. Parturition prediction and timing of canine pregnancy. Theriogenology 2007;68:1177–82.
7. PW C. Canine pregnancy: predicting parturition and timing events of gestation. International Veterinary Information Service.
8. Rendano VT. Radiographic evaluation of fetal development in the bitch and fetal death in the bitch and queen. Current Veterinary Therapy. vol. VIII. Philadelphia: WB Saunders; 1983. p. 947–52.
9. Toal RL, Walker MA, Henry GA. A comparison of real-time ultrasound, palpation and radiography in pregnancy detection and litter size determination in the bitch. Vet Radiol 1986;27:102–8.
10. Boyd JS. The radiographic identification of the various stages of pregnancy in the domestic cat. J Small Anim Pract 1971;12:501–6.
11. Tiedemann K, Henschel E. Early radiographic diagnosis of pregnancy in the cat. J Sm An Pr 1973;14:567–72.
12. Haney DR, Levy JK, Newell SM, et al. Use of fetal skeletal mineralization for prediction of parturition date in cats. J Am Vet Med Assoc 2003;223(11):4–6.
13. Root CR, Spaulding KA. Diagnostic imaging in companion animal theriogenology. Semin Vet Med Surg (Small Anim) 1994;9(1):7–27.
14. Kim B, Son C. Time of initial detection of fetal and extra-fetal structures by ultrasonographic examination in Miniature Schnauzer bitches. J Vet 2007;8(3):289–93.
15. Nyland TJ, Mattoon JS. Ovaries and uterus. Small Anim Diagn Ultrasound. Philadelphia: WB Saunders; 2002. p. 231–49.
16. England GCW, Allen WE. Studies on canine pregnancy using B-mode ultrasound: diagnosis of early pregnancy and the number of conceptuses. J Small Anim Pract 1990;31:321–3.
17. Yeager AE, Concannon PW. Association between the preovulatory luteinizing hormone surge and the early ultrasonographic detection of pregnancy and fetal heartbeats in Beagle dogs. Theriogenology 1990;34(4):656–65.
18. England GCW, Allen WE, Porter DJ. Studies on canine pregnancy using B-mode ultrasound: development of the conceptus and determination of gestational age. J Sm An Pr 1990;31:324–9.
19. Yeager AE, Mohammed HO, Meyers-Wallen V, et al. Ultrasonographic appearance of the uterus, placenta, fetus, and fetal membranes throughout accurately timed pregnancy in Beagles. Am J Vet Res 1992;53:342–51.

20. Kutzler MA, Yeager AE, Mohammen HO, et al. Accuracy of canine parturition date prediction using fetal measurements obtained by ultrasonography. Theriogenology 2003;60:1309–17.

21. Beccaglia M, Luvoni GC. Comparison of the accuracy of two ultrasonographic measurements in predicting the parturition the parturition date in the bitch. J Sm An Pr 2006;47:670–3.

22. Luvoni GC, Beccaglia M. The prediction of parturition date in canine pregnancy. Reprod Domest Anim 2006;41:27–32.

23. Cartee RE, Rowles T. Preliminary study of the ultrasonographic diagnosis of pregnancy and fetal development in the dog. Am J Vet Res 1984;45:1259–65.

24. Luvoni GC, Grioni A. Determination of gestational age in medium and small size bitches using ultrasonographic fetal membranes. J Sm An Pr 2000;41:292–4.

25. Son C, Jeong K, Kim J, et al. Establishment of the prediction table of parturition day with ultrasonography in small pet dogs. J Vet Med Sci 2001;63:715–21.

26. Levstein-Volanski R. Evaluation of tests commonly used to predict parturition date in the bitch. Guelph (ON): University of Guelph; 2008.

27. Groppetti D, Vegetti F, Bronzo V, et al. Breed-specific fetal biometry and factors affecting the prediction of whelping date in the German shepherd dog. Anim Reprod Sci 2015;152:117–22.

28. Beccaglia M, Faustini M, Luvoni GC. Ultrasonographic study of deep portion of diencephalo-telencephalic vesicle for the determination of gestational age of the canine foetus. Reprod Dom Anim 2008;43:367–70.

29. Beccaglia M, Luvoni GC. Ultrasonographic study during pregnancy of the growth of an encephalic portion in the canine foetus. Vet Res Commun 2004;28:161–4.

30. Okkens AC, Teunissen JM, Van Osch W, et al. Influence of litter size and breed on the duration of gestation in dogs. J Reprod Fertil Suppl 2001;57:193–7.

31. Okkens AC, Hekerman TWM, DeVogel JW, et al. Influence of litter size and breed on variation in length of gestation in the dog. Vet Q 1993;15:160–1.

32. Bobic Gavrilovic B, Andersson K, Linde Forsberg C. Reproductive patterns in the domestic dog - a retrospective study of the Drever breed. Theriogenology 2008; 70(5):783–94.

33. Eilts BE, Davidson AP, Thompson RA, et al. Factors influencing gestation length in the bitch. Theriogenology 2005;64:242–51.

34. Davidson AP, Acvim D, Baker TW. Reproductive ultrasound of the bitch and queen. Top Companion Anim Med 2009;24(2):55–63.

35. Zambelli D, Caneppele B, Bassi S, et al. Ultrasound aspects of fetal and extrafetal structures in pregnant cats. J Feline Med Surg 2002;4(2):95–106.

36. Topie E, Bencharif D, Briand L, et al. Early pregnancy diagnosis and monitoring in the queen using ultrasonography with a 12.5 MHz probe. J Feline Med Surg 2015;17(2):87–93.

37. Zambelli D, Prati F. Ultrasonography for pregnancy diagnosis and evaluation in queens. Theriogenology 2006;66:135–44.

38. Zambelli D, Castagnetti C, Belluzzi S, et al. Correlation between fetal age and ultrasonographic measurements during the second half of pregnancy in domestic cats (Felis catus). Theriogenology 2004;62:1430–7.

39. Beck KA, Baldwin CJ, Bosu WT. Ultrasound prediction of parturition in queens. Vet Radiol 1990;31(1):32–5.

40. Socha P, Janowski T. Predicting the parturition date in bitches of different body weight by ultrasonographic measurements of inner chorionic cavity diameter and biparietal diameter. Reprod Domest Anim 2014;49:292–6.

41. Lenard ZM, Hopper BJ, Lester NV, et al. Accuracy of prediction of canine litter size and gestational age with ultrasound. Aust Vet J 2007;85(6):222–5.
42. Beccaglia M, Anastasi P, Grimaldi E, et al. Accuracy of the prediction of parturition date through ultrasonographic measurement of fetal parameters in the queen. Vet Res Commun 2008;32(Suppl 1):S99–101.
43. Gil EMU, Garcia DAA, Froes TR. In utero development of the fetal intestine: sonographic evaluation and correlation with gestational age and fetal maturity in dogs. Theriogenology 2015;84(5):681–6.
44. Maldonado AL, Araujo Júnior E, Mendonça DS, et al. Ultrasound determination of gestational age using placental thickness in female dogs: an experimental study. Vet Med Int 2012;2012:850867.
45. Zambelli D, Castagnetti C, Belluzzi S, et al. Correlation between the age of the conceptus and various ultrasonographic measurements during the first 30 days of pregnancy in domestic cats (Felis catus). Theriogenology 2004;57: 1981–7.
46. Davidson AP, Nyland TG, Tsutsui T. Pregnancy diagnosis with ultrasound in the domestic cat. Vet Radiol 1986;27(4):109–14.
47. Miranda SA, Domingues SFS. Conceptus ecobiometry and triplex Doppler ultrasonography of uterine and umbilical arteries for assessment of fetal viability in dogs. Theriogenology 2010;74(4):608–17.
48. Nautrup P. Doppler ultrasonography of canine maternal and fetal arteries during normal gestation. J Reprod Fertil 1998;112:301–14.
49. Gil EMU, Garcia DAA, Giannico AT, et al. Use of B-mode ultrasonography for fetal sex determination in dogs. Theriogenology 2015;84(6):875–9.
50. Davidson A. Uterine monitoring during pregnancy. Annual Proc Soc Theriogenology. 1998. p. 123–5.
51. Verstegen JP, Silva LD, Onclin K, et al. Echocardiographic study of heart rate in dog and cat fetuses in utero. J Reprod Fertil Suppl 1993;47:175–80.
52. Zone MA, Wanke MM. Diagnosis of canine fetal health by ultrasonography. J Reprod Fert 2001;57:215–9.
53. Gil EMU, Garcia DAA, Giannico AT, et al. Canine fetal heart rate: do accelerations or decelerations predict the parturition day in bitches? Theriogenology 2014; 82(7):933–41.
54. Alonge S, Mauri M, Faustini M, et al. Feto-maternal heart rate ratio in pregnant bitches: effect of gestational age and maternal size. Reprod Domest Anim 2016;51(5):688–92.

Pyometra in Small Animals

Ragnvi Hagman, DVM, PhD

KEYWORDS

- Endometritis • Cystic endometrial hyperplasia • *Escherichia coli* • Endotoxemia
- Aglepristone • Prostaglandin • Cabergoline • Bromocriptine

KEY POINTS

- Pyometra foremost affects middle-aged to older intact bitches and queens, usually within 4 months after estrus.
- Hormonal and bacterial factors are involved in the pathogenesis, and progesterone plays a key role.
- Cystic endometrial hyperplasia (CEH) is a predisposing factor, but pyometra and CEH can develop independently.
- Pyometra induces endotoxemia and sepsis, and early diagnosis and treatment increase the chances of survival.
- Diagnosis is based on clinical signs and findings on physical examination, hematology and biochemistry laboratory tests, and diagnostic imaging identifying intrauterine fluid.
- Surgical ovariohysterectomy is the safest and most effective treatment, as the source of infection is removed and recurrence prevented. Medical treatment can be an alternative in young and otherwise healthy breeding animals with open cervix and without other uterine or ovarian pathologies.

 Video content accompanies this article at http://www.vetsmall.theclinics.com.

INTRODUCTION

Pyometra, literally meaning "pus-filled uterus," is a common illness in adult intact female dogs and cats and a less frequent diagnosis in other small animal species.[1,2] The disease is characterized by an acute or chronic suppurative bacterial infection of the uterus post estrum with accumulation of inflammatory exudate in the uterine lumen and a variety of clinical and pathologic manifestations, locally and systemically.[3] The disease develops during the luteal phase, and progesterone plays a key role for the establishment of infection with ascending opportunistic bacteria. The pathogen most often isolated from pyometra uteri is *Escherichia coli*.[4–6] A wide range of clinical signs are associated with the disease, which can be life-threatening in severe cases. It is important to seek

The author has nothing to disclose.
Department of Clinical Sciences, Swedish University of Agricultural Sciences, PO Box 7054, Uppsala SE-75007, Sweden
E-mail address: Ragnvi.Hagman@slu.se

Vet Clin Small Anim 48 (2018) 639–661
https://doi.org/10.1016/j.cvsm.2018.03.001
0195-5616/18/© 2018 Elsevier Inc. All rights reserved.

immediate veterinary care when pyometra is suspected because a patient's status may deteriorate rapidly and early intervention increases chances of survival. The diagnosis is generally straightforward but can be challenging when there is no vaginal discharge and obscure clinical signs. Surgical ovariohysterectomy (OHE) is the safest and most efficient treatment, but purely medical alternatives may be an option in some cases.

EPIDEMIOLOGY AND RISK FACTORS

Pyometra is an important disease, particularly in countries where elective neutering of healthy dogs and cats is not generally performed.[1,2,7] In Sweden, in average 20% of all bitches are diagnosed before 10 years of age and more than 50% in certain high-risk breeds. The disease generally affects middle-aged to older bitches, with a mean age at diagnosis of 7 years, and has been reported in dogs from 4 months to 18 years of age. The overall incidence rate is 199 per 10,000 dog-years at risk.[7] In cats, pyometra is not as common, which is believed to depend on less progesterone dominance due to seasonality and induced ovulation. In queens, 2.2% are diagnosed with the disease before 13 years of age, with an incidence rate of 17 cats per 10,000 cat-years at risk.[2] The mean age at diagnosis is 5.6 years, with an age range of 10 months to 20 years, and the incidence increases with age and markedly over 7 years of age.[2,8–10] A higher incidence in some dog and cat breeds indicates that they may have a genetic predisposition.[1,2,7,9] Exogenous treatment with steroid hormones, such as progestogens, or estrogen compounds that increase the response to progesterone, are associated with increased risk of the disease.[11,12] Pregnancy is slightly protective in dogs, an effect that is also influenced by breed.[13] Cystic endometrial hyperplasia (CEH) is believed to increase the uterine susceptibility for infection.[14,15] In cats, little is known about risk factors and protective factors but previous hormone therapy (ie, exogenous progesterone) is associated with an increased risk.[16]

ETIOLOGY AND PATHOGENESIS

The complex pathogenesis of pyometra is not yet completely understood but involves both hormonal and bacterial factors. Although most studies have been done in dogs, the development is believed similar in cats. The uterine environment during the luteal phase is suitable for pregnancy but also for microbial growth. Progesterone stimulates growth and proliferation of endometrial glands, increased secretion, cervical closure, and suppression of myometrial contractions.[14] The local leukocyte response and uterine resistance to bacterial infection also become decreased.[17–19] Circulating concentrations of estrogen and progesterone are not usually abnormally elevated in pyometra, and increased numbers and sensitivity of hormone receptors are believed to initiate an amplified response.[20,21] Simultaneous corpora lutea and follicular cysts are more often found in bitches with pyometra, supporting a synergistic hormonal effect.[22]

Progesterone-mediated pathologic proliferation and growth of endometrial glands and formation of cysts (ie, cystic endometrial hyperplasia [CEH]) is believed to predispose for pyometra but the 2 disorders can develop independently (**Fig. 1**).[23] Sterile fluid may accumulate in the uterine lumen, with or without CEH, which is defined as hydrometra or mucometra or, more rarely, hemometra, depending on the type of fluid and its mucin content. Clinical signs are generally subclinical or mild when there is no bacterial infection of the uterus.[3,24,25]

E coli is the predominant pathogen isolated from pyometra uteri, but other species may also occur (**Table 1**).[4,26–29] More than 1 bacterial species can be involved, and cultures are sometimes negative.[28,29] Emphysematous pyometra is caused by gas-producing bacteria.[30] A healthy uterus eliminates bacteria that have entered during

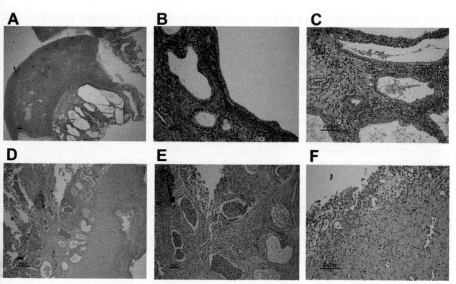

Fig. 1. Images of histologic examination findings in uterine tissues examples from dogs with CEH/pyometra. (A) CEH; (B) larger magnification of (A); (C) CEH–endometritis; (D) pyometra; (E) larger magnification of (D); (F) pyometra–atrophic endometrium.

cervical opening, but the clearance capacity varies depending on the estrus cycle stage. Experimental *E coli* infection during the luteal phase more often leads to CEH/pyometra compared with in other estrus cycle stages.[31] The infection is most likely ascending because the same strains are present in the gastrointestinal tract, but hematogenic spread could possibly also occur.[6,32,33] *E coli* are natural inhabitants

Table 1
Bacterial species isolated from the uterus in bitches and queens with pyometra

Organism	Proportion in Bitches (%)	Proportion in Queens (%)
Escherichia coli	65–90	71
Staphylococcus spp	2–15	8
Streptococcus spp	4–23	19
Pseudomonas spp	1–8	—
Proteus spp	1–4	—
Enterobacter spp	1–3	—
Nocardia spp	1	0
Pasteurella spp	1–2	<1
Klebsiella spp	2–14	<1
Mixed culture	4–16	—
No growth	10–26	20
Mycoplasma spp, *Enterococcus* spp, *Clostridium perfringens*, *Corynebacterium* spp, *Citrobacter* spp, *Moraxella* spp, *Edwardsiella* spp, and others	<1	<1

Data from Refs.[4,5,8–10,28,30,47,52–54,93]

of the vaginal flora[34] and have an increased ability to adhere to specific receptors in a progesterone-stimulated endometrium.[5] Certain serotypes of E coli are more common and often exhibit the same virulence traits as isolates from urinary tract infections.[35–37] The same bacterial clone can frequently be isolated from the uterus and the urinary bladder in pyometra.[5,6,33]

Bacteria and bacterial products are potent inducers of local and systemic inflammation. Endotoxin, lipopolysaccharide components of Gram-negative bacteria, such as E coli, are released into the circulation during bacterial disintegration and induces fever, lethargy, tachycardia, and tachypnea.[38] Higher endotoxin concentrations may cause fatal shock, disseminated intravascular coagulation, and generalized organ failure.[39,40] Pyometra has been associated with endotoxemia[40,41] and bacteremia,[42] and disseminated infection may affect various organs.[43,44] Approximately 60% of bitches and 86% of queens with pyometra suffer from sepsis (ie, life-threatening organ dysfunction caused by a dysregulated host response to an infectious process).[45,46] The illness is considered a medical emergency and it is important to seek immediate veterinary care because a patient's health status may deteriorate rapidly.

CLINICAL PRESENTATION

Typically, middle-aged to older animals are presented up to 2 months to 4 months after estrus with a history of various signs associated with the genital tract and systemic illness (**Table 2**). A continuous or intermittent mucopurulent to hemorrhagic vaginal discharge is often present but can be absent if the cervix is closed.[47] The systemic illness is often more severe if the cervix is closed, and the uterus may become severely

Table 2	
History data and clinical signs in bitches with pyometra	
Case History and Clinical Signs	**In Percentage (%)**
Vaginal discharge[a]	57–88
Lethargy/depression[a]	63–100
Inappetence/anorexia[a]	42–87
Polydipsia[a]	28–89
Polyuria[a]	34–73
Vomiting	13–38
Diarrhea	0–27
Abnormal mucous membranes	16–76
Dehydration	15–94
Palpable enlarged uterus	19–40
Pain on abdominal palpation	23–80
Lameness	16
Distended abdomen	5
Fever	32–50
Hypothermia	3–10
Tachycardia	23–28
Tachypnea	32–40
Systemic inflammatory response syndrome	57–61

[a] Usually in greater than 50% of the bitches.
Data from Refs.[24,25,48,49,53,93,107]

distended.[48] Classic systemic signs are anorexia, depression/lethargy, polydipsia, polyuria, tachycardia, tachypnea, weak pulse quality, and abnormal visible mucous membranes. Fever, dehydration, vomiting, abdominal pain on palpation, anorexia, gait abnormalities, and diarrhea are present in approximately 15% to 30% of bitches with the disease.[47,49] The most common clinical signs in queens are vaginal discharge, lethargy, and gastrointestinal disturbances, such as anorexia, vomiting, and diarrhea (**Fig. 2**).[8,10] Vaginal discharge may absent or concealed by fastidious cleaning habits in up to 40% of affected queens.[9] Weight loss, dehydration, polydipsia/polyuria, tachycardia, tachypnea, abdominal pain on palpation, abnormal mucous membranes (pale, hyperemic, or toxic), and unkept appearance are other findings associated with feline pyometra.

DIAGNOSIS

The disease is easy to recognize in classic cases but can be more challenging when there is no vaginal discharge (ie, closed cervix), and the history and clinical picture are obscure. Pyometra should be a differential diagnosis in bitches and queens admitted with signs of illness after estrus, but the disease can occur at any time during the estrus cycle. The preliminary diagnosis is based on history and findings on physical and gynecologic examinations, hematology and blood biochemistry analyses, and ultrasonography and/or radiography of the abdomen. Bacteriologic culturing of the vaginal discharge is not helpful for the diagnosis because the same microbes are present in the vagina in healthy animals.[50] Careful abdominal palpation, to avoid rupture of a fragile uterus, may identify an enlarged uterus. Diagnostic imaging is valuable for determining the uterine size and to rule out other causes of uterine enlargement (**Fig. 3**A–G). Radiography frequently identifies a large tubular structure in the caudoventral abdomen. Ultrasonography has the advantage of detecting intrauterine fluid, even when the uterine diameter is within the normal range, and of revealing additional pathologic changes of the uterine tissue and ovaries, such as ovarian cysts or CEH, which may affect the outcome of medical treatment negatively (**Fig. 4**, Video 1). More advanced diagnostic imaging techniques are seldom necessary. Differential diagnoses include mucometra, hydrometra, and hemometra that may have similar clinical presentation and ultrasonography findings.[51] Vaginal cytology usually shows severe leukocyte degeneration, neutrophils and some macrophages, plasmacytes, and lymphocytes but bacterial phagocytosis is not always visible.[52] Vaginoscopy is

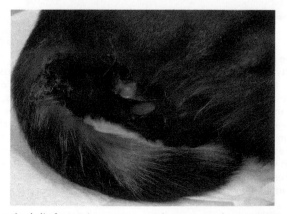

Fig. 2. Purulent vaginal discharge in a queen with open cervix pyometra.

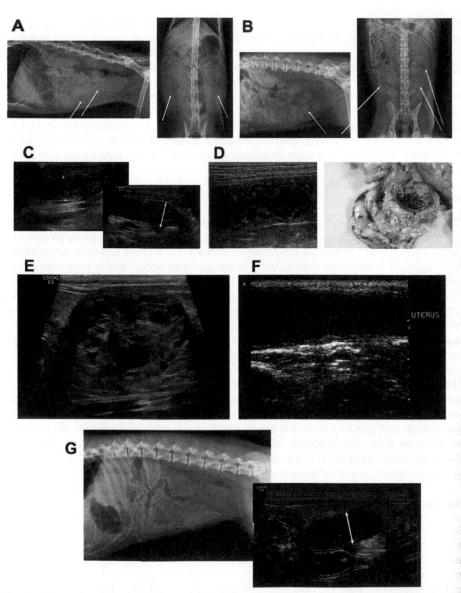

Fig. 3. (A) Uterine enlargement in a cat; diagnosis: pyometra. Tubular structures of soft tissue/fluid opacity (arrows). (B) Uterine enlargement in a dog; diagnosis: CEH. Tubular structures of soft tissue/fluid opacity (arrows). (C) Ultrasound images of CEH in a dog. Thickening of the uterine wall with multiple anechoic cystic structures, no intraluminal fluid. Uterine diameter was 2 cm. Cervix located between double-headed arrow. (D) CEH and pyometra—thickening of the uterine wall with multiple anechoic cystic structures; the intraluminal fluid was purulent. Both images in (D) are of the same uterus. The uterine diameter was 2 cm. (E) CEH in a rabbit. (F) Atrophic wall pyometra: enlarged uterus with a thin wall and echogenic intraluminal fluid. (G) Uterus or small intestines of the same diameter (radiograph to the left). Uterus between white double-headed arrows, CEH. Small intestine with typical layered appearance between black double-headed arrows.

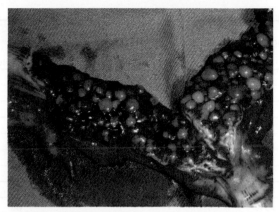

Fig. 4. Canine uterus with CEH and purulent appearance of the fluid in some cysts.

helpful for determining the origin of a vaginal discharge and to exclude other pathologies but is usually not performed in the emergent clinical setting. The diagnosis pyometra is verified by postoperative macroscopic and histologic examination of the uterus and ovaries, and microbiological examination of the uterine content.

CLINICOPATHOLOGIC TESTING—LABORATORY PARAMETERS

Hematology and biochemistry parameter abnormalities are generally investigated,[49,53] with additional tests performed depending on the health status (**Table 3**). Leukocytosis, with neutrophilia and left shift, and monocytosis are characteristic findings in pyometra together with normocytic, normochromic regenerative anemia. Renal dysfunction is common, to which endotoxemia, glomerular dysfunction, renal tubular damage and decreased response to antidiuretic hormone contribute.[54,55] Concomitant cystitis and proteinuria usually resolve after treatment of the pyometra, but severe proteinuria that remains may predispose for renal failure.[54] Circulating inflammatory mediators and acute phase proteins are generally increased.[56] A hypercoagulable state is usually present.[57]

TREATMENT ALTERNATIVES

Surgical treatment, OHE, is safest and most effective because the source of infection and bacterial products are removed and recurrence prevented.[53] Laparoscopically assisted techniques have been developed but are not commonly used and only in mild cases.[58] Medical management (solely pharmacologic) may be possible in young and otherwise healthy breeding animals or in a patient for which anesthesia and surgery is hazardous. In patients with serious illness or when complications, such as peritonitis or organ dysfunctions, are present or the cervix is closed, medical treatment is not recommended and surgery is the treatment of choice. Candidates for medical treatment need to be carefully selected for best prognosis for recovery and subsequent fertility.[59] Microbiological culturing and sensitivity testing are prerequisites for optimal selection of antimicrobial therapy, for which samples are obtained from the cranial vagina or postoperatively from the uterus.

SURGICAL TREATMENT

Prior to surgery, the patient is stabilized with adequate intravenous fluid therapy to correct hypotension, hypoperfusion, shock, dehydration, acid-base balance and

Table 3
Laboratory findings in bitches with pyometra

Abnormality	In No. of Bitches (%)
Leukopenia	4
Leukocytosis	61
Neutropenia	4
Neutrophilia	55
Monocytopenia	3
Monocytosis	60
Anemia	55
Band neutrophils	40
Band neutrophils >3%	83
Trombocytopenia	37
Toxic changes present	9
Increased ALAT	22
Hypoalbuminemia	33
Decreased ALP	49
Increased ALP	37
Increased AST	64
Cholesterolemia	74
Hypernatremia	29
Hypochloremia	2
Hypochloremia	33
Azotemia	5
BUN decreased	10
BUN increased	5
Bile acids increased	21
Hypoglycemia	6
Hyperglycemia	4
Hypokalemia	4
Hypercalcemia	6
Hypokalemia	25
Hyperlactatemia	10
Urine enzymes increased	42
Bacteruria	25

Abbreviations: ALAT, alanine aminotransferase; ALP, alkaline phosphatase; AST, aspartate transaminase; BUN, blood urea nitrogen.
Data from Refs.[24,49,54]

electrolyte abnormalities, coagulation disturbances, and organ dysfunctions.[60] Monitoring and intervention in critically ill patients following parameters according to the "rule of 20" is recommended.[61] In moderately severely and severely ill patients, or if sepsis or serious complications are identified, intravenous broad-spectrum bactericidal antimicrobials are administered to prevent systemic effects of bacteremia and sepsis.[62] The initial choice of antimicrobial drug should be effective against the most common pathogen E coli and adjusted after culture and sensitivity results to a narrow-spectrum alternative.[62] The drug should not be nephrotoxic, and the dose route, and frequency of administration adjusted to ascertain optimal effect. In 1 study, 90% of *E coli* pyometra isolates were sensitive to ampicillin.[4] The frequency of antimicrobial resistance, however, may differ by geographic location, which needs to be considered, and national regulations concerning restriction of antimicrobial usage in pets should be followed.[27,32] In life-threatening peritonitis, severe sepsis, or septic shock, a combination of antimicrobials is usually recommended for covering a wider range of pathogens.[62] If the health status is close to normal or only mildly depressed and without complications or concurrent diseases, OHE is curative for pyometra per se, and antimicrobials not included in the perioperative supportive treatment.

Removal of the infection is key, and surgery should not be unnecessarily delayed due to the risk of endotoxemia and sepsis when the uterus remains in situ. Anesthesia and perioperative management are focused on maintaining hemodynamic function, gastrointestinal function and protection, pain management, cellular oxygenation, nutrition, and nursing care.[63] Certain drugs may alleviate the inflammatory response.[64] A standard OHE is performed with some modifications.[16,65] The uterus may be large, friable, and prone to rupture, and it is important to handle the tissues carefully (**Figs. 5–9**). The abdominal cavity should be protected from accidental leakage of pus via uterine laceration or the fallopian tubes/ovarian bursa opening by packing off the uterus with moistened laparotomy swabs (see **Fig. 9**). Vessels in the broad ligament are usually ligated. Purulent material is completely removed from the remaining cervical tissue stump, which is not oversewn. Urine for bacterial culturing can be obtained by cystocentesis when the bladder is exposed. The abdomen is routinely closed but if contaminated with pus this should be removed and the abdomen rinsed with several liters of warmed physiologic saline solution and a closed suction (or open) drainage considered.[63,65] Samples for bacterial culturing are acquired before abdominal closure if needed. For verification of the diagnosis, macroscopic and histopathologic examination of the uterus and ovaries is performed.

Intensive postoperative monitoring is essential, and in uncomplicated cases 1 day to 2 days of postoperative hospitalization is usually sufficient. The need for continued supportive care and antimicrobial therapy is evaluated several times daily on a case-by-case basis.[49] Antimicrobial therapy is discontinued as soon as possible. The overall health status and most laboratory abnormalities improve rapidly after surgery and often normalize within 2 weeks.[56,66]

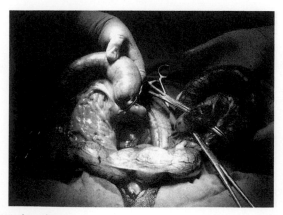

Fig. 5. Canine pyometra uterus.

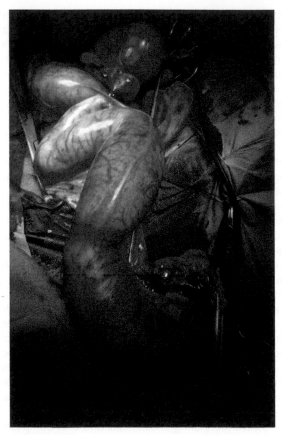

Fig. 6. Canine pyometra uterus.

Considering the seriousness of pyometra, the prognosis for survival is good and mortality rates relatively low, 3% to 20%.[1,9,49,67] If more severe systemic illness or complications, such as uterine rupture, peritonitis, or septic shock, develop, however, mortality rates can be considerably higher.[9,62,68] In queens with pyometra and uterine

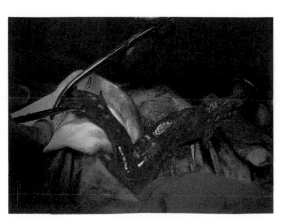

Fig. 7. Feline pyometra uterus.

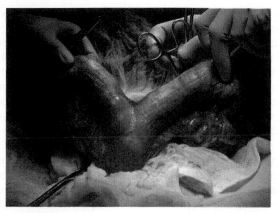

Fig. 8. Canine pyometra uterus.

rupture, a mortality rate of 57% has been reported.[8] Complications develop in approximately 20% of pyometra patients, the most common peritonitis, in 12%.[9,43,44,49,69] Other reported complications include uveitis, urinary tract infection, intracranial thromboemboli, bacterial osteomyelitis, pericarditis, myocarditis, septic arthritis, incisional swelling, dehiscence, urethral trauma, recurrent estrus, uterine stump pyometra, fistulous tracts, and urinary incontinence.[43,44,54]

MEDICAL (NONSURGICAL) TREATMENT

For purely medical management, careful patient selection is central to ensure the best possible outcome (ie, resolution of clinical illness and maintained fertility). Suitable candidates are young and otherwise healthy breeding bitches and queens with open cervix and that have no ovarian cysts. It is important that the patients are stable and not critically ill, because it may take up to 48 hours until treatment effect for some drugs used.[70] Contraindications include systemic illness, fever or hypothermia, intrauterine fetal remains, organ dysfunctions, or complications, such as peritonitis or sepsis. Adverse drug effects may occur, and endotoxemia and sepsis can quickly transform a clinically stable pyometra to an emergency. Hospitalization is, therefore,

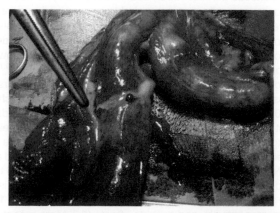

Fig. 9. Canine pyometra uterus with rupture and leakage of pus showing at the tip of the lamp.

recommended to allow close monitoring, supportive treatments, and rapid intervention. Clinical signs, reduction, and clearing of the vaginal discharge, the uterine size, and laboratory abnormalities gradually normalize in 1 week to 3 weeks.[71] OHE may be necessary without delay if complications arise or the general health status deteriorates and in refractory cases. Antimicrobials alone for treatment of pyometra may reduce the disease and prevent its progression but does not result in uterine healing.

The strategies of medical treatment are to minimize effects of progesterone by preventing its production and/or action, eliminate the uterine infection, promote relaxation of the cervix and expulsion of the intraluminal pus, and facilitate uterine healing. Commonly used drugs are natural prostaglandin $F_{2\alpha}$ ($PGF_{2\alpha}$) or its synthetic analog cloprostenol, dopamine agonists (cabergoline and bromocriptine), or progesterone-receptor blockers (aglepristone)[72] (**Tables 4** and **5**). The available protocols include systemic antimicrobial therapy, often recommended for 2 weeks or more.[73] The shortest effective duration of adjunctive antimicrobial therapy, however, has not been determined, and 5 days and 6 days were sufficient in 2 studies using aglepristone.[70,74] The antimicrobial drug and administration protocol should be based on bacterial culturing, sensitivity tests, and pharmacokinetics/pharmacodynamics for achieving optimal effect. Additional supportive treatment, including intravenous fluids and electrolyte supplementation, is provided depending on physical examinations and laboratory tests results.

$PGF_{2\alpha}$ is luteolytic and uterotonic and stimulates smooth musculature. Side effects, such as hypothermia, frequent defecation, diarrhea, salivation, vomiting, restlessness, shivering, and depression, are common and dose dependent and may last for approximately 1 hour after administration.[75] $PGF_{2\alpha}$ should be administrated far from feeding to reduce the risk of vomiting. Treatment with metoclopramide or walking the bitch for 15 minutes to 20 minutes after administration has been suggested to lessen nausea and vomiting.[72,76] Serious adverse effects of the drug ($PGF_{2\alpha}$), such as death, shock, and ventricular tachycardia, have been reported and the therapeutic window is narrow, which is why dosage calculations should be done meticulously. It is therefore very important to chose the lowest possible effective dose and hospitalize patients during treatment for monitoring and immediate intervention if severe side-effects develop. Brachycephalic breeds may be predisposed to bronchospasm, making $PGF_{2\alpha}$ contraindicated.[73,76] Owner consent, with information of potential risks, is necessary to obtain prior to extra-label drug usage. Several protocols are still considered experimental, because efficiency and optimal dosages have not yet been established. For natural $PGF_{2\alpha}$, ie, dinoprost tromethamine, subcutaneous administration of 0.1 mg/kg every 12 hours to 24 hours until resolution is the dose generally recommended in bitches and queens. Despite at the lower end of the recommended range and administered once daily, this dose is associated with many undesired side effects (the recommended range includes higher doses, following evaluation of the effect of a lower dose), which is why other lower dose alternatives and drug combinations are becoming more commonly used.[75,77] Other authors suggest starting by giving 10 µg/kg subcutaneously 5 times on the first day, gradually increasing the dose to 25 µg/kg 5 times on the second day, and reaching 50 µg/kg by day 3. Doses of 50 µg/kg were then given 3 times to 5 times daily from day 3 and onward over the treatment period, a regime resulting in side effects in 15% of treated bitches.[72] A dose of 100 µg/kg natural $PGF_{2\alpha}$ administered subcutaneously once daily for 7 days resulted in recovery in 7 bitches, but many side-effects were observed and lower doses are preferable.[78] Natural $PGF_{2\alpha}$, 20 µg/kg, was given intramuscularly 3 times daily on up to 8 consecutive days in 1 study, and 30 µg/kg was given subcutaneously twice daily for 8 days in another study, resulting in resolution of the illness in 70% of 10 bitches and in 100% of 7 bitches, respectively, and no side effects.[79,80] More recent low dose protocols, recommend subcutaneous administration of natural $PGF_{2\alpha}$ at a dose of 10-50µg/

Table 4
Examples of studies of medical treatment protocols for open cervix pyometra in dogs

Drug	N	Protocol and Dosage	Outcome and Side Effects	Reference
Aglepristone	24	Aglepristone 10 mg/kg SC q 24 h on day 2, 7 and 14	Recovery in 100%; recurrence after up to 54 months 12%; fertility in 12% of 17 bitches mated	Jurka et al,[84] 2010
Aglepristone	28	Aglepristone 10 mg/kg SC q 24 h on days 1, 2, 7, 15, and 23, 29 if not cured	Recovery in 75% (resolution of clinical signs); recurrence: 48% after up to 6 y; fertility in 69% of 13 mated bitches	Ros et al,[85] 2014
Aglepristone	52	Aglepristone 10 mg/kg SC q 24 h on days 1, 2, and 7	Recovery in 92%; recurrence: 10% after 3 months, 19% in 37 bitches followed up to 1 y; fertility in 83% (5/6 mated bitches)	Trasch et al,[83] 2003
Aglepristone	13	Aglepristone 10 mg/kg SC q 24 h on days 1, 2, 7, and 14	Recovery in 46%	Gurbulak et al,[82] 2005
Aglepristone	20	Aglepristone 10 mg/kg SC q 24 h on days 1, 2, and 8 and if not cured on day 15	Recovery in 60%	Fieni,[70] 2006
Aglepristone + cloprostenol	32	Aglepristone 10 mg/kg SC q 24 h on days 1, 2, and 8 and if not cured on days 14 and 28 + cloprostenol: 1 µg/kg SC q 24 h on days 3–7	Recovery in 84%; no side effect of cloprostenol in 45% of the bitches; in 56% some side effects were noted: loss of appetite, lethargy, vomiting, nausea; 19% recurrence; in closed cervix pyometra cases: recovery in 76.5%, in open cervix pyometra recovery in 74.3%; 1 euthanasia due to declining health, 1 death; Follow-up time: 90 d and up to 2 y in 23 bitches; fertility in 80% (4/5 mated bitches)	Fieni,[70] 2006

(continued on next page)

Table 4
(continued)

Drug	N	Protocol and Dosage	Outcome and Side Effects	Reference
Aglepristone	73	Traditional protocol: aglepristone 10 mg/kg SC q 24 h on days 1, 2, and 7 (26 bitches) Modified protocol: aglepristone 10 mg/kg SC q 24 h on days 1, 3, 6, and 9 (47 bitches)	Recovery with traditional protocol in 88%; recurrence: 17%; fertility in 86% Resolution of clinical signs of pyometra with modified protocol, in 100%; recurrence: 0%; fertility in 78% Follow-up after 2 y	Contri et al,[74] 2015
Aglepristone + cloprostenol	15	Aglepristone 10 mg/kg SC q 24 h on days 1, 3, 8, and 15 (if not cured) + cloprostenol: a. 1 μg/kg SC q 24 h on days 3 and 8 (N = 8) b. 1 μg/kg, SC q 24 h on days 3, 5, 8 10, 12, and 15 (N = 7)	Recovery in 100%, recurrence: 20% by the next estrus cycle (in all 15 bitches); fertility in 100% (1 bitch mated); no side effects reported	Gobello et al,[91] 2003
Cabergoline + cloprostenol	29	Cabergoline 5 μg/kg PO q 24 h + cloprostenol 1 μg/kg SC q 24 h for 7–14 d	Recovery in 83% by day 14, recurrence: 21%; fertility in 1/2 mated bitches. Mild side effects noted.	Corrada et al,[81] 2006
Cabergoline + cloprostenol	22	Cabergoline 5 μg/kg PO q 24 h + cloprostenol 5 μg/kg every third day SC for 7–13 d	Recovery in 90.5% by day 13; recurrence: 20%; fertility in 64% of 11 bitches mated; side effects: retching, vomiting, mild abdominal straining, diarrhea, and panting up to 60 min after administration	England et al,[71] 2007

All protocols combined with and systemic antimicrobial therapy. See the original reference for the most accurate information and more details.
Abbreviations: N, number of bitches; PO, per os; PG, prostaglandin; recovery, resolution of pyometra; SC, subcutaneous.

Table 5
Selected studies of medical treatment protocols for open cervix pyometra in cats

Drug	N	Protocol and Dosage	Outcome and Side Effects	Reference
PGF$_{2\alpha}$ (natural)	21	0.1 mg/kg SC q 12–24 h for 3–5 d (6 queens); 0.25 mg/kg was used in 15 queens but was not more effective	Resolution of signs of pyometra and return to cyclicity in 95%; treatment was repeated in 1 queen; fertility in 81%; no difference between the 2 different dosages (ie, the lower dosage recommended); transient side effects observed in 76%: vocalization, panting, restlessness, grooming, tenesmus, salivation, diarrhea, kneading, mydriasis, emesis, urination, and lordosis lasting up to 60 min. Recurrence of pyometra in 14% (3 cats)	Davidson et al,[8] 1992
Prostaglandin F$_{2\alpha}$ (synthetic analog cloprostenol)	5	5 µg/kg SC q 24 h for 3 consecutive days	Resolution of signs of pyometra in 100%; no recurrence after 1 y; fertility in 40%; transient side effects: diarrhea, vomiting, vocalization	Garcia Mitacek et al,[92] 2014
Progesterone receptor blocker (aglepristone)	10	10 mg/kg SC q 24 h on days 1, 2, and 7 and on day 14 (if not cured)	Resolution of signs of pyometra in 90%; no recurrence after 2-y follow-up; no side effects observed	Nak et al,[87] 2009

See the original reference for the most accurate information and more details.
Abbreviations: IM, intramuscular administration; q, every; N, number of cats; PO, oral administration; SC, subcutaneous administration.

kg every 4-6 hours.[73] The synthetic PGF$_{2\alpha}$ analog cloprostenol is administered at a notably lower dose than for natural PGF$_{2\alpha}$,[78] and accurate calculations are crucial to avoid serious side-effects or fatalities. For cloprostenol, subcutaneous administration of 1 µg/kg to 3 µg/kg every 12 hours to 24 hours to resolution/effect is the recommended dose for bitches and queens.[75] Subcutaneous administration of low-dose cloprostenol, 1 µg/kg, once daily was effective in 100% of 7 bitches in 1 study but with a high recurrence rate, 85%, and subsequent fertility rate of 14%.[78]

The dopamine agonists cabergoline and bromocriptine are effectively luteolytic from day 25 after estrus because of their antiprolactin effects and have been used together with PGF$_{2\alpha}$ for augmented treatment of pyometra.[71,72] Cabergoline usually causes less vomiting than bromocriptine, which is an advantage.[72,73,76] Cabergoline combined with a low dose of cloprostenol led to resolution of the illness in 90.5% of 22 treated bitches with pyometra in 1 study.[71] In another study using cabergoline and cloprostenol, 83% of 29 bitches recovered from the illness.[81] This combination was also shown the most effective compared with only low-dose cloprostenol or natural PGF$_{2\alpha}$.[78] For treatment of pyometra in cats, no clinical studies have been published on cabergoline and bromo-criptine, but similar doses and regimes as for dogs have been suggested.[16]

The progesterone blocker aglepristone is commonly used in Europe for treatment of pyometra (see **Tables 4** and **5**) but is not currently approved for use in North America. Aglepristone binds to progesterone receptors effectively and competitively and without stimulating any of the hormone's effects. Side effects are usually rare and not severe, and cervical relaxation induced within 48 hours.[70,74,82–85] According to the recommended protocol, 10 mg/kg aglepristone is administered subcutaneously once daily on days 1, 2, and 7 or 8 and on days 14 and 28 if not cured. This protocol results in success rates of 46% to 100%, recurrence rates 0% to 48% and subsequent fertility rates of 69% to 85%.[86] Aglepristone was administered more frequently (on days 1, 3, 6, and 9) in a modified protocol, which resulted in resolution of the illness in all 47 treated bitches and with no reported recurrence for up to 2 years.[74] Treatment with aglepristone resulted in resolution of pyometra in 9 of 10 queens, with no recurrence reported after 2 years and no side effects observed (see **Table 5**).[87]

Local treatment methods of pyometra have been shown effective but are not yet commonly used in clinical practice in bitches and have not been reported in cats.[88] Intravaginal infusion of prostaglandins and antimicrobials yielded successful result in 15 of 17 treated bitches, without side effects or recurrence after 12 months.[89] Aglepristone in combination with intrauterine antimicrobials was successful in 9 of 11 bitches.[82] Intra-uterine drainage through transcervical catheters may facilitate recovery in refractory cases.[88] Surgical drainage and intrauterine lavage resulted in fertility in 100% of 8 treated bitches.[90] Whether prostaglandin E_2, administered intravaginally or orally, gives a cervical relaxation that is beneficial in medical treatment protocols remains to be studied.[73,76]

PROGNOSIS AFTER MEDICAL TREATMENT

The prognosis for survival and fertility is considered guarded to good. Breeding on the subsequent estrus cycle is consistently recommended after medical treatment, to avoid recurrence. The mean reported long-term success (resolution of clinical illness) of medical treatment is approximately 86% (range 46%–100%) in dogs[67,70,71,74,78,81–83,85,91] and in cats 95% (range 90%–100%)[8,87,92] (see **Tables 4** and **5**). The prognosis for fertility after medical treatment is generally considered good, with a mean fertility rate of 70% (range 14%–100%) reported in dogs and of 60% in cats. The mean recurrence rate reported in dogs is 29% (range 0%–85%), and 0% to 14% in cats. Fertility rates after aglepristone treatment are higher in younger (<5 years) bitches and those that have no other uterine or ovarian pathology.[84,85]

PREDICTIVE MARKERS

Of clinical and laboratory parameters investigated, leukopenia has been associated with both presence of peritonitis and increased postoperative hospitalization in surgically treated bitches with pyometra.[49] Concentrations of the acute-phase proteins, C-reactive protein and serum amyloid A, are increased in sepsis.[69,93] Concentrations of C-reactive protein and $PGF_{2\alpha}$ have been linked with length of postoperative hospitalization.[25,69] Acute-phase proteins concentrations decrease gradually during postoperative recovery, and maintained or increased concentrations may indicate complications.[56] Persistent proteinuria and urinary protein-creatinine indicate renal disease that requires special attention.[54] Central venous oxygen saturation and base-deficit and lactate levels were valuable for determining outcome in bitches with pyometra and sepsis.[94] Band neutrophil concentrations, lymphopenia and monocytosis, blood urea nitrogen greater than 30 mg/dL, and creatinine concentrations greater than 1.5 mg/dL have been associated with death.[95] Certain inflammatory variables may be clinically useful for prognostication if cageside tests become available.[96] In queens, white blood cell counts, neutrophils, band neutrophils, monocytes, and the percentage band neutrophils were positively, and albumin concentrations negatively, associated with postoperative hospitalization.[10]

DIFFERENTIATION OF PYOMETRA AND MUCOMETRA OR HYDROMETRA

Fluid in the uterine lumen is present in both pyometra and mucometra/hydrometra, and their clinical manifestations can be similar. In pyometra, however, life-threatening complications may develop because of the bacterial infection, and differentiation of these disorders is thus important to optimize treatments. Ultrasonographic examination of the uterus illustrating the fluid echogenicity and hemodynamic parameters may be helpful in some cases but is not diagnostic.[51] The health status is more depressed and lethargy and gastrointestinal disturbances more frequently observed in pyometra. More than 3 clinical signs of illness and a more pronounced inflammatory response are also indicative of pyometra as opposed to mucometra/hydrometra.[24,25]

PREVENTION

To diagnose and treat CEH and pyometra early is favorable, and noninvasive diagnostic methods are warranted.[97,98] Elective OHE has the advantage of being performed in a healthy animal and preventing pyometra and other uterine diseases. Because there are many negative side effects of spaying, all pros and cons of such intervention, need to be thoroughly evaluated in each individual.[99] Breeding on the first estrus after medical treatment is not possible, close monitoring is advisable to rule out abnormalities that may emerge during the luteal phase. Progesterone receptor blockers or prostaglandins may prevent the development of pyometra in high-risk patients.[97] Some investigators recommend postponing the subsequent estrus after medical treatment of pyometra, to promote uterine healing.[72]

STUMP PYOMETRA

A stump pyometra is when pyometra develops in residual uterine tissue in incompletely spayed bitches and queens, most often because of hormone-producing ovarian remnants.[100] The clinical presentation is similar, except for a history of previous spay. Ultrasonography usually shows areas of local fluid accumulation at the tissue stump, but it may be difficult to localize the ovarian remnant tissue unless follicles are present (Fig. 10). Incomplete resection is the leading cause, but ectopic or revascularized

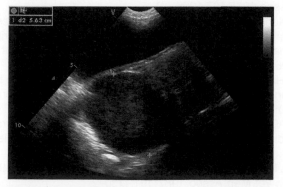

Fig. 10. Stump pyometra due to ovarian remnant.

ovarian tissue separated from the ovary during surgery have also been proposed.[100] Treatment includes surgical resection of remaining uterine and ovarian tissue, in combination with supportive treatments and antimicrobials, if indicated.

Pyometra has been described in many other small animals, such as rabbits (see **Fig. 3**), rodents, guinea pigs, hamsters, gerbils, ferrets, and chipmunks.[101–104] The causative microbes often differ from isolates in dogs and cats with the disease. Ultrasonography and cytology are helpful to confirm a presumptive diagnosis based on clinical signs and physical examination, and the preferred treatment is OHE. Aglepristone combined with antibiotics has been used successfully for medical treatment in a golden hamster and a guinea pig.[105,106]

ACKNOWLEDGMENTS

The author is very grateful for the following experts' contributions: Dr Fredrik Södersten, DVM, PhD, Swedish University of Agricultural Sciences, performed histopathology examinations and provided the images in **Fig. 1**. Dr George Mantziaras, DVM, PhD, VetRepro, Athens, Greece, provided the ultrasonography Video 1 supplementary files and the stump pyometra ultrasonography image for **Fig. 10**. Associate Professor, Kerstin Hansson, DVM, PhD, Diplomate ECVDI, Swedish University of Agricultural Sciences and the University Animal Hospital, Swedish University of Agricultural Sciences provided the diagnostic imaging and text in **Fig. 3**.

SUPPLEMENTARY DATA

Supplementary data related to this article can be found online at https://doi.org/10.1016/j.cvsm.2018.03.001.

REFERENCES

1. Egenvall A, Hagman R, Bonnett BN, et al. Breed risk of pyometra in insured dogs in Sweden. J Vet Intern Med 2001;15:530–8.
2. Hagman R, Strom Holst B, Moller L, et al. Incidence of pyometra in Swedish insured cats. Theriogenology 2014;82:114–20.
3. Dow C. The cystic hyperplasia-pyometra complex in the bitch. J Comp Pathol 1959;69:237–50.
4. Hagman R, Greko C. Antimicrobial resistance in Escherichia coli isolated from bitches with pyometra and from urine samples from other dogs. Vet Rec 2005;157:193–6.
5. Sandholm M, Vasenius H, Kivisto AK. Pathogenesis of canine pyometra. J Am Vet Med Assoc 1975;167:1006–10.
6. Wadås B, Kuhn I, Lagerstedt AS, et al. Biochemical phenotypes of Escherichia coli in dogs: comparison of isolates isolated from bitches suffering from pyometra and urinary tract infection with isolates from faeces of healthy dogs. Vet Microbiol 1996;52:293–300.
7. Jitpean S, Hagman R, Strom Holst B, et al. Breed variations in the incidence of pyometra and mammary tumours in Swedish dogs. Reprod Domest Anim 2012;47(Suppl 6):347–50.
8. Davidson AP, Feldman EC, Nelson RW. Treatment of pyometra in cats, using prostaglandin F2 alpha: 21 cases (1982-1990). J Am Vet Med Assoc 1992;200:825–8.
9. Kenney KJ, Matthiesen DT, Brown NO, et al. Pyometra in cats: 183 cases (1979-1984). J Am Vet Med Assoc 1987;191:1130–2.

10. Hagman R, Karlstam E, Persson S, et al. Plasma PGF 2 alpha metabolite levels in cats with uterine disease. Theriogenology 2009;72:1180–7.
11. Niskanen M, Thrusfield MV. Associations between age, parity, hormonal therapy and breed, and pyometra in Finnish dogs. Vet Rec 1998;143:493–8.
12. Von Berky AG, Townsend WL. The relationship between the prevalence of uterine lesions and the use of medroxyprogesterone acetate for canine population control. Aust Vet J 1993;70:249–50.
13. Hagman R, Lagerstedt AS, Hedhammar A, et al. A breed-matched case-control study of potential risk-factors for canine pyometra. Theriogenology 2011;75: 1251–7.
14. Cox JE. Progestagens in bitches: a review. J Small Anim Pract 1970;11:759–78.
15. England GC, Moxon R, Freeman SL. Delayed uterine fluid clearance and reduced uterine perfusion in bitches with endometrial hyperplasia and clinical management with postmating antibiotic. Theriogenology 2012;78:1611–7.
16. Hollinshead F, Krekeler N. Pyometra in the queen: to spay or not to spay? J Feline Med Surg 2016;18:21–33.
17. Wijewardana V, Sugiura K, Wijesekera DP, et al. Effect of ovarian hormones on maturation of dendritic cells from peripheral blood monocytes in dogs. J Vet Med Sci 2015;77:771–5.
18. Rowson LE, Lamming GE, Fry RM. Influence of ovarian hormones on uterine infection. Nature 1953;171:749–50.
19. Hawk HW, Turner GD, Sykes JF. The effect of ovarian hormones on the uterine defense mechanism during the early stages of induced infection. Am J Vet Res 1960;21:644–8.
20. Chaffaux S, Thibier M. Peripheral plasma concentrations of progesterone in the bitch with pyometra. Ann Rech Vet 1978;9:587–92.
21. Prapaiwan N, Manee-In S, Olanratmanee E, et al. Expression of oxytocin, progesterone, and estrogen receptors in the reproductive tract of bitches with pyometra. Theriogenology 2017;89:131–9.
22. Strom Holst B, Larsson B, Rodriguez-Martinez H, et al. Prediction of the oocyte recovery rate in the bitch. J Vet Med A Physiol Pathol Clin Med 2001;48:587–92.
23. De Bosschere H, Ducatelle R, Vermeirsch H, et al. Cystic endometrial hyperplasia-pyometra complex in the bitch: should the two entities be disconnected? Theriogenology 2001;55:1509–19.
24. Fransson BA, Karlstam E, Bergstrom A, et al. C-reactive protein in the differentiation of pyometra from cystic endometrial hyperplasia/mucometra in dogs. J Am Anim Hosp Assoc 2004;40:391–9.
25. Hagman R, Kindahl H, Fransson BA, et al. Differentiation between pyometra and cystic endometrial hyperplasia/mucometra in bitches by prostaglandin F2alpha metabolite analysis. Theriogenology 2006;66:198–206.
26. Børresen B, Naess B. Microbial immunological and toxicological aspects of canine pyometra. Acta Vet Scand 1977;18:569–71.
27. Coggan JA, Melville PA, de Oliveira CM, et al. Microbiological and histopathological aspects of canine pyometra. Braz J Microbiol 2008;39:477–83.
28. Fransson B, Lagerstedt AS, Hellmen E, et al. Bacteriological findings, blood chemistry profile and plasma endotoxin levels in bitches with pyometra or other uterine diseases. Zentralbl Veterinarmed A 1997;44:417–26.
29. Grindlay M, Renton JP, Ramsay DH. O-groups of Escherichia coli associated with canine pyometra. Res Vet Sci 1973;14:75–7.
30. Hernandez JL, Besso JG, Rault DN, et al. Emphysematous pyometra in a dog. Vet Radiol Ultrasound 2003;44:196–8.

31. Nomura K, Yoshida K, Funahashi H, et al. The possibilities of uterine infection of Escherichia coli inoculated into the vagina and development of endometritis in bitches. Japanese Journal of Reproduction 1988;34:199–203.

32. Agostinho JM, de Souza A, Schocken-Iturrino RP, et al. Escherichia coli strains isolated from the uteri horn, mouth, and rectum of bitches suffering from pyometra: virulence factors, antimicrobial susceptibilities, and clonal relationships among strains. Int J Microbiol 2014;2014:979584.

33. Hagman R, Kuhn I. Escherichia coli strains isolated from the uterus and urinary bladder of bitches suffering from pyometra: comparison by restriction enzyme digestion and pulsed-field gel electrophoresis. Vet Microbiol 2002;84:143–53.

34. Watts JR, Wright PJ, Whithear KC. Uterine, cervical and vaginal microflora of the normal bitch throughout the reproductive cycle. J Small Anim Pract 1996;37:54–60.

35. Mateus L, Henriques S, Merino C, et al. Virulence genotypes of Escherichia coli canine isolates from pyometra, cystitis and fecal origin. Vet Microbiol 2013;166: 590–4.

36. Siqueira AK, Ribeiro MG, Leite Dda S, et al. Virulence factors in Escherichia coli strains isolated from urinary tract infection and pyometra cases and from feces of healthy dogs. Res Vet Sci 2009;86:206–10.

37. Chen YM, Wright PJ, Lee CS, et al. Uropathogenic virulence factors in isolates of Escherichia coli from clinical cases of canine pyometra and feces of healthy bitches. Vet Microbiol 2003;94:57–69.

38. Van Miert ASJ, Frens J. The reaction of different animal species to bacterial pyrogens. Zentralbl Veterinarmed A 1968;15:532–43.

39. McAnulty JF. Septic shock in the dog: a review. J Am Anim Hosp Assoc 1983;19: 827–36.

40. Okano S, Tagawa M, Takase K. Relationship of the blood endotoxin concentration and prognosis in dogs with pyometra. J Vet Med Sci 1998;60:1265–7.

41. Hagman R, Kindahl H, Lagerstedt AS. Pyometra in bitches induces elevated plasma endotoxin and prostaglandin F2alpha metabolite levels. Acta Vet Scand 2006;47:55–67.

42. Karlsson I, Wernersson S, Ambrosen A, et al. Increased concentrations of C-reactive protein but not high-mobility group box 1 in dogs with naturally occurring sepsis. Vet Immunol Immunopathol 2013;156:64–72.

43. Marretta SM, Matthiesen DT, Nichols R. Pyometra and its complications. Probl Vet Med 1989;1:50–62.

44. Wheaton LG, Johnson AL, Parker AJ, et al. Results and complications of surgical treatment of pyometra: a review of 80 cases. J Am Anim Hosp Assoc 1987; 25:563–8.

45. Singer M. The new sepsis consensus definitions (Sepsis-3): the good, the not-so-bad, and the actually-quite-pretty. Intensive Care Med 2016;42:2027–9.

46. Brady CA, Otto CM, Van Winkle TJ, et al. Severe sepsis in cats: 29 cases (1986-1998). J Am Vet Med Assoc 2000;217:531–5.

47. Børresen B. Pyometra in the dog. II.–A pathophysiological investigation. II.–Anamnestic, clinical and reproductive aspects. Nord Vet Med 1979;31:251–7.

48. Jitpean S, Ambrosen A, Emanuelson U, et al. Closed cervix is associated with more severe illness in dogs with pyometra. BMC Vet Res 2017;13:11.

49. Jitpean S, Strom-Holst B, Emanuelson U, et al. Outcome of pyometra in female dogs and predictors of peritonitis and prolonged postoperative hospitalization in surgically treated cases. BMC Vet Res 2014;10:6.

50. Bjurstrom L. Aerobic bacteria occurring in the vagina of bitches with reproductive disorders. Acta Vet Scand 1993;34:29–34.

51. Bigliardi E, Parmigiani E, Cavirani S, et al. Ultrasonography and cystic hyperplasia-pyometra complex in the bitch. Reprod Domest Anim 2004;39:136–40.
52. Vandeplassche M, Coryn M, De Schepper J. Pyometra in the bitch: cytological, bacterial, histological and endocrinological characteristics. Vlaams Dierge-neeskd Tijdschr 1991;60:207–11.
53. Hardy RM, Osborne CA. Canine pyometra: pathophysiology, diagnosis and treatment of uterine and extra-genital lesions. J Am Anim Hosp Assoc 1974;10:245–67.
54. Maddens B, Heiene R, Smets P, et al. Evaluation of kidney injury in dogs with pyometra based on proteinuria, renal histomorphology, and urinary biomarkers. J Vet Intern Med 2011;25:1075–83.
55. Asheim A. Renal function in dogs with pyometra. 8. Uterine infection and the pathogenesis of the renal dysfunction. Acta Pathol Microbiol Scand 1964;60:99–107.
56. Dabrowski R, Kostro K, Lisiecka U, et al. Usefulness of C-reactive protein, serum amyloid A component, and haptoglobin determinations in bitches with pyometra for monitoring early post-ovariohysterectomy complications. Theriogenology 2009;72:471–6.
57. Dorsey TI, Rozanski EA, Sharp CR, et al. Evaluation of thromboelastography in bitches with pyometra. J Vet Diagn Invest 2018;30(1):165–8.
58. Becher-Deichsel A, Aurich JE, Schrammel N, et al. A surgical glove port technique for laparoscopic-assisted ovariohysterectomy for pyometra in the bitch. Theriogenology 2016;86:619–25.
59. Fieni F, Topie E, Gogny A. Medical treatment for pyometra in dogs. Reprod Domest Anim 2014;49(Suppl 2):28–32.
60. Fantoni D, Shih AC. Perioperative fluid therapy. Vet Clin North Am Small Anim Pract 2017;47:423–34.
61. Kirby R. An introduction to SIRS and the rule of 20. In: Kirby R, Linklater A, editors. Monitoring and intervention for the critically ill small animal. Ames (IA): Wiley Blackwell; 2017. p. 1–8.
62. DeClue A. Sepsis and the systemic inflammatory response syndrome. In: Ettinger SJ, Feldman EC, Cote E, editors. Textbook of veterinary internal medicine: diseases of the dogs and cat. 8th edition. St Louis (MO): Elsevier; 2016. p. 554–60.
63. Devey JJ. Surgical considerations in the emergent small animal patient. Vet Clin North Am Small Anim Pract 2013;43:899–914.
64. Liao PY, Chang SC, Chen KS, et al. Decreased postoperative C-reactive protein production in dogs with pyometra through the use of low-dose ketamine. J Vet Emerg Crit Care (San Antonio) 2014;24:286–90.
65. Tobias KM, Wheaton LG. Surgical management of pyometra in dogs and cats. Semin Vet Med Surg (Small Anim) 1995;10:30–4.
66. Bartoskova A, Vitasek R, Leva L, et al. Hysterectomy leads to fast improvement of haematological and immunological parameters in bitches with pyometra. J Small Anim Pract 2007;48:564–8.
67. Feldman EC, Nelson RW. Cystic endometrial hyperplasia/pyometra complex. In: Feldman EC, Nelson RW, editors. Endocrinology and reproduction. 3rd edition. St Louis (MO): Saunders; 2004. p. 852–67.
68. Fantoni DT, Auler Junior JO, Futema F, et al. Intravenous administration of hypertonic sodium chloride solution with dextran or isotonic sodium chloride solution for treatment of septic shock secondary to pyometra in dogs. J Am Vet Med Assoc 1999;215:1283–7.
69. Fransson BA, Lagerstedt AS, Bergstrom A, et al. C-reactive protein, tumor necrosis factor alpha, and interleukin-6 in dogs with pyometra and SIRS. J Vet Emerg Crit Care 2007;17:373–81.

70. Fieni F. Clinical evaluation of the use of aglepristone, with or without cloproste-nol, to treat cystic endometrial hyperplasia-pyometra complex in bitches. Ther-iogenology 2006;66:1550–6.

71. England GC, Freeman SL, Russo M. Treatment of spontaneous pyometra in 22 bitches with a combination of cabergoline and cloprostenol. Vet Rec 2007;160: 293–6.

72. Verstegen J, Dhaliwal G, Verstegen-Onclin K. Mucometra, cystic endometrial hyperplasia, and pyometra in the bitch: advances in treatment and assessment of future reproductive success. Theriogenology 2008;70:364–74.

73. Lopate C. Pyometra, cystic endometrial hyperplasia (hydrometra, mucometra, hematometra). In: Greco DS, Davidson AP, editors. Blackwell's five-minute vet-erinary consult clinical companion, small animal endocrinology and reproduc-tion. Hoboken (NJ): Wiley-Blackwell; 2017. p. 53–62.

74. Contri A, Gloria A, Carluccio A, et al. Effectiveness of a modified administration protocol for the medical treatment of canine pyometra. Vet Res Commun 2015; 39:1–5.

75. Davidson A. Female and male infertility and subfertility. In: Nelson RW, Couto CG, editors. Small Animal Internal Medicine. 5th edition. St Louis (MO): Elsevier; 2014. p. 951–65.

76. Greer M. Canine reproduction and neonatology - a practical guide for veterinar-ians, veterinary staff and breeders. Jackson (WY): Teton Newmedia; 2015.

77. BSAVA small animal formulary. 8th edition. Gloucester (United Kingdom): British Small Animal Veterinary Association; 2014.

78. Jena B, Rao KS, Reddy KCS, et al. Comparative efficacy or various therapeutic protocols in the treatment of pyometra in bitches. Vet Med 2013;58:271–6.

79. Arnold S, Hubler M, Casal M, et al. Use of low dose prostaglandin for the treat-ment of canine pyometra. J Small Anim Pract 1988;29:303–8.

80. Sridevi P, Balasubramanian S, Devanathan T, et al. Low dose prostaglandin F2 alpha therapy in treatment of canine pyometra. Indian Vet J 2000;77:889–90.

81. Corrada Y, Arias D, Rodriguez R, et al. Combination dopamine agonist and prostaglandin agonist treatment of cystic endometrial hyperplasia-pyometra complex in the bitch. Theriogenology 2006;66:1557–9.

82. Gurbulak K, Pancarci M, Ekici H, et al. Use of aglepristone and aglepristone + intrauterine antibiotic for the treatment of pyometra in bitches. Acta Vet Hung 2005;53:249–55.

83. Trasch K, Wehrend A, Bostedt H. Follow-up examinations of bitches after con-servative treatment of pyometra with the antigestagen aglepristone. J Vet Med A Physiol Pathol Clin Med 2003;50:375–9.

84. Jurka P, Max A, Hawrynska K, et al. Age-related pregnancy results and further examination of bitches after aglepristone treatment of pyometra. Reprod Domest Anim 2010;45:525–9.

85. Ros L, Holst BS, Hagman R. A retrospective study of bitches with pyometra, medically treated with aglepristone. Theriogenology 2014;82:1281–6.

86. Gogny A, Fieni F. Aglepristone: a review on its clinical use in animals. Therioge-nology 2016;85:555–66.

87. Nak D, Nak Y, Tuna B. Follow-up examinations after medical treatment of pyo-metra in cats with the progesterone-antagonist aglepristone. J Feline Med Surg 2009;11:499–502.

88. Lagerstedt A-S, Obel N, Stavenborn M. Uterine drainage in the bitch for treat-ment of pyometra refractory to prostaglandin F2α. J Small Anim Pract 1987; 28:215–22.

89. Gabor G, Siver L, Szenci O. Intravaginal prostaglandin F2 alpha for the treatment of metritis and pyometra in the bitch. Acta Vet Hung 1999;47:103–8.
90. De Cramer KG. Surgical uterine drainage and lavage as treatment for canine pyometra. J S Afr Vet Assoc 2010;81:172–7.
91. Gobello C, Castex G, Klima L, et al. A study of two protocols combining aglepristone and cloprostenol to treat open cervix pyometra in the bitch. Theriogenology 2003;60:901–8.
92. Garcia Mitacek MC, Stornelli MC, Tittarelli CM, et al. Cloprostenol treatment of feline open-cervix pyometra. J Feline Med Surg 2014;16:177–9.
93. Jitpean S, Pettersson A, Hoglund OV, et al. Increased concentrations of Serum amyloid A in dogs with sepsis caused by pyometra. BMC Vet Res 2014;10:273.
94. Conti-Patara A, de Araujo Caldeira J, de Mattos-Junior E, et al. Changes in tissue perfusion parameters in dogs with severe sepsis/septic shock in response to goal-directed hemodynamic optimization at admission to ICU and the relation to outcome. J Vet Emerg Crit Care (San Antonio) 2012;22:409–18.
95. Kuplulu S, Vural MR, Demirel A, et al. The comparative evaluation of serum biochemical, haematological, bacteriological and clinical findings of dead and recovered bitches with pyometra in the postoperative process. Acta Veterinaria-Beograd 2009;59:193–204.
96. Hagman R. Diagnostic and prognostic markers for uterine diseases in dogs. Reprod Domest Anim 2014;49(Suppl 2):16–20.
97. Mir F, Fontaine E, Albaric O, et al. Findings in uterine biopsies obtained by laparotomy from bitches with unexplained infertility or pregnancy loss: an observational study. Theriogenology 2013;79:312–22.
98. Christensen BW, Schlafer DH, Agnew DW, et al. Diagnostic value of transcervical endometrial biopsies in domestic dogs compared with full-thickness uterine sections. Reprod Domest Anim 2012;47(Suppl 6):342–6.
99. Artl S, Wehrend A, Reichler IM. Kastration der Hundin - neue und alte Erkenntnisse zu Vor- und nachteilen. Tierärztliche Praxis Kleintiere 2017;45:253–63.
100. Ball RL, Birchard SJ, May LR, et al. Ovarian remnant syndrome in dogs and cats: 21 cases (2000-2007). J Am Vet Med Assoc 2010;236:548–53.
101. Kondert L, Mayer J. Reproductive medicine in guinea pigs, chinchillas and degus. Vet Clin North Am Exot Anim Pract 2017;20:609–28.
102. Martorell J. Reproductive disorders in pet rodents. Vet Clin North Am Exot Anim Pract 2017;20:589–608.
103. Mancinelli E, Lord B. Urogenital system and reproductive disease. Glouchester (United Kingdom): BSAVA; 2016.
104. Heap RB. Prostaglandins in pyometrial fluid from the cow, bitch and ferret. Br J Pharmacol 1975;55:515–8.
105. Engelhardt AB. Behandlung des Endometritis/Pyometrakomplexes eines Meerschweinchens - ein Fallbericht. Prakt Tierarzt 2006;87:14–6.
106. Pisu MC, Andolfatto A, Veronesi MC. Pyometra in a six-month-old nulliparous golden hamster (Mesocricetus auratus) treated with aglepristone. Vet Q 2012; 32:179–81.
107. Nelson RW, Feldman EC. Pyometra. Vet Clin North Am Small Anim Pract 1986; 16(3):561–76.

Periparturient Diseases in the Dam

Kristine Gonzales, DVM

KEYWORDS

- Periparturient • Lactation • Dam • Diseases • Neonates

KEY POINTS

- Understanding the physiologic, physical, and hormonal changes that occur in the dam around the time of delivery helps identify and treat reproductive diseases during this unique time.
- All pharmacologic therapy prescribed for a dam affects her offspring, often creating a challenge in balancing her medical needs with the health of the neonates.
- Early recognition of disease relies on daily evaluation of the dam's attitude, body condition, appetite, and maternal behavior.

INTRODUCTION

This article provides an overview of some of the most common diseases affecting the dam in the periparturient period, including disorders of lactation, inappropriate maternal behavior, mastitis, metritis, and eclampsia. The dam experiences hormonal, physiologic, and physical changes during pregnancy, parturition, and lactation. Obtaining a detailed history and performing a thorough physical examination are essential for accurately diagnosing and treating the dam during this unique time. A particular challenge exists when identifying problems in the periparturient period because all medications and aspects of management impact the health of both the dam and her offspring.

AGALACTIA

Agalactia is a failure of the dam to provide milk to the neonates. Primary agalactia is rare and results from an anatomic or physiologic abnormality causing a lack of mammary gland development and milk production.[1] A defect in the pituitary ovarian mammary gland axis is suspected to be the cause.[2] Secondary agalactia results from low milk production or decreased let down of milk into the teat canal.[3] Often the lack of milk supply is identified within 2 to 3 days postpartum when the neonates fail to

The author has nothing to disclose.
Veterinary Services, Guide Dogs for the Blind, 350 Los Ranchitos Road, San Rafael, CA 94903, USA
E-mail address: kgonzales@guidedogs.com

Vet Clin Small Anim 48 (2018) 663–681
https://doi.org/10.1016/j.cvsm.2018.02.010
0195-5616/18/© 2018 Elsevier Inc. All rights reserved.

gain 5% to 10% of body weight daily. Normally, mammary gland development is evident by day 45 of gestation and milk secretion starts at or shortly after parturition.[4] Prolactin hormone plays a pivotal role in milk production. During late gestation when progesterone is decreasing, prolactin increases and subsequently increases again when the neonates start to suckle.[4] Prolactin production receives both inhibitory and stimulatory signals. Dopamine is a main inhibitory factor of prolactin[5] and the relationship is important for modulating milk production with drug therapy. At parturition, the dam produces, thick, yellow colostrum. With the stimulus of neonates nursing, milk production increases to reach peak lactation at 3 to 4 weeks. Early intervention to correct agalactia will ensure that the neonates receive adequate nutrition.

Physical Examination and Diagnosis

Primary agalactia is atypical and is characterized by an absence of mammary gland development and milk production.[6] Secondary agalactia is more common and results from either a lack of milk let down or poor milk production.[3] Mammary glands may be developed, but milk production is low or milk cannot be readily expressed owing to a lack of milk ejection from the teat sphincters.[2,7] There are several possible causes for agalactia.[3,8]

- Concurrent medical conditions: malnutrition, systemic illness, premature parturition, progesterone therapy, mastitis, metritis, endotoxemia, stress, and pain from a cesarean delivery.[1,3]
- The dam is highly nervous and anxious and the production of adrenalin blocks the release of oxytocin from the pituitary.[7]
- The dam has a large litter with high lactational demands.
- The dam has poor appetite and is unwilling to consume adequate nutrition.

Pharmacologic Treatment

Primary agalactia does not respond to medical therapy.[3] Medical therapy for secondary agalactia, including lack of milk ejection and milk production, focuses on treating and resolving any concurrent diseases, relaxing the anxious dam, and/or providing a stimulus for milk ejection and production.

- Administer intravenous or subcutaneous fluids to dams that are ill, dehydrated, or have a poor appetite.
- Oxytocin stimulates milk ejection by causing contractions in the myoepithelium surrounding alveolar ducts; however, it lacks galactopoietic properties.[5]
  - If lack of ejection is noticed early, give oxytocin 0.25 to 1 U (per dam) subcutaneously (SQ) every 2 to 4 hours for 1 to 2 days. Neonates are removed for 30 minutes after injection, and then returned to suckle, or gentle stripping of the glands can be performed and neonates are bottle or tube fed.[2,9]
  - Oxytocin nasal sprays have anecdotally been reported to enhance milk let down and also improve maternal behavior in dams.[3,10]
- Metoclopramide is an antiemetic; however, it antagonizes dopamine at receptor sites and promotes an increase in prolactin and milk production.[6]
  - Give metoclopramide 0.1 to 0.2 mg/kg SQ or orally (PO) every 8 to 12 hours.[2] A response is typically noted in 24 to 48 hours[2] and therapy continues for 2 days beyond desired milk production. Extrapyramidal side effects, such as restlessness, agitation, and ataxia, are more common at higher dosages and the dose should be reduced if there is concern about a dam's behavior and safety with her litter.[5]

- Domperidone is a peripheral dopamine receptor antagonist and also increases prolactin and milk production; however, it is less permeable to the blood–brain barrier than metoclopramide and central nervous system effects are unlikely.[5]
  - Give domperidone (Equidone domperidone oral gel 110 mg/mL) 2.2 mg/kg PO every 8 to 12 hours[5,9,11] and continue for 2 days beyond desired milk production. Diarrhea is a reported side effect in the bitch.[5]
- Acepromazine is a phenothiazine agent that blocks postsynaptic dopamine receptors in the central nervous system.[12] It may decrease anxiety in the dam and increase prolactin release.[9] Thus, it may calm an anxious dam, allowing the neonates to nurse.
  - Give acepromazine 0.01 to 0.02 mg/kg SQ.[2] If used with metoclopramide, it may increase its extrapyramidal effects.[12]

Nonpharmacologic Treatment

- Add water to meals and provide an energy-dense diet approved for reproduction and lactation, consisting of 30% protein, 20% fat, and 20% to 30% carbohydrate on dry matter basis.[13,14]
- House the dam in a quiet and traffic-free room.
- Use a dog-appeasing pheromone plug-in diffuser, spray, or collar (ADAPTIL, Ceva Sante Animale, Libourne, France), which provides a synthetic equivalent of the calming pheromone produced by dams when they are reassuring their pups.
- Acupuncture for stimulating milk production: using SI1 and LI4 with dry needles and the addition of electroacupuncture stimulation if needed, has been reported to be successful.[15]

Treatment for Neonates That May Lack Passive Immune Transfer

If neonates fail to ingest colostrum, they will lack passive immune protection[16] because the endotheliochorial placenta transfers only 5% to 10% of maternal immunoglobulins (Ig).[17] Colostrum provides essential nutrients, water, growth factors, digestive enzymes, and maternal IgG, IgA, and IgM,[18] protecting the neonate against sepsis, a frequent cause of neonatal death.[19,20] The window of absorption of maternal IgG is short; in 1 study, neonatal intestinal barrier closure was determined to begin as early as 4 hours after birth and to be completed by 16 to 24 hours.[21] Gillette and Filkins[22] showed that neonates fed hyperimmune serum 8 hours postpartum had optimum absorption of antibodies followed by a decrease in absorption when serum was fed 12 hours of age or later. The study by Bouchard and associates[23] also showed that intestinal absorption of Igs was minimal after 12 hours and the route of administration of immune protection, other than oral, should be considered after this time. The intake of colostrum is maximized by assisting any weak neonates to latch, suckle, and ingest colostrum every 2 hours. The nursing also provides further stimulation for a dam's natural oxytocin release and milk ejection. If a dam is unable to provide colostrum to her young, cross-fostering neonates to a surrogate dam with colostrum is an option. Alternatively, oral immune protection can be given by feeding fresh or previously frozen colostrum or immune serum or plasma to the neonate before intestinal barrier closure. By 16 to 24 hours, intestinal absorption of IgG is near complete,[9,21] and subcutaneous injection of plasma or serum must be considered.[9]

PROTOCOLS
Oral Immune Protection

- A protocol for collection, freezing, thawing, and oral administration of high immune quality colostrum from a dam is outlined in **Box 1**.[19]

Box 1
Protocol for collection, freezing, and thawing of high immune quality colostrum from a dam and administration to a neonate

Store colostrum from bitches living in same kennel or household.

Collect colostrum from donor dam approximately 24 hours postpartum. Timing is a compromise to allow donor to supply sufficient antibodies to her neonates before donating to the bank.

Clean skin and collect by gentle teat massage.

One- to 5-mL samples are stored in polypropylene or glass tubes and immediately frozen at −20°C.

Before administration, warm colostrum to 30°C to 35°C with baby bottle warmer (avoid microwave, which destroys immunoglobulin G).

Administer minimum of 1.5 mL/100 g of body weight within the first 8 hours of life.

Data from Mila H, Grellet A, Mariani C, et al. Natural and artificial hyperimmune solutions: impact on health in puppies. Reprod Domest Anim 2017;52 Suppl 2:164.

- A dose for providing serum or plasma orally, preferably within 12 hours of birth, is 22 mL/kg.[17,24] Eight hours postpartum is reported to have optimal absorption.[22]

Parenteral Immune Protection

Various dosages have been published for giving serum or plasma parentally, including 16 mL/neonate divided SQ over 24 hours[23,25] and 22 mL/kg divided SQ over 24 hours.[16,17] Subcutaneous pooling of serum and subsequent skin necrosis have been reported in the literature[19] and monitoring injection sites is recommended.

GALACTOSTASIS

Galactostasis occurs when there is a delay in passage of milk from the mammary gland cisterns into the teat canals, resulting in engorged and uncomfortable mammary glands.[1,3,26] Enlarged glands may seems to be similar to septic mastitis, yet the dam is not systemically ill. Because prolonged galactostasis can progress to septic mastitis,[1,6] treatment is directed at reducing engorgement and increasing comfort to the dam.[1]

Patient History

Galactostasis occurs shortly after parturition or after a dam has weaned from pups or lost a litter. It can also be associated with a dam nursing a small litter that has produced a large amount of milk or when neonates are weak or not rotating to nurse all glands.[6]

Physical Examination and Diagnosis

- Evaluate for the presence of anatomic abnormalities of the teat canal or orifices, such as inverted or imperforate teats[3,9] (**Fig. 1**).
- Glands are firm, enlarged, and may be uncomfortable on palpation without any redness or heat. The dam is afebrile and milk is difficult to express.
- Rarely occurs during pseudopregnancy.
- Cytologic examination of milk often contains neutrophils, eosinophils, and macrophages with engulfed milk fat within the cytoplasm.[3,10] Milk must be

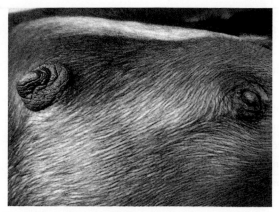

Fig. 1. Normal (*left*) and inverted teat (*right*) in a lactating dam.

differentiated from septic mastitis milk that contains degenerate neutrophils and bacteria.[27,28]

Treatment for Dams Nursing Neonates

- Confirm neonates' ability to effectively suckle and dam's acceptance to nursing the litter.[26]
- Cool compress hard and engorged glands and alternate with warm compresses to gently soften. Massage the glands frequently, relieving pressure and eliciting milk ejection.[9] Neonates nursing immediately after the application of warm compresses will maximize the emptying of glands.
- When glands soften and milk ejection occurs, assist nurse neonates to further stimulate milk let down.

Treatment for Dams Weaned from Neonates

- Reduce food intake[10,27] and physically separate the dam from the pups.
- Apply cool compresses 10 minutes 3 times per day to engorged glands.
- Give nonsteroidal analgesics for pain relief.
- If necessary, the dopamine agonist cabergoline reduces prolactin secretion and milk production: give 2.5 to 5 µg/kg/d for 4 to 6 days.[5,27]

INAPPROPRIATE MATERNAL BEHAVIOR

Desirable maternal behavior for a dam includes cleaning, nursing, and protecting of the neonates. A dam's general health and environment influences her maternal behavior in the postpartum period. The maternal behavior is strengthened by the peptide hormone oxytocin, which is produced from the posterior pituitary in response to neurologic stimulation (Ferguson's reflex and suckling).[29] Its production in the periparturient period strengthens a dam's maternal bonding and stimulates milk let down. The first 24 to 72 hours after vaginal or cesarean delivery, a dam may seem to be unsettled, necessitating close monitoring to prevent injury to the litter. If a dam fails to groom neonates, they will not receive the stimulus for reflex urination and defecation, and will suffer health problems. On rare occasions, a dam may cannibalize the litter, which is termed kronism.[29] There are many reasons for inappropriate maternal behavior (**Box 2**) and treatment is variable and depends on the cause(s).[1,30]

Box 2
Common reasons for inappropriate maternal behavior

Anesthetic drugs

Pain associated with cesarean delivery

Primiparous dam

Anxious and agitated

Unfamiliar environment

Environment overcrowded with humans/animals

Strong human bond with caretaker

Medical conditions
  Metritis
  Mastitis
  Hypocalcemia

Genetic predisposition

Patient History and Diagnosis

History and physical examination findings allow an assessment to be made about the underlying etiology. If a medical condition is diagnosed, prompt treatment for that condition will optimize the health of the dam and the litter. If there are not any abnormalities on physical examination consider a complete blood count (CBC), biochemistry profile, and total and ionized calcium levels to screen for hypoglycemia, hypocalcemia, leukocytosis, and anemia. Monitoring the rectal temperature at least every 8 to 12 hours allows the identification of any slight change in the dam's condition.

Pharmacologic and Nonpharmacologic Treatments

- For nervous dams
  - Maintain a quiet and safe whelping box.
  - Acepromazine 0.01 to 0.02 mg/kg SQ at lowest effective dose.[1,2]
  - Supervise and assist nurse neonates every 2 to 3 hours and muzzle the dam if necessary.
  - To aid in calming the dam, use a dog appeasing pheromone plug-in diffuser, spray, or collar (ADAPTIL, Ceva Sante Animale).
  - Anecdotal use of oxytocin nasal spray to improve maternal behavior has been reported.
- For a lack of maternal behavior after a cesarean delivery, save placentas and amniotic fluid and rub on puppies to improve acceptance.
- For maternal behaviors characterized by dazed appearance, aggression toward neonates, and overall inattentiveness, there have been anecdotal accounts of successful resolution after administration of calcium supplementation.

MASTITIS

Mastitis is complication of lactation that results in septic inflammation of 1 or more of the mammary glands[1,10,26] and it is most commonly diagnosed in the postpartum dam. It is rarely seen before parturition or in dams exhibiting pseudopregnancy.[31] Primarily bacteria and rarely fungal organisms invade the mammary tissue.[32]

Patient History

Dams nursing large litters may be predisposed to acquiring mastitis because neonates frequently are nursing multiple glands and the orifices are repeatedly open, predisposing to ascending bacterial infection. Dams nursing small litters are also susceptible because excess milk pools in the glands, providing a nutrient source for bacteria. Potential routes of infection include cutaneous, hematogenous, and exogenous, such as rearing a litter in unsanitary conditions.[1,26] Neonates also may fail to thrive because of a dam's poor mothering behavior and her diminishing milk supply.

Physical Examination

Mild mastitis

Early in the disease, the dam may be afebrile and have mild mammary discomfort and firm palpable tissue within the mammary gland. Discolored milk from teat orifices may be present, but if symptoms are subtle, obtaining a milk sample from a suspected gland will aid with the diagnosis and reveal degenerative neutrophils and bacteria.[1,9,30]

Moderate to severe mastitis

A mild mastitis may progress into a moderate to severe form, or the dam may present with an acute and fulminant mastitis, characterized by fever exceeding 103.5° F, anorexia, depression, trembling, vomiting, and reluctance to nurse or lie down.[1,26] The affected gland(s) are hot, enlarged, and painful with associated cutaneous erythema, edema, and inflammation. Discolored milk may drain from 1 or more orifices on a teat and may appear brown, green, or yellow (**Fig. 2**). Glands that are difficult

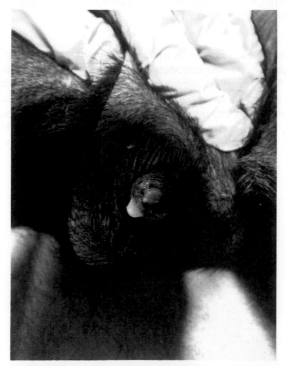

Fig. 2. Milk at 2 teat orifices after a mammary gland was expressed. Note the normal-appearing (*left*) and purulent milk drops (*right*).

to express are frequently blood tinged. Dams with abscessed and gangrenous (necrotic dark skin) mastitis often present septic (**Fig. 3**).

Diagnosis

The clinical presentation usually confirms a diagnosis; however, further diagnostics are often necessary to select appropriate treatment.

- A CBC may be normal early in the disease process and then change to a leukocytosis with left shift.[26,30] Platelet abnormalities have been reported with gangrenous mastitis.[33]
- Culture and sensitivity of milk is obtained by aseptically handling and cleaning the teat and skin with alcohol and expressing abnormal milk. The first drop is discarded and milk is directly swabbed for submission to the laboratory.
- Cytologic examination of milk from a septic gland is evaluated for free and intracellular bacteria and high numbers of degenerate neutrophils and macrophages,[26,27] and must be differentiated from normal milk, which may contain lower numbers of neutrophils and macrophages.[3,26]
- Ultrasound examination of glands is helpful in identifying abnormal changes in echogenicity within mammary tissue and fluid associated with abscessation.

Pharmacologic Treatments

Fluid therapy

Administer intravenous or subcutaneous fluids to dams that are lethargic and anorexic in an effort to maintain milk production.

Antibiotics

Common bacteria isolated from milk includes *Escherichia coli*, staphylococcal spp, streptococcal spp,[6,10,34] *Pseudomonas* spp, *Klebsiella* spp, *Pasteurella* spp, and *Clostridium* spp.[9] Treatment is aimed at choosing an appropriate antibiotic that is safe for the dam and her nursing neonates. Initial selection is based on milk cytology pending culture and sensitivity results. Final antibiotic selection is based on antimicrobial susceptibility results and a 7- to 14-day course is typical. In acute mastitis, many antibiotics enter the mammary secretions because the milk–plasma barriers are

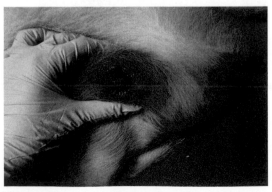

Fig. 3. An inflamed mammary gland that developed a ruptured abscess near the teat, draining purulent fluid.

interrupted.[10,31] As inflammation subsides, antibiotics do not enter the milk glands as readily and attention to culture and sensitivity, pH portioning, and lipid solubility factors need to be considered.[10] US Food and Drug Administration classification of antibiotics used during pregnancy and lactation in women are based on human epidemiologic studies and laboratory animal investigations. Extrapolated data provide the basis for the listing of antibiotics that are considered safe for dams during pregnancy and lactation (**Table 1**).[6,35]

Clavulanic acid–potentiated amoxicillin 14 mg/kg PO every 8 to 12 hours[1,3,6] and cephalexin 10 to 20 mg/kg PO every 8 to 12 hours[2,36] are good initial choices. Final antimicrobial sensitivity and clinical symptoms dictate final antibiotic selection, some of which may be toxic to neonates. When necessary, the clinician must weigh the risks and benefits of antibiotics and determine when nursing should cease and neonates should be hand reared.

Antibiotics that should be used cautiously owing to neonatal toxicity include:

- Tetracyclines (discoloration of teeth).[6,26]
- Fluoroquinolones (impaired cartilage development).[6] Controversy surrounds its use in neonatal/pediatric populations; however, the benefits may outweigh the risk of cartilage abnormalities.[37] The risk may be low in non–weight-bearing neonates less than 3 weeks of age, but informed consent with the client is recommended.
- Sulfas (autoimmune disorders and bone marrow suppression).[6]
- Chloramphenicol (safety to neonates has been questioned owing to its association with toxicity in infants,[3] although it has good penetration into milk).

Analgesia

Studies confirming the efficacy and safety of using analgesics during lactation are sparse. The clinician must weigh risks and benefits of their use.

- Opioids are used to control pain for perioperative procedures in lactating dams and their short-term use has been reported to be safe.[38] In an effort to minimize side effects, avoid nursing neonates during peak drug levels and, when possible, time nursing before the next dose.[38]
- Tramadol HCL is a centrally acting opiate-like agonist that has primarily μ-receptor activity, but also inhibits reuptake of serotonin and norepinephrine.[37] These actions contribute to its analgesic properties. Sedation is a side effect and efficacy for pain control remains controversial. This author has not observed side effects in neonates.

Table 1
Antibiotics considered safe to use in pregnancy and lactation

Antibiotic	Lactation
Ampicillin Amoxicillin Cephalosporins (cefazolin, cefpodoxime, cephalexin) Clavulanic acid-amoxicillin Penicillin Ticarcillin/clavulanate	Excreted in milk in low concentrations
Erythromycin	Excreted into milk in moderate concentrations
Azithromycin	Accumulate in milk because of ion trapping

- Nonsteroidal antiinflammatory drugs provide effective pain relief to the dam with mastitis; however, the neonates' exposure in milk is a concern.[9] Until studies evaluate the effect on renal maturation of the neonate, it is recommended that nonsteroidal antiinflammatory drugs be used cautiously and short term.[38]

Nonpharmacologic treatments

- Moist hot packing of gland(s) softens mammary tissue and allows the expression of infected milk. Frequency depends on inflammation, but initially every 4 to 6 hours is ideal.
- Apply rinsed, cool cabbage leaves to engorged glands after hot packing. Cabbage contains antibiotic and anti-irritant properties.[39]
- If painful, apply a bandage or loose fitting shirt on the dam to protect gland from trauma and prevent nursing of the affected gland.
- When necessary for the dam's comfort, separate the dam from litter during initial healing and only allow nursing with supervision.
- The dam may continue to nurse neonates, even on the infected glands, unless the infected glands become too painful, abscessed, or gangrenous, or the dam is receiving medication that neonates should not consume in milk.

Surgical Treatment

Surgical debridement is necessary if there is necrotic, abscessed, or gangrenous mammary tissue (**Figs. 4–6**).

ACUTE METRITIS

Metritis is an acute infection involving the endometrium and the myometrium of the uterus and typically occurs 1 to 7 days after whelping.[3,40] Bacteria ascend into the uterus during parturition when the cervix is dilated.

Patient History

Dams are at greater risk of developing metritis when there has been retention of fetuses, placentas, and fetal tissues during parturition, or if the dam delivered a large litter, had a prolonged labor, underwent obstetric manipulations, or developed secondary uterine inertia.[41,42] Dams with metritis are ill and prompt medical care will optimize the outcome.

Physical Examination

Clinical symptoms support the diagnosis. The dam is lethargic and febrile, and often has a temperature exceeding 103.5° F.[3] She usually has malodorous, voluminous, purulent, and frequently blood-tinged uterine discharge. Palpation of the abdomen and uterus may elicit a pain response. Milk production may decrease and the neonates' daily weight gains may decrease to less than 5% to 10%.

Diagnosis

- A CBC reveals leukocytosis with a left shift.[43]
- Cytologic examination of uterine fluid shows large numbers of degenerate neutrophils, red blood cells, bacteria, and debris.[44]
- Fluid is obtained from the cranial vagina using a double guarded vaginal culture swab and submitted for culture and sensitivity (**Figs. 7 and 8**).
- Abdominal radiographs allow for the evaluation of the uterus and the presence of any retained fetuses.

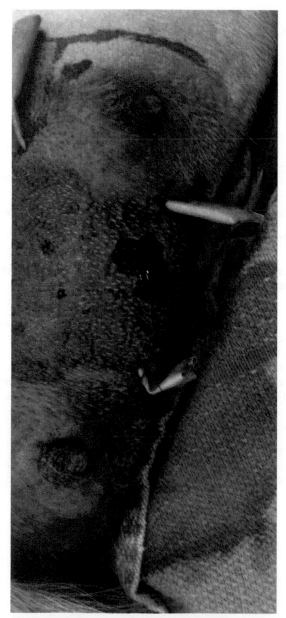

Fig. 4. Gangrenous mastitis characterized by swelling, deep ulceration, and necrosis of the skin. Drains were removed and surgical debridement performed.

- Abdominal ultrasound examination allows for the evaluation of retained placentas, uterine fluid, uterine lumen/walls, and for any free abdominal fluid. The uterus is easily identified after parturition[45] and the lumen may be of mixed echogenicity. There is a lack of a progressive decrease in uterine lumen and horn width with metritis.[46] Uterine involution is not normally complete on ultrasound imaging until 15 weeks postpartum.[45]

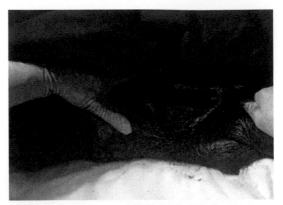

Fig. 5. Appearance of surgical site after necrotic mammary tissue has been excised.

Pharmacologic Treatments

Fluid therapy

Intravenous or subcutaneous fluid therapy is often necessary to stabilize the dam with metritis that is febrile, septic, and lethargic.

Antibiotics

E coli is the most common bacteria cultured in metritis[6,26,44]; however, other bacteria that are often present are *Klebsiella* spp, *Pseudomonas* spp., *Pasteurella* spp,[9] *Staphylococcus* spp, *Streptococcus* spp, and *Proteus* spp.[6,9]

If the dam is nursing, safe immediate antimicrobial therapy includes ampicillin, amoxicillin, cefazolin, or ticarcillin/clavulanic acid.[6] Aminoglycosides, fluoroquinolones, and third-generation cephalosporins are bactericidal against *E coli*,[6] but the final choice of antibiotics is based on the final antimicrobial sensitivity and should be tailored to the safety of the dam and neonates.

Prostaglandin therapy

Prostaglandin F2α (PGF2α; Dinoprost Tromethamine, Lutalyse) is a natural prostaglandin that effectively promotes uterine evacuation. It is preferred over the use of

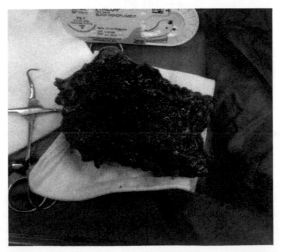

Fig. 6. Appearance of necrotic mammary tissue excised from gangrenous mastitis.

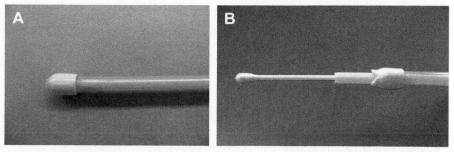

Fig. 7. A double-guarded vaginal culture swab that can be eased into vagina using a speculum, obtaining fluid from cranial vagina. Before (*A*) and after release (*B*) of culture swab.

oxytocin when it has been more than 24 hours post partum, owing to the variable amount of expression of oxytocin receptors on the uterus after parturition.[6,47] The therapeutic index for PGF2α in dogs is narrow, with a lethal dose for natural prostaglandins of 5.15 mg/kg.[48] An awareness of the side effects and complications associated with prostaglandin therapy must be considered and the clinician should decide on appropriateness of its use for each patient. Side effects include tachycardia, panting, anxiety, hypersalivation, diarrhea, vomiting, and urination,[12,49,50] and are known to be dose dependent and to diminish with repetition.[49] Effects are usually evident within 30 minutes after an injection and persist for 20 to 30 minutes.[12] Uterine rupture, peritonitis, coagulopathies, and sepsis are also potential complications.[27] PGF2α is contraindicated if there is an increased concern for uterine rupture. There are many published doses for prostaglandin therapy and the clinician can tailor the dose and frequency of administration for each patient. This author suggests considering the lower dose therapy initially because it is often effective with minimal side effects. Therapy is typically given for 3 to 5 days until there is diminished fluid in the uterus. Serial ultrasound examinations of uterus confirm resolution.

- 10 to 50 µg/kg SQ 3 to 5 times per day[49]
- 50 µg/kg SQ every 12 or 24 hours (frequently effective in author's experience)
- 100 µg/kg SQ every 12[51] or 24 hours[52]

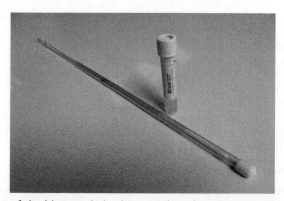

Fig. 8. Entire view of double-guarded culture swab and transport media.

Nonpharmacologic treatments

- Frequent baths remove infected uterine fluids off the tail and perineum, and prevent bacterial contamination of the neonates
- Short walks promote uterine drainage and minimize side effects of PGF2α therapy.

Surgical Treatment

- If medical management does not evacuate a retained fetus or fetal parts, surgical removal is necessary.
- Ovariohysterectomy is indicated in severe cases.

PUERPERAL ECLAMPSIA (HYPOCALCEMIA)

Clinical symptoms of eclampsia are related to low levels of ionized calcium in the extracellular space,[3,53] which alters cell membrane potentials and allows spontaneous discharge of nerve fibers to induce tonic or tonoclonic contractions.[27] The demand for calcium is high postpartum and the cause for hypocalcemia may be related to the ossification of fetal skeletons, production of milk, poor gastrointestinal absorption of dietary calcium, and parathyroid atrophy caused by improper nutrition and supplementation.[42,53]

Patient History

Eclampsia typically occurs during the first 4 weeks of lactation[1]; however, symptoms may arise prenatally on rare occasions.[42] Although small breed dams with large litters are typical,[54] any size and breed of dog may develop the condition.[55] Calcium supplementation or ingesting calcium containing foods during gestation inhibits parathyroid hormone secretion, predisposing the dam to eclampsia during lactation.[56] A dam with heavy lactational demands[53] or one that is reluctant to maintain adequate nutrition[57] is also at risk.

Physical Examination

The clinical signs may initially be nonspecific behavior changes; however, symptoms can quickly progress to a life-threatening condition. The most common clinical signs of eclampsia are listed in **Box 3**.[1,9,42,55,56]

Diagnosis

History, signalment, and physical examination findings are usually sufficient to diagnose eclampsia; however, obtaining ionized and total serum calcium levels will confirm the diagnosis. CBC and biochemistry profiles will help to assess for any concurrent problems such as hypoglycemia,[9,27,57] hypophosphatemia,[9,57] hypomagnesemia,[57,58] and metabolic acidosis.[55] Because normal calcium values vary among reference and in-clinic laboratories, clinicians must consider the symptoms of the dam and the calcium values obtained using their own laboratories when making a diagnosis. In general, published guidelines for diagnosing hypocalcemia in dams include total serum calcium of less than 9 mg/dL[9,53,59] and ionized calcium of less than 1.00 mmol/L.[53,59] In a retrospective study, all dams but one presenting with clinical eclampsia had ionized calcium values less than or equal to 0.8 mmol/L with reference range of 1.13 to 1.33 mmol/L.[55]

Immediate Pharmacologic Treatment

Immediate treatment is a slow intravenous infusion of 10% calcium gluconate to effect at a dose of 5 to 15 mg/kg elemental calcium, corresponding with 0.54 to 1.61 mL/kg

---

Box 3
Common symptoms of eclampsia (hypocalcemia)

Restlessness

Poor mothering

Facial pruritis

Hyperthermia

Hypersalivation

Panting

Anxiousness/whining

Muscle fasciculation

Stiffness

Staggering

Dilated pupils

Tachycardia

Opisthotonos

Collapse/lateral recumbency

Involuntary tremors/twitching

Seizures

---

over 10 to 30 minutes.[12,36] Lower dose ranges have also been published and the average volumes ranges from 1 to 20 mL per dam intravenously.[1,27,56] During the calcium infusion, there is close monitoring of pulse, heart rate, and rhythm with a stethoscope and electrocardiography.[9,30] If bradycardia, arrhythmias, or vomiting occurs, the administration is discontinued until heart rate, rhythm, and electrocardiograph are normal.[27,53,56] Infusion can resume at a slower rate.[42]

A dam exhibiting seizure-type activity may be given diazepam (1-5 mg IV) or barbiturates to control symptoms.[30,53] Hypoglycemia, hyperthermia, or cerebral edema should be treated as necessary.[6] Corticosteroids are contraindicated, because they are calciuric.[6]

Stabilization

Once life-threatening symptoms are controlled, a SQ infusion of 10% calcium gluconate (not calcium chloride) diluted 50%[6,40] or 1:2[59] with physiologic saline is given and repeated every 8 hours until the dam is stable and able to receive oral supplementation.[6,59] The SQ infusion volume is based on the amount of calcium gluconate IV required during treatment of symptomatic hypocalcemia.[59] Oral calcium carbonate supplementation is continued throughout lactation at a dose of 25 to 50 mg/kg/d (elemental calcium)[6] or generally 0.5 g (toy breeds) to 4 g (giant breeds) of elemental calcium orally per day.[37] Each 500-mg calcium carbonate tablet (TUMS, GlaxoSmithKline, Middlesex, UK) supplies 200 mg of elemental calcium.

Nonpharmacologic Treatment

- Remove the dam from neonates for 12 to 24 hours, or permanently, depending on the dam's response to initial treatment and oral supplementation.

- If the dam is receiving adequate nutrition and is recovered, then gradually allow neonates to nurse while providing commercial milk supplementation.
- Optimize the nutrition of dam and feed a balanced diet while providing her with frequent opportunities to be away from the litter to eat and drink.[42]

Prevention

- Avoid oral calcium supplementation during pregnancy[59] and feeding diets high in legumes that contain phytates that could bind dietary calcium.[60]
- If the dam had previous eclampsia, recurrence may possibly be prevented by providing oral calcium supplementation only postpartum, but not during pregnancy.[27]
- Supplement large litters with milk replacer.[42]

SUMMARY

The dam experiences hormonal, physical, and behavioral changes during pregnancy, parturition, and lactation. As a result, there is an array of disorders that occur during the periparturient period. The conditions may be minor or severe, have a gradual or acute onset, and frequently pose a challenge to the clinician considering the dam's well-being directly affects the health of her offspring. With methodical and judicious evaluation, appropriate therapy can be instituted, resulting in a very rewarding outcome for the dam and her litter.

REFERENCES

1. Wallace M, Davidson AP. Abnormalities in pregnancy, parturition, and the periparturient period. In: Ettinger S, Feldman E, editors. Textbook of veterinary internal medicine. 4th edition. Philadelphia: W.B. Saunders; 1995. p. 1614–24.
2. Davidson AP. Postpartum disorders in the bitch and queen. 81st Western Veterinary Conference held at Las Vegas (NV), February 15–19, 2009. Available at: https://www.vin.com/doc/?id=3985422. Accessed April 24, 2017.
3. Johnston S, Root Kustritz M, Olson P. Periparturient disorders in the bitch. In: Kersey R, LeMelledo D, editors. Canine and feline theriogenology. Philadelphia: WB Saunders Co; 2001. p. 129–45.
4. Concannon PW. Understanding and monitoring canine pregnancy. Paper presented at the 30th World Congress of the World Small Animal Veterinary Association. Mexico City, Mexico, May 11–14, 2005.
5. Romagnoli S, Lopate C. Control of mammary gland function in the bitch and queen: a review. Clin Theriogenology 2012;4(3):196–205.
6. Wiebe VJ, Howard JP. Pharmacologic advances in canine and feline reproduction. Top Companion Anim Med 2009;24(2):71–99.
7. Argyle D. The mammary gland. In: Simpson G, England GCW, Harvey M, et al, editors. BSAVA manual of small animal reproduction and neonatology. Cheltenham (United Kingdom): British Small Animal Veterinary Association; 1998. p. 53–9.
8. Traas A, O'Connor C. Postpartum emergencies. Paper presented at the International Veterinary Emergency and Critical Symposium. Chicago (IL): September 9–13, 2009.
9. Lopate C. Reproductive physiology of canine pregnancy and parturition and conditions of the periparturient period. In: Lopate C, editor. Management of pregnant and neonatal dogs, cats, and exotic pets. Ames (IA): Wiley-Blackwell; 2012. p. 25–41.

10. Olson J, Olson PN. Disorders of the canine mammary gland. In: Morrow DA, editor. Current therapy in theriogenology: diagnosis, treatment, and prevention of reproductive diseases in small and large animals. 2nd edition. Philadelphia: Saunders; 1986. p. 506–9.

11. Hess M. Agalactia. In: VIN, editor. Canine Associate: VIN; 2014. Available at: https://www.vin.com/Members/Associate/Associate.plx?DiseaseId=555. Accessed April 1, 2018.

12. Plumb DC. Plumb's veterinary drug handbook. 8th edition. Stockholm (WI): Wiley Blackwell; 2015.

13. Greco DS. Nutritional supplements for pregnant and lactating bitches. Theriogenology 2008;70(3):393–6.

14. Johnson CA. Pregnancy management in the bitch. Theriogenology 2008;70(9): 1412–7.

15. Freshman JL. Look sharp! acupuncture in canine reproduction. Clin Theriogenology 2017;9(3):267–76.

16. Root Kustritz MV. History and physical examination of the neonate. In: Peterson ME, Kutzler MA, editors. Small animal pediatrics: the first 12 months of life. 1st edition. St Louis (MO): Saunders/Elsevier; 2011. p. 20–7.

17. Poffenbarger E, Olson P, Chandler M, et al. Use of adult dog serum as a substitute for colostrum in the neonatal dog. Am J Vet Res 1991;52(8):1221–4.

18. Kirk CA. New concepts in pediatric nutrition. Vet Clin North Am Small Anim Pract 2001;31(2):369–92.

19. Mila H, Grellet A, Mariani C, et al. Natural and artificial hyperimmune solutions: impact on health in puppies. Reprod Domest Anim 2017;52(Suppl 2):163–9.

20. Lawler DF. Neonatal and pediatric care of the puppy and kitten. Theriogenology 2008;70(3):384–92.

21. Chastant-Maillard S, Freyburger L, Marcheteau E, et al. Timing of the intestinal barrier closure in puppies. Reprod Domest Anim 2012;47(Suppl 6):190–3.

22. Gillette DD, Filkins M. Factors affecting antibody transfer in the newborn puppy. Am J Physiol 1966;210(2):419–22.

23. Bouchard G, Plata-Madrid H, Youngquist RS, et al. Absorption of an alternate source of immunoglobulin in pups. Am J Vet Res 1992;53(2):230–3.

24. Lopate C. Canine neonatal physiology, behavior, and socialization. In: Lopate C, editor. Management of pregnant and neonatal dogs, cats, and exotic pets. Ames (IA): Wiley-Blackwell; 2012. p. 93–127.

25. Greer ML. Neonatal and pediatric care. In: Cann CC, editor. Canine reproduction and neonatology: a practical guide for veterinarians, veterinary staff, and breeders. Jackson (WY): Teton NewMedia; 2015. p. 140–215.

26. White R. Diseases of the mammary glands. In: Morgan R, editor. Handbook of small animal practice. 5th edition. St Louis (MO): Elsevier; 2008. p. 593–602.

27. Feldman EC, Nelson RW. Periparturient diseases. In: Feldman E, Nelson RW, editors. Canine and feline endocrinology and reproduction. 3rd edition. St Louis (MO): W.B. Saunders; 2004. p. 808–34.

28. Olson PN, Olson AL. Cytologic evaluation of canine milk. Vet Medicine Small Anim Clinician 1984;(79):641–6.

29. Root Kustritz MV. Reproductive behavior of small animals. Theriogenology 2005; 64(3):734–46.

30. Greer ML. Managing the immediate postpartum period in the bitch. In: Cann CC, editor. Canine reproduction and neonatology: a practical guide for veterinarians, veterinary staff, and breeders. Jackson (WY): Teton NewMedia; 2015. p. 128–38.

31. Root Kustritz MV. Mammary disorders. The practical veterinarian small animal theriogenology. St Louis (MO): Butterworth-Heinemann; 2003. p. 421–46.
32. Murai A, Maruyama S, Nagata M, et al. Mastitis caused by Mycobacterium kansasii infection in a dog. Vet Clin Pathol 2013;42(3):377–81.
33. Hasegawa T, Fujii M, Fukada T, et al. Platelet abnormalities in a dog suffering from gangrenous mastitis by Staphylococcus aureus infection. J Vet Med Sci 1993; 55(1):169–71.
34. Sager M, Remmers C. Perinatal mortality in dogs. Clinical, bacteriological and pathological studies. Tierarztl Prax 1990;18(4):415–9 [in German].
35. Papich M. Effects of drugs on pregnancy. In: Kirk R, editor. Current veterinary therapy X. Small animal practice. WB Saunders; 1989. p. 1291–9.
36. Jutkowitz LA. Reproductive emergencies. Vet Clin North Am Small Anim Pract 2005;35(2):397–420, vii.
37. Plumb DC. Drugs in neonates: principles and guesses. Paper presented at the SFT Annual Conference & SFT/ACT Symposia. Lexington, Kentucky, August 4–7, 2004.
38. Mathews KA. Pain management for the pregnant, lactating, and neonatal to pediatric cat and dog. Vet Clin North Am Small Anim Pract 2008;38(6): 1291–308, vi-vii.
39. Davls M, IBCLC. The cabbage cure. Paper presented at the Therio Conference, Canine Seminar and Wet Lab. Asheville, NC, 2016.
40. Macintire DK. Emergencies of the female reproductive tract. Vet Clin North Am Small Anim Pract 1994;24(6):1173–88.
41. Olson PN, Jones RL, Mather EC. The use and misuse of vaginal cultures in diagnosing reproductive diseases in the bitch. In: Morrow D, editor. Current therapy in theriogenology. Philadelphia: WB Saunders; 1986. p. 469–75.
42. Johnson C. Postpartum and mammary disorders. In: Nelson RW, Couto GC, editors. Small animal internal medicine. 5th edition. St Louis (MO): Mosby/Elsevier; 2009. p. 944–9.
43. Smith FO. Postpartum diseases. Vet Clin North Am Small Anim Pract 1986;16(3): 521–4.
44. Simpson G, England GCW, Harvey M. British small animal veterinary association. Parturition. In: Simpson G, editor. BSAVA manual of small animal reproduction and neonatology. Cheltenham (United Kingdom): British Small Animal Veterinary Association; 1998. p. 127–42.
45. England G, Yeager A, Concannon PW. Ultrasound imaging of the reproductive tract of the bitch. In: Concannon PW, England G, Verstegen III J, et al, editors. Recent advances in small animal reproduction. Ithaca (NY): International Veterinary Information Service; 2003. Document No. A1203.0703. Available at: http://www.ivis.org/ advances/Concannon/england/chapter.asp?LA=1. Accessed April 1, 2018.
46. Davidson AP, Baker TW. Reproductive ultrasound of the bitch and queen. Top Companion Anim Med 2009;24(2):55–63.
47. Grundy SA, Davidson AP. Theriogenology question of the month. Acute metritis secondary to retained fetal membranes and a retained nonviable fetus. J Am Vet Med Assoc 2004;224(6):844–7.
48. Sokolowski JH, Geng S. Effect of prostaglandin F2alpha-THAM in the bitch. J Am Vet Med Assoc 1977;170(5):536–7.
49. Verstegen J, Dhaliwal G, Verstegen-Onclin K. Mucometra, cystic endometrial hyperplasia, and pyometra in the bitch: advances in treatment and assessment of future reproductive success. Theriogenology 2008;70(3):364–74.
50. Henderson RT. Prostaglandin therapeutics in the bitch and queen. Aust Vet J 1984;61(10):317–9.

51. Freshman J. Pyometra and beyond: presentation and treatment of uterine infection in the bitch. Paper presented at the ACVIM Forum Proceedings. Dallas (TX), May 29-June 1, 2002.
52. Davidson A. Update: therapeutics for reproductive disorders in small animal practice. Paper presented at the ACVIM Forum Proceedings. Minneapolis (MN), June 9–12, 2004.
53. Davidson AP. Reproductive causes of hypocalcemia. Top Companion Anim Med 2012;27(4):165–6.
54. Austad R, Bjerkas E. Eclampsia in the bitch. J Small Anim Pract 1976;17(12): 793–8.
55. Drobatz KJ, Casey KK. Eclampsia in dogs: 31 cases (1995-1998). J Am Vet Med Assoc 2000;217(2):216–9.
56. Biddle D, Macintire DK. Obstetrical emergencies. Clin Tech Small Anim Pract 2000;15(2):88–93.
57. Jackson PGG. Postparturient problems in the dog and cat. Handbook of veterinary obstetrics. 2nd edition. New York: Saunders; 2004. p. 233–7.
58. Aroch I, Srebro H, Shpigel NY. Serum electrolyte concentrations in bitches with eclampsia. Vet Rec 1999;145(11):318–20.
59. Nelson R, Couto GC. Electrolyte imbalances. In: Nelson R, Couto G, editors. Small animal internal medicine. 5th edition. St Louis (MO): Mosby/Elsevier; 2009. p. 864–83.
60. Olson P. Periparturient diseases of the bitch. Paper presented at the Proceedings of the Society for Theriogenology, September 16–17, 1988. p. 19–35.

Small Animal Neonatal Health

Robyn R. Wilborn, DVM, MS

KEYWORDS

- Neonate • Apgar • Viability • Puppy • Kitten

KEY POINTS

- Adequate warmth for neonates is essential and is often overlooked.
- Glucose levels and hydration status must be maintained by frequent feedings or medical intervention.
- Fetal viability score sheets and neonatal weight charts are easy to use and provide critical information for both the owner and the medical team.
- The single best indicator of neonatal well-being for owners is steady weight gain.

INTRODUCTION
Educating the Veterinary Team

Depending on the veterinary college you attended, small animal neonatology may or may not have even been part of the curriculum. The teaching of small animal theriogenology topics in the veterinary curriculum has evolved significantly over the last 20 years. In fact, one could argue that what is taught on this particular subject has changed more during that time than any other discipline within our profession.

Those who graduated before 1990 were likely taught a great deal about theriogenology and the basic care of neonates because they were accustomed to seeing patients who were sexually intact, having either planned or unplanned litters that required care. In contrast, those who graduated between 1990 and 2005 were likely taught very little small animal theriogenology except to neuter every dog and cat, in a concerted effort to control the pet overpopulation problem at that time. Overall, this group of veterinarians is the least likely to have basic knowledge of neonatal care simply because most of their patients were not intact.

For those who have graduated since 2005, there has been a major shift in the mindset of both pet owners and also our profession. Therefore, we are all beginning to question and investigate when, and even *whether*, some pets should be

Disclosure Statement: The author has nothing to disclose.
Department of Clinical Sciences, Bailey Small Animal Teaching Hospital, Auburn University, 1220 Wire Road, Auburn, AL 36849-5540, USA
E-mail address: wilborn@auburn.edu

Vet Clin Small Anim 48 (2018) 683–699
https://doi.org/10.1016/j.cvsm.2018.02.011
0195-5616/18/© 2018 Elsevier Inc. All rights reserved.

vetsmall.theclinics.com

gonadectomized. The veterinarians who are graduating now will be the ones to encounter this paradigm shift in pet ownership as it relates to the decision of neutering and, thus, will likely see more intact dogs and cats and, consequently, more neonates, throughout their career.

This same trajectory of reproductive and neonatal knowledge can be extrapolated to the veterinary support staff as well. It should never be assumed that support staff, even those who are credentialed, are trained in neonatal care. Both veterinarians and support staff in the veterinary hospital can benefit from a periodic review of basic principles of neonatal clinical care. *With both veterinary students and support staff, the author repeatedly emphasizes the most common threats to newborns: hypothermia, hypoglycemia, and dehydration.* Adding an annual training session in basic neonatology for staff can pay big dividends in client retention/satisfaction as well as improve outcomes for your patients. This is one area of veterinary medicine where having a strong knowledge base of simple physiology and common clinical presentations for neonates (hypothermia, hypoglycemia, dehydration) can often mitigate adverse outcomes.

Educating Owners

In contrast to the veterinary team, owners are often armed with vast experience in caring for neonates. In these situations, both veterinarians and support staff can benefit from learning useful tips and tricks from experienced breeders. In the author's clinic, approximately half of the clients are experienced breeders. Consequently, that also means that the other half are novice breeders and require more help from the hospital team. The author has discovered that once the support staff is comfortable, they actually enjoy educating owners.

The author has also discovered that owners enjoy the interaction with the support staff (vs the doctors) because they are more comfortable asking questions and clarifying instructions. These educational sessions with clients are time consuming for the support staff but are of utmost importance with novice owners. The author commonly sees neonates lost to poor mothering/husbandry, and many of these situations can be avoided by educating owners to the early warning signs of neonates that are failing to thrive.

Steady weight gain is the author's number one parameter that is stressed to owners. To emphasize this point, the author's clinic records birth weights and sends home a weight chart for owners to complete for the first week of neonatal life (**Fig. 1**). The owners are instructed to purchase a small scale that measures in grams or ounces and to record the weight of the neonates twice daily on the chart. These scales are inexpensive and readily available on the kitchen aisle of local retail stores (**Fig. 2**). Steady weight gain is the number one indication of well-being in neonates. Failure to gain weight is often the first indication of a problem and can be noted by astute owners even before development of clinical signs, such as lethargy or inappetence. Encourage all hospital staff to reinforce with owners the 3 most important threats to neonates: hypothermia, hypoglycemia, and dehydration.

Key Points for Both Owners and the Veterinary Team

- Warmth first
- Nutrition second (*body temperature >95°F before feeding*)
- Stimulate urination/defection if dam does not
- Steady weight gain is single best indicator of neonatal well-being

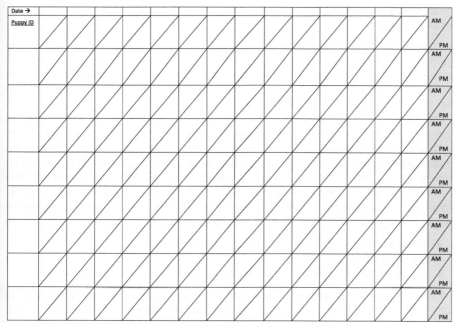

Date →																
Puppy ID																AM
																PM
																AM
																PM
																AM
																PM
																AM
																PM
																AM
																PM
																AM
																PM
																AM
																PM
																AM
																PM
																AM
																PM

Please weigh the puppies twice daily

Fig. 1. Example of a neonatal weight chart.

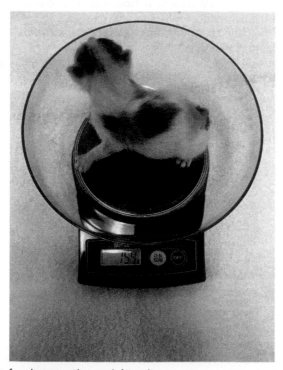

Fig. 2. Gram scale for documenting weight gain.

EVALUATION AT BIRTH
Resuscitation

Neonatal resuscitation in the veterinary hospital is most often done during Cesarean delivery but may also be performed following natural delivery. In the case of a Cesarean delivery, the doctor will still be in surgery while staff members perform the resuscitation of the puppies or kittens. Thus, staff training and confidence in these procedures is of paramount importance.

The obvious difference in neonates born via Cesarean delivery versus natural delivery is the effect of anesthetic drugs on the neonate. If an opioid is used as a pre-medication, naloxone may be given to neonates to reverse those effects. Preferred induction agents are propofol (2–6 mg/kg intravenously [IV]) or alfaxalone (1–2 mg/kg IV) with isoflurane or sevoflurane gas inhalation for maintenance. Although one study demonstrated transient improvement in neonate viability scores using alfaxalone, there was no overall difference in puppy survival; this author sees no significant benefit in using one versus the other.[1,2] The overarching goals for Cesarean delivery are

- Safety for dam and neonates, with minimal stress to both
- Efficiency of the clinical team
- Selection of anesthetic drugs/protocols that are short-acting or reversible

Aside from the use of naloxone, the resuscitation principles discussed later apply to both Cesarean and natural deliveries. In general, neonates from natural deliveries require less assistance and resuscitation.

For resuscitation of neonates, consider the following points:

- *Warm, well-lit workspace for resuscitation efforts:* A wet table filled with hot water and covered with a towel makes a nice, warm workspace for this purpose (**Fig. 3**). All of the necessary tools (light, oxygen, and so forth) are within reach; the shape of the table allows several staff members to work on the same litter together, in contrast to a countertop workstation.
- *Vigorous rubbing:* It is no longer recommended to swing puppies/kittens; vigorous rubbing and gentle tilting in a downward direction is safer and more effective.
- *Suction mouth and nasal passages:*
  - The author prefers the use of a DeLee catheter (also called a neonatal mucus trap; **Fig. 4**).

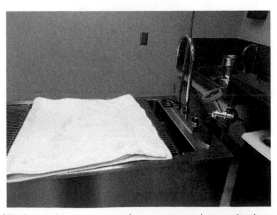

Fig. 3. Wet table filled with hot water used as a neonatal resuscitation workspace.

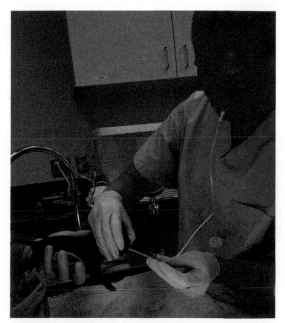

Fig. 4. Use of a mucous trap for clearing neonatal airways.

- ○ The DeLee is inexpensive, user friendly, and can suction more effectively in narrow airways. One can also quantify the volume of secretions that are removed (**Fig. 5**), which is another advantage of the DeLee versus a traditional bulb syringe.
- *Acupuncture*: If no spontaneous respirations are noted, a 25-gauge needle placed in the nasal philtrum (Governing vessel [GV] 26) (**Fig. 6**) will help stimulate breathing.[3]
- *Mask:* If needed, provide oxygen via a small, well-fitted mask.
  - ○ Flow-by methods are acceptable, but a small mask is preferred. One can provide some degree of positive-pressure ventilation using a small mask (20–30 breaths per minute).
  - ○ In the author's hospital, intubation is a last resort. It is somewhat difficult to perform and can cause trauma. The author prefers a 5F to 6F red rubber catheter for intubation, but a 12-gauge to 16-gauge IV catheter can be used as well.
- *No response:* If there is no response with the aforementioned measures, consider the following:
  - ○ Perform chest compressions at 1 to 2 beats per second using the thumb and forefinger.
  - ○ The author uses the aforementioned methods for 1 to 2 minutes before using medications. All medications listed next can be given either IV (jugular or umbilical vein) or sublingually:
    - Naloxone (0.1 mg/kg): if the dam was given an opioid as a premedication, naloxone will reverse those effects; it is not necessary in all cases.[4]
    - Doxapram (0.1 mL) is ineffective if the brain is hypoxic. Use the aforementioned methods first; the neonate needs to be alive greater than 15 minutes for doxapram to be effective. It was once used routinely but is now used as a last resort.[5,6]

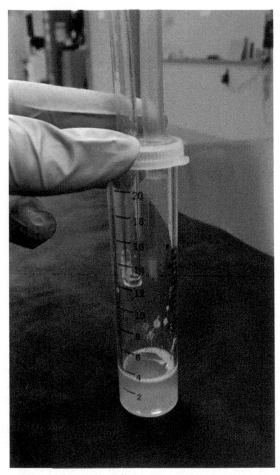

Fig. 5. Quantifying volume of aspirated fluid.

- Atropine is ineffective in neonates less than 14 days of age.[7]
- Epinephrine (0.1 mg/kg) is usually ineffective but used as a last resort; continue ventilation and chest compressions while administering.[8]

Apgar and Fetal Viability Scoring

Once immediate resuscitation is successful, attention of the veterinary team can then be directed toward an objective measurement of fetal well-being using a scoring system for each neonate. This step is often overlooked. However, it is simple for hospital staff to perform, takes very little time, and provides an objective assessment of each neonate. These findings can then guide the veterinary team to focus on the neonates that may need more clinical support in the first few hours.

Most people are conversationally familiar with the Apgar scoring method used in human medicine to assess infants. The term *Apgar* is derived from the name of the physician, Dr Virginia Apgar, who developed the scoring system in 1953. Since that time, the word *Apgar* has also been used as an acronym to help medical staff remember *A*ppearance, *P*ulse, *G*rimace, *A*ctivity, and *R*espiration. Dr Apgar's method involved assigning a score of 0 to 2 in each of the 5 following categories, performed 60 minutes

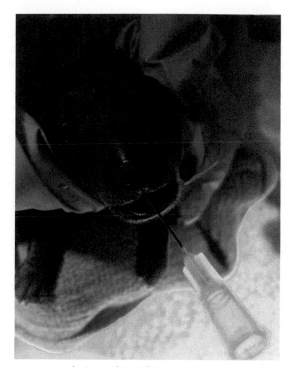

Fig. 6. Use of acupuncture techniques (GV 26) to stimulate neonatal respiration.

after birth of the infant: heart rate, spontaneous breathing, reflex irritability (response to a stimulus), muscle tone, and color of mucous membranes. A total score of 0 to 10 is obtained, with higher scores representing better neonatal viability and lower scores representing neonates that require increased medical support and have high mortality rates.[9,10]

Apgar scoring has been presented for use in a variety of animal species, including canine and feline neonates. Several variations of this scoring system have been adapted for use in veterinary medicine, with some scores ranging from 0 to 10[11] and other scores ranging from 0 to 14.[12] Outcomes have been assessed in several studies in recent years using the concept of Apgar scoring in canine neonates, and it has been found to be a good predictor of neonatal survivability. With scoring most commonly based on the 0 to 10 scale, scores of 6 or lower within the first 8 hours of life were associated with the highest neonatal mortality rate.[13–15]

In our hospital, we choose to use the Modified Apgar scoring system (range: 0–10) developed by Veronesi and colleagues[11] because of its simplicity, ease of use, and its similarity to the human model. Using this system, a score of 7 to 10 indicates no distress; 4 to 6 indicates moderate distress; 0 to 3 indicates severe distress. Parameters are self-explanatory and easily assessed by veterinary support staff, with the exception of reflex irritability (response to a stimulus). This response can be achieved several ways, but the author's preferred method is a light toe pinch or scruffing (pinching) of the nape of the neck to elicit a response.

In addition to Apgar scoring, assigning a fetal viability score for small animal neonates has also been described,[13] which includes an Apgar score combined with other reflexes indicating fetal viability. Rooting behavior (searching for teat), righting reflex, and suckle reflex should all be present at birth in vigorous newborn puppies and kittens. The author's hospital has developed a neonatal examination form (**Fig. 7**) that uses the Modified Apgar scoring system[11] and also includes aspects of the fetal viability reflexes (rooting and suckle) for an overall clinical assessment of each neonate.

The author recommends performing an Apgar score as soon as satisfactory resuscitation of the litter is achieved (~5 minutes after birth) and then again at 30 minutes and 1 to 2 hours. No matter the scoring system used or the time frame performed, hospital staff quickly learn the system and appreciate having an objective assessment of

Litter DOB:________________

Bitch's Patient Sticker/Info

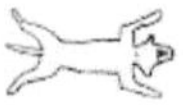

Color:________________ ID:________________

Sex:________________ Wt:________________

PE: Hard and soft palate ☐ Anus ☐ Urogenital ☐ Umbilicus ☐ Auscultation ☐ Abnormalities: ________________

	0	1	2	Score: 5 min	30 min	2 h
Mucous Membrane color	Cyanotic	pale	pink			
Heart Rate	<180 bpm	180–220 bpm	>220 bpm			
Respiratory effort/rate	No crying/ <6 rpm	Mild crying/ 6–15 rpm	Crying/ >15 rpm			
Reflex irritability	Absent	Feeble reaction (grimace)	Vigorous Reaction (grimace/vocalization)			
Mobility, muscle tone	Flaccid	Some tone in extremities	Active Movements			
Suckling (scored as -, +, ++)						
Rooting (scored as -, +, ++)						

Score: 7–10 = No distress; 4–6 = Moderate distress; 0–3 = severe distress Totals: ______ ______ ______

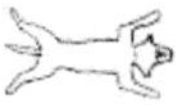

Color:________________ ID:________________

Sex:________________ Wt:________________

PE: Hard and soft palate ☐ Anus ☐ Urogenital ☐ Umbilicus ☐ Auscultation ☐ Abnormalities: ________________

	0	1	2	Score: 5 min	30 min	2 h
Mucous Membrane color	Cyanotic	pale	pink			
Heart Rate	<180 bpm	180–220 bpm	>220 bpm			
Respiratory effort/rate	No crying/ <6 rpm	Mild crying/ 6–15 rpm	Crying/ >15 rpm			
Reflex irritability	Absent	Feeble reaction (grimace)	Vigorous Reaction (grimace/vocalization)			
Mobility, muscle tone	Flaccid	Some tone in extremities	Active Movements			
Suckling (scored as -, +, ++)						
Rooting (scored as -, +, ++)						

Score: 7 –10 = No distress; 4–6 = Moderate distress; 0–3 = severe distress Totals: ______ ______ ______

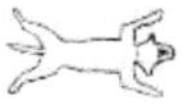

Color:________________ ID:________________

Sex:________________ Wt:________________

PE: Hard and soft palate ☐ Anus ☐ Urogenital ☐ Umbilicus ☐ Auscultation ☐ Abnormalities: ________________

	0	1	2	Score: 5 min	30 min	2 h
Mucous Membrane color	Cyanotic	pale	pink			
Heart Rate	<180 bpm	180–220 bpm	>220 bpm			
Respiratory effort/rate	No crying/ <6 rpm	Mild crying/ 6–15 rpm	Crying/ >15 rpm			
Reflex irritability	Absent	Feeble reaction (grimace)	Vigorous Reaction (grimace/vocalization)			
Mobility, muscle tone	Flaccid	Some tone in extremities	Active Movements			
Suckling (scored as -, +, ++)						
Rooting (scored as -, +, ++)						

Score: 7–10 = No distress; 4–6 = Moderate distress; 0–3 = severe distress Totals: ______ ______ ______

Fig. 7. Example of a neonatal examination form.

each newborn to help focus clinical efforts on the neonates needing the most assistance.

Neonatal Examination Checklist

The neonatal examination form used in the author's hospital (see **Fig. 7**) also includes a simple physical examination checklist for each newborn puppy or kitten. Several congenital defects can be detected immediately after birth, but one must be systematic and ensure that each newborn is examined carefully. Many of these congenital defects warrant euthanasia because of a poor prognosis, and this decision is best made at birth rather than discovering the problem later. A normal palate is illustrated in **Fig. 8** in comparison with a severe cleft palate, or palatoschisis, in **Fig. 9**. Examples of other common congenital defects can be seen in **Figs. 10–13**. This body systems checklist on the neonatal examination form provides a good reminder for hospital staff to confirm that each neonate has been examined and did not get missed.

Birthweights are also recorded at this time, and puppies or kittens are identified using a reliable method. Owners often prefer colored collars for identification; but if those are not yet available, then the author's clinic will use a very small dot of fingernail polish in different colors applied to the dorsum of each puppy to serve as temporary identification. Of course this is particularly important for large litters of solid-colored breeds (eg, Golden retrievers), whereby the neonates are indistinguishable from one another. One must stress to owners the importance of reliable identification for the purposes of weighing the neonates twice daily for the first several days.

Create your own neonatal assessment form or use the template provided in **Fig. 7** and adapt it to your needs. Forms should include the following for each neonate:

- Apgar and viability scoring system of your choice
- Neonatal examination checklist for congenital defects

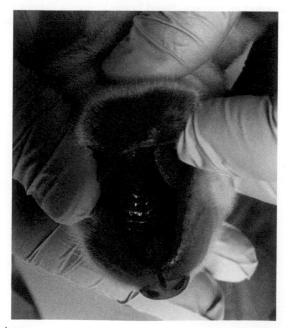

Fig. 8. Normal palate.

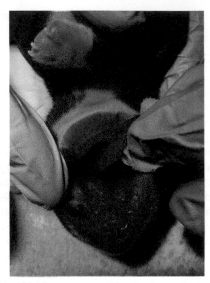

Fig. 9. Cleft palate (palatoschisis).

- Birth weight
- Sex and identification (color of collar/paint)

CONSIDERATIONS FOR THE FIRST WEEK OF LIFE
Feeding/Daily Weight Gain

Steady weight gain is the single best indicator of fetal well-being and can be easily measured and recorded by owners. Send home a simple weight chart (see **Fig. 1**) for owners to record body weights twice daily using a kitchen scale that measures

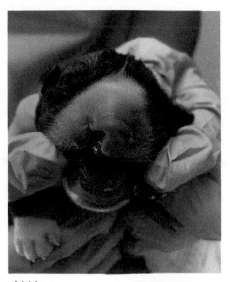

Fig. 10. Cleft lip (cheiloschisis).

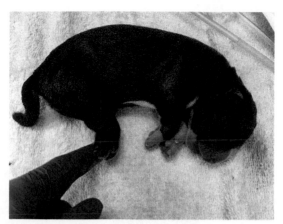

Fig. 11. Severe bilateral ankylosis of rear limbs.

in either grams or ounces (see **Fig. 2**). Low birth weight is the single greatest risk factor in neonatal mortality[16]; thus, it is imperative that smaller neonates have diligent care, including accurate records of weight gain. After the first 24 hours of life, all neonates should gain steadily. A good rule of thumb is a weight gain of 10% per day as a minimum. Failure to gain weight is often noticed even before the development of clinical signs of illness, and early medical intervention is paramount with neonates.

Failure to adequately gain weight in the first week could be due to several reasons. One common reason is poor mothering, with failure of the dam to adequately stimulate urination/defection or failure of the dam to allow adequate nursing sessions because of nervousness or inexperience. Once identified, these challenges can be managed

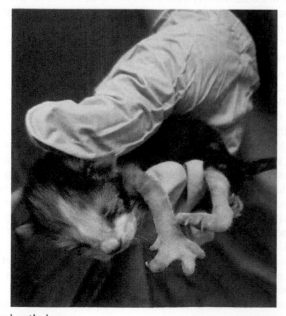

Fig. 12. Phalangeal pathology.

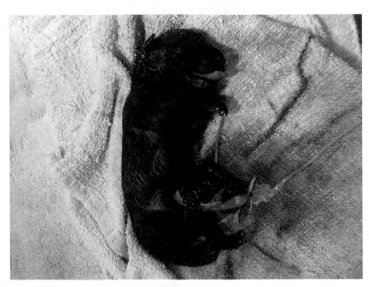

Fig. 13. Gastroschisis in a schnauzer neonate.

by the owner by limiting stress to the dam, encouraging time spent in the whelping box, and using a warm, wet cloth on the genital area of the neonates several times daily to stimulate evacuation. The appetite of constipated neonates will improve quickly following stimulated evacuation.

Another common reason is agalactia in the dam. If agalactia is suspected, treatment can be initiated using either domperidone (0.1 mg/kg by mouth twice a day) or metoclopramide (0.2–0.4 mg/kg by mouth 3 times a day); puppies will require supplemental feedings (ie, tube or bottle feeding between nursing sessions) for a few days until milk production increases.[17] *With supplemental feedings, remember that neonates must be warmed to a normal body temperature (95°F–99°F for neonates <1 week of age) before feeding to avoid gastrointestinal ileus.* Keeping neonates warm with ambient temperatures between 98°F and 101°F will help prevent proliferation of canine herpesvirus and consequent fading puppy syndrome.

Agalactia is also an important consideration in patients undergoing elective cesarean delivery. In these patients, neonates are delivered surgically approximately 12 to 36 hours sooner than Mother Nature would have preferred; it is common for dams to be agalactic in the first few hours. Although there have been anecdotal reports of using oxytocin to hasten this process, it is the author's experience that these dams will begin a normal lactation within 24 hours without any treatment and the puppies can easily be managed with supplemental tube feeding in the interim. Puppies and kittens not nursing actively from the dam within 12 hours after birth are at risk of failure of passive transfer and subsequent septicemia and should be supplemented with oral colostrum, serum, or plasma if they are less than 12 hours old or subcutaneous (SQ) serum or plasma if they are greater than 12 hours old (see discussion later).

Certainly there are more severe causes for lack of weight gain and failure to thrive that are not as easily managed as those described earlier. These causes include neonatal septicemia from bacterial pathogens and debilitation from viral pathogens, such as herpesvirus; these are discussed in detail elsewhere and generally carry a much poorer prognosis.

Thermoregulation, Hypothermia, and Hyperthermia

It should be emphasized that physical examination of a canine or feline neonate will differ from that of an adult animal in several ways. The first and most important aspect is thermoregulation. Neonates are unable to regulate their body temperature and depend on a warm environment and close contact with the dam to maintain adequate body temperature. When they are away from the dam for veterinary examinations and other reasons, one must take great care to keep them warm and in close contact with littermates whenever possible. This requirement cannot be overemphasized, especially with veterinary staff or owners who may be inexperienced with neonates.

Normal body temperature for neonates less than 1 week of age is 95°F to 99°F. When sick or limp neonates are presented to the hospital, they must be warmed carefully and slowly (~2°F/h). *Body temperature must increase to 95°F or greater before feeding in order to avoid gastrointestinal ileus, which can become serious and life threatening.*[18] It is also important to remember that neonates are unable to move away from heat sources, so extreme caution should be exercised to ensure that they do not overheat, especially when using sources such as heating lamps and heating pads. Unfortunately, this is a common mistake of inexperienced owners. Depending on the severity of the hyperthermia and length of exposure, those situations are often associated with high mortality rates for the puppies or kittens.

Hypoglycemia and Dehydration

Unlike adult animals, neonates are unable to use glycogen stores and are unable to maintain adequate blood glucose levels without frequent feedings. Blood glucose can easily be measured, just as with an adult animal. However, when presented with a sick, limp neonate, hypoglycemia is most commonly assumed and treatment is often initiated even without blood glucose measurement. Dextrose solutions can be used orally in a weak neonate that still maintains a suckle reflex. For more debilitated patients, the IV or intraosseous route is preferred.

In addition to hypoglycemia, newborn puppies and kittens are also very susceptible to dehydration. The clinical tools used for determining dehydration in an adult animal, such as skin turgor/tent and packed cell volume, are not reliable in neonates. A quick and useful technique is to gently stimulate urination and subjectively assess the color of the urine. Urine in a normal, well-hydrated neonate should be almost colorless. Thus, neonatal urine that is yellow is often an indirect indication of dehydration. As with hypoglycemia discussed earlier, dehydration is usually assumed rather than diagnosed when presented with a sick neonate. Oral fluids can be given if depression is mild and a suckle reflex present, but IV or intraosseous fluids are preferred. Isotonic solutions without dextrose may be given SQ, although the response will be slower. No matter the route of fluid/dextrose administration, remembering to warm the solution first will help to avoid iatrogenic heat loss and subsequent hypothermia.

Administration of Serum or Plasma in the Absence of Colostrum

If owners are uncertain of colostrum intake, serum or plasma can be administered to newborn puppies and kittens in an effort to provide antibodies. The serum or plasma can be harvested from any well-vaccinated adult animal. The author prefers to use another animal from the same household whenever possible to provide the maximum protection for pathogens specific to that environment. When the litter is large, or in cats and small-breed dogs, the author avoids using the dam, as the amount of required blood may be large. Pooling serum from different donors, especially in the case of cats, has been practiced in the author's clinic. Evidence-based guidelines for administration of serum or plasma to neonates are lacking, but **Table 1** describes common practices regarding volume and route of administration.

For canine neonates, research has shown that gut closure begins as early as 4 to 8 hours after birth, with complete closure occurring between 16 to 24 hours. In that study, puppies who ingested colostrum between birth and 4 hours had the highest immunoglobulin absorption rate.[19] Thus, the ideal window for oral administration of colostrum/serum/plasma is within the first 12 hours of life. If neonates are less than12 hours old, the serum or plasma may be given orally via tube-feeding techniques. If they are more than 12 hours old, then SQ administration is preferred.

It should be emphasized that colostrum is always the best source of antibodies. Some owners mistakenly think that administering serum or plasma is preferable to colostrum, but this is simply not the case. In a 2015 study by Mila and colleagues,[20] antibody concentrations were compared between serum and colostrum of the same dams. Immunoglobulin G concentration was found to be an average of 2.8 times greater in the colostrum than in the serum, confirming that colostrum is always preferable when available.

Postoperative Pain Medication Following Cesarean Delivery: Potential Risk to Neonates

Postoperative pain management for the dam is a highly debated topic among both veterinarians and owners. Many different opinions exist, but there remain very little data. Most veterinarians agree that the dam would benefit from medications to control pain and inflammation after such an invasive surgery. However, it is known that almost all drugs are passed in the milk of the lactating dam, some to a higher degree than others. The ultimate goal is to achieve adequate pain control for the dam, while not making her drowsy and unable to care for the puppies and to also do no harm to the nursing neonates.

Drugs that have historically been used for pain control postoperatively include tramadol, butorphanol, fentanyl, and gabapentin. Collectively, these medications have questionable efficacy for pain control in dogs and cats and a variable half-life and produce some level of sedation. All of these drugs also have concerns with client safety, accountability, and potential abuse. Given these current challenges, the author chooses to not use any of these for postoperative pain control in cesarean delivery patients.

The use of nonsteroidal antiinflammatory drugs (NSAIDs) in lactating dams has been debated. Human studies indicate very low passage of NSAIDs in breastmilk but also indicate that NSAIDs are contraindicated when human infants are born premature because cyclooxygenase 2 enzymes are important for renal development in the infant.[21,22] Because puppies normally have immature renal function until 6 to 8 weeks of age, there is some concern over NSAID use in these cases. However, ongoing but unpublished research in this area indicates that carprofen has been used safely

Table 1			
Common practices regarding volume and route of administration of serum or plasma to neonates			
	Volume of Serum or Plasma to Be Given	**Route of Administration**	**Notes**
Puppies	10 mL/lb	PO if <12 h SQ if >12 h	Can be given at once; no more than 5 mL per site if SQ
Kittens	15 mL total	PO if <12 h SQ if >12 h	Given in 5 mL boluses at birth, 12 h and 24 h

in more than 300 litters and offspring have been followed to maturity without any apparent adverse effects.[23]

In most cases of cesarean delivery, this author's preference is to administer hydromorphone (0.1 mg/kg IV) and carprofen (4.4 mg/kg SQ) either intraoperatively after puppies have been delivered or on recovery and then dispense oral carprofen to be given at home (2.2 mg/kg by mouth twice daily) for no more than 3 days' duration. Of course, this is assuming a healthy animal that was also well hydrated with IV fluids during surgery and the immediate recovery period. In these routine cases, the author's preference is to discharge patients and the new litter within 1 to 2 hours of recovery. With the use of an epidural and the intraoperative/postoperative hydromorphone and carprofen, the author has been very pleased with the comfort and mothering ability of the dams during the first few hours and days post partum and have not seen any adverse effects in the neonates when using this short-term NSAID therapy on the dams.

SUMMARY

Table 2 briefly summarizes the most common conditions of neonates (listed from most to least common at the author's hospital) and their relative prognosis. Be encouraged that the most common conditions are easily treatable with simple veterinary intervention, do not require specialized skills or equipment, and carry a good prognosis if treatment occurs in a reasonable time frame. Although some causes of neonatal morbidity and mortality are infectious in nature, most neonatal losses are related to husbandry, management, or poor mothering ability of the dam and are preventable.

When presented with neonatal puppies or kittens, it cannot be stressed enough that 'the common things happen commonly.' Send home simple weight charts to remind owners that steady weight gain is the most reliable sign of neonatal well-being. Education of veterinary staff and clients is paramount in preventing most problems,

Table 2
Common clinical conditions of neonates

Common Neonatal Conditions	Treatment	Prognosis/Survivability
Hypothermia	Safe, steady warmth	Good to excellent
Hypoglycemia	Dextrose (oral, IV, or IO)	Good to excellent
Dehydration	Fluid support (IV or IO preferred; oral or SQ as well)	Good to fair
Failure to gain weight: loss of appetite caused by constipation from poor mothering	Gentle stimulation of anogenital area with warm, wet cotton ball	Good to excellent
Failure to gain weight: agalactia of dam	Oral domperidone or metoclopramide for dam; tube feeding of neonates	Good to excellent
Septicemia	Supportive care, antibiotics	Fair to poor
Herpesvirus	Supportive care, +/− antiviral medications	Fair to poor
Hyperthermia from an external heat source	Removal of heat source; gradual return to normal temperature	Fair to poor

Abbreviation: IO, intraosseous.

especially discussions reinforcing when to seek veterinary attention. Take the time to educate veterinary staff on the basics of neonatal examination and care, perhaps using this as a topic to revisit annually for a hospital staff meeting. It is vital to have well-trained staff that can then reinforce the principles of neonatal care with clients.

REFERENCES

1. De Cramer KGM, Joubert KE, Nöthling JO. Puppy survival and vigor associated with the use of low dose medetomidine premedication, propofol induction and maintenance of anesthesia using sevoflurane gas-inhalation for cesarean section in the bitch. Theriogenology 2017;96:10–5.
2. Doebeli A, Michel E, Bettschart R, et al. Apgar score after induction of anesthesia for canine cesarean section with alfaxalone versus propofol. Theriogenology 2013;80(8):850–4.
3. Janssens L, Altman S, Rogers PA. Respiratory and cardiac arrest under general anaesthesia: treatment by acupuncture of the nasal philtrum. Vet Rec 1979; 105(12):273–6.
4. Moon PF, Massat BJ, Pascoe PJ. Neonatal critical care. Vet Clin North Am Small Anim Pract 2001;31:343–67.
5. Holladay JR. Routine use of doxapram hydrochloride in neonatal pups delivered by cesarean section. Vet Med Small Anim Clin 1971;66(1):28.
6. Vliegenthart R, Ten Hove C, Onland W, et al. Doxapram treatment for apnea of prematurity: a systematic review. Neonatology 2017;111(2):162–71.
7. Grundy SA. Clinically relevant physiology of the neonate. Vet Clin North Am Small Anim Pract 2006;36:443–59.
8. Traas A. Resuscitation of canine and feline neonates. Theriogenology 2008;70: 343–8.
9. Apgar V. A proposal for a new method of evaluation of the newborn infant. Curr Res Anesth Analg 1953;32(4):260–7.
10. Apgar V, James LS. Further observations of the newborn scoring system. Am J Dis Child 1962;104:419–28.
11. Veronesi MC, Panzani S, Faustini M, et al. An Apgar scoring system for routine assessment of newborn puppy viability and short-term survival prognosis. Theriogenology 2009;72(3):401–7.
12. Groppettia D, Pecilea A, Del Carroa AP, et al. Evaluation of newborn canine viability by means of umbilical vein lactate measurement, Apgar score and uterine tocodynamometry. Theriogenology 2010;7:1187–96.
13. Vassalo FG, Simões CR, Sudano MJ, et al. Topics in the routine assessment of newborn puppy viability. Top Companion Anim Med 2015;30(1):16–21.
14. Batista M, Moreno C, Vilar J, et al. Neonatal viability evaluation by Apgar score in puppies delivered by cesarean section in two brachycephalic breeds (English and French bulldog). Anim Reprod Sci 2014;146(3–4):218–26.
15. Mila H, Grellet A, Delebarre M, et al. Monitoring of the newborn dog and prediction of neonatal mortality. Prev Vet Med 2017;143(1):11–20.
16. Mila H, Grellet A, Chastant-Maillard S. Prognostic value of birth weight and early weight gain on neonatal and pediatric mortality: a longitudinal study on 870 puppies. In: Program and presented at the 7th International Symposium on Canine and Feline Reproduction. Whistler, Canada, July 26–29, 2012. p. 163–4.
17. Greer M. Canine reproduction and neonatology. Jackson (WY): Teton New Media; 2015.

18. Kustritz MV. History and physical examination of the neonate. In: Peterson M, Kutzler M, editors. Small animal pediatrics: the first 12 months of life. St Louis (MO): Elsevier-Saunders; 2011. p. 20–7.

19. Chastant-Maillard S, Freyburger L, Marcheteau E, et al. Timing of the intestinal barrier closure in puppies. Reprod Domest Anim 2012;47(Suppl. 6):190–3.

20. Mila H, Feugier A, Grellet A, et al. Immunoglobulin G concentration in canine colostrum: evaluation and variability. J Reprod Immunol 2015;112:24–8.

21. Rigourd V, Meritet JF, Seraissol P, et al. Rapid and sensitive analysis of polymorphisms from breastmilk shows that ibuprofen is safe during certain stages of breastfeeding. Acta Paediatr 2015;104(9):e420–1.

22. Bloor M, Paech M. Nonsteroidal anti-inflammatory drugs during pregnancy and the initiation of lactation. Anesth Analg 2013;116(5):1063–75.

23. Escobar S, Kolster K. Analgesia for canine cesarean section recovery. Proceedings of the Society for Theriogenology Annual Conference. Asheville, NC, August 27–30, 2016.

Canine Prostate Disease

Bruce W. Christensen, DVM, MS

KEYWORDS

- Prostate • Benign prostatic hyperplasia (BPH) • Prostatitis • Prostatic neoplasia
- Canine prostate-specific arginine esterase (CPSE)

KEY POINTS

- All intact, male dogs eventually develop benign prostatic hyperplasia and a subset will develop clinical signs associated with subfertility, discomfort, or infection.
- Any male dog may develop neoplasia associated with the prostate, with a higher proportion of neutered males being affected.
- Ultrasound imaging and prostatic tissue cytology remain the most reliable diagnostic tests for canine prostate disease, but canine prostate-specific arginine esterase shows value as a supporting diagnostic test.
- Older recommendations to treat prostatitis for 4 to 8 weeks with appropriate antibiotics have been updated to now recommend a truncated 4-week treatment regime for acute cases.
- Medical treatments for benign prostatic hyperplasia have variable effects on prostate size and function, and may affect androgen production.

 Video content accompanies this article at http://www.vetsmall.theclinics.com/.

INTRODUCTION

The prostate is the only accessory sex organ in dogs. Diseases of the canine prostate are relatively common. The canine prostate is constantly developing and growing under androgenic influence throughout the life of the intact male dog. This androgenic influence seems to have a protective effect in the case of neoplastic disease,[1–3] but the increase in size under androgens also predisposes the canine prostate to infection and cystic disease.[4–6] The consequences of these diseases range from mild discomfort to varying effects on semen quality to very painful or life-threatening illness. An evolving understanding of the way the canine prostate functions has led to expanded diagnostic options and recent changes in treatment recommendations for some of these conditions. Each prostatic condition is discussed separately.

The author has nothing to disclose.
Kokopelli Assisted Reproductive Services, Franklin Ranch Pet Hospital, 10207 Franklin Boulevard, Elk Grove, CA 95757, USA
E-mail address: kokopellivet@gmail.com

Vet Clin Small Anim 48 (2018) 701–719
https://doi.org/10.1016/j.cvsm.2018.02.012

vetsmall.theclinics.com

PROSTATIC ANATOMY AND PHYSIOLOGY

The prostate in the dog is a bilobed, oval to spherical-shaped organ with both a dorsal and ventral sulcus that sits in the cranial pelvic canal or in the caudal abdomen. The proximal urethra runs through the prostate between the 2 lobes. Testosterone is converted to dihydrotestosterone (DHT) via the enzyme 5α-reductase and it is this androgen, DHT, that stimulates prostatic development, growth, and secretions.[7] The enzyme 5α-reductase is found in 2 isoenzymes in the body, types 1 and 2. Each isoenzyme is encoded by a different chromosome, but common coding sequences indicate a common evolutionary precursor. Isoenzyme type 1 is found throughout the body, including the skin, liver, and prostate. Isoenzyme type 2 is found predominantly in the prostate and other genital tissue. Testosterone and DHT both bind to the same androgen receptors and cause the same effects. The binding of DHT to the androgen receptor, however, is much tighter and of longer duration than that of testosterone. The resultant effect is that lower concentrations of DHT cause an amplified response compared with testosterone.[8,9] This mechanism is important to consider when discussing medical treatment of BPH elsewhere in this article.

Benign Prostatic Hyperplasia

The disorder consists of both cellular hyperplasia and hypertrophy.[10] The prostate exhibits continual, androgen-dependent growth, eventually exhibiting hyperplasia and hypertrophy that is, sensitive to estrogens, which increase androgen receptors, leading to more hyperplasia.[11,12] Although benign prostatic hyperplasia (BPH) can be present as early as 1 year of age, it does become increasingly more prevalent as intact dogs age (**Table 1**).[13] Approximately one-half of intact male dogs will have histologic signs of BPH by 4 years of age and more than 90% by 8 years of age. Most dogs with BPH do not show any clinical signs and, therefore, require no immediate treatment, although preventative treatment has been advocated and is discussed elsewhere in this article. Clinical signs may include sanguinous prostatic fluid dripping from the prepuce, hematospermia, hematuria, dysuria, constipation, or tenesmus.[14]

Dogs with BPH will show signs of subfertility, often accompanied by a marked number of red blood cells in the prostatic fluid. Spermatozoa from dogs with BPH have

Table 1 Prevalence of BPH by age	
Age Range (y)	**Total Prevalence of Canine, n/N BPH (%)**
0.1–1.0	0/25 (0)
1.1–2.0	3/19 (16)
2.1–3.0	8/25 (32)
3.1–4.0	9/21 (43)
4.1–5.0	5/9 (56)
5.1–6.0	34/39 (87)
6.1–7.0	15/18 (83)
7.1–8.0	9/10 (90)
8.1–9.0	27/28 (96)
9.1–10+	25/27 (93)

Abbreviation: BPH, benign prostatic hyperplasia.

Modified from Berry SJ, Strandberg JD, Saunders WJ, et al. Development of canine benign prostatic hyperplasia with age. Prostate 1986;9(4):363–73; with permission.

increased DNA fragmentation and increased numbers of primary morphologic defects.[15] Dogs with BPH are predisposed to prostatitis and cystic disease (discussed elsewhere in this article); indeed, these conditions are extremely rare in neutered male dogs with smaller prostates.

BENIGN PROSTATIC HYPERPLASIA DIAGNOSIS

The prostate should be digitally, transrectally palpated. In some dogs with advanced BPH, the prostate will have fallen cranially into the abdomen and cannot be palpated initially transrectally. In these cases, it is often helpful to gently lift up on the caudal abdomen to push the prostate back into the pelvis where it can be reached transrectally with the clinician's finger. Each of the 2 lobes of the prostate should be symmetric in size and shape. The consistency should be firm, but not hard. Gentle palpation of the prostate should not be painful to the dog with simple BPH. In this way, it is possible to gain a subjective opinion about the size, shape, and consistency of the prostate.

Objective measurements must be done with transabdominal ultrasound evaluation. Three-dimensional measurements can be taken of length, width, and height. A linear or curvilinear probe (5.0–8.0 mHz) may be used (**Fig. 1**, Video 1). Clipping is usually not necessary because of the scarcity of hair in the inguinal region. Acoustic gel and alcohol should be applied to obtain diagnostic images. The dog may be in a standing position, but can also be placed in lateral or dorsal recumbency. The probe is placed lateral to the prepuce in both transverse and sagittal orientations to obtain length (sagittal), width (transverse), and height (both transverse and sagittal) measurements. Accurate sagittal images are confirmed by observing the hypoechoic urethral tract. At least 3 views in each orientation should be obtained and the average measurement for each dimension used. The volume of the prostate may then be calculated by using the ellipsoid formula of length × width × height × 0.523 (where height is the average of the transverse and sagittal measurements). Normal prostatic measurements for dogs of

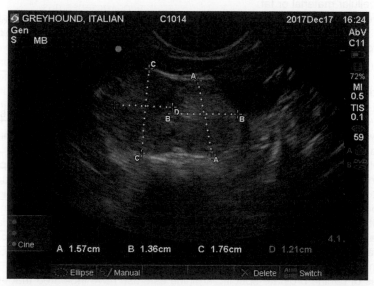

Fig. 1. Cross-sectional view of the prostate from a 6-year-old, intact Italian Greyhound. The bladder is visible to the right. The prostate is enlarged, but homogeneously echogenic, consistent with benign prostatic hyperplasia.

different ages and weights have been published.[16,17] The maximum predicted value (containing 97.5% of the normal population) for prostate volume may be calculated by using the following formula,[16] where BW is body weight and A is age:

$$V = (0.867 \times BW) + (1.885 \times A) + 15.88$$

The echogenic texture and uniformity should also be evaluated with ultrasound imaging. Normal prostatic parenchyma is uniformly echogenic throughout the organ (see **Fig. 1**). The hypoechoic urethra may be located between the 2 lobes. Any distinct hyperechoic or hypoechoic areas should be evaluated closely and likely indicate pathologic changes, like neoplasia, inflammation, or cystic disease. Enlargement of the prostate with a uniformly echogenic parenchyma is consistent with BPH.

Prostatic fluid evaluation is highly diagnostic for prostatic disease.[18] Prostatic fluid may be obtained through massage and aspiration or through collection and fractionation of an ejaculate. Fluid may be obtained by passing a lubricated, flexible catheter, such as a red rubber catheter, up the urethra to the level of the prostate (palpable transrectally). Then, 1 to 2 mL of sterile saline are infused slowly while the prostate is massaged transrectally and then aspirated back into the syringe.

Simply collecting and fractionating an ejaculate can obtain an even more voluminous sample with greater concentration of potentially diagnostic material. The canine ejaculate consists of 3 fractions. The second fraction comes from the epididymis and is the sperm-rich fraction. The first and third fractions come from the prostate, with the third fraction being the greatest in volume. Most intact, male dogs can be stimulated to ejaculate with manual stimulation into either an artificial vagina or into funnels, although males with painful prostatic conditions may be reluctant to ejaculate. The artificial vagina or funnel should have a plastic reservoir attached for collecting the fluid. By switching the collection device after each subsequent stage of ejaculation, the prostatic portion of the ejaculate may be separated from the sperm-rich fraction. The third fraction from a normal prostate is clear. Any detectable turbidity or color indicates cellular material or fat.

Recovered fluid is centrifuged at $1000 \times g$ for 10 minutes and the resultant pellet can be used for both culture and cytology. The culture sample should be submitted for both aerobic growth. The portion used for cytology can be rolled gently onto a slide, air dried, and stained with a Romanowsky stain, such as Diff-Quik. Normal prostatic cytology will have parabasal epithelial cells usually with very low numbers of red blood cells and neutrophils (typically ≤ 5 red blood cells or polymorphonuclear neutrophils per high-power field) and spermatozoa from the second fraction. Dogs with BPH may have dramatically increased numbers of RBC's (>20 per high-power field) in semen, which generally appears pinkish to red before centrifugation. Large numbers of prostatic epithelial cells are obtained and have a mosaic appearance.[19]

If cytology samples cannot be obtained via ejaculation or massage and aspiration, ultrasound-guided fine needle aspiration can also be used to obtain prostatic samples for histologic analysis.[18] Concerns for spreading infection or neoplastic cells are often raised, but there is a lack of evidence of this actually occurring in either human or veterinary literature. This technique is commonly used because many veterinarians are comfortable with ultrasound examinations, but lack experience in manual collection of ejaculates. Evidence also suggests that prostatic tissue sample culture is more specific than culture of prostatic fluid.[20]

Studies of canine prostate-specific arginine esterase have indicated that elevated serum concentrations of this enzyme correlate well with histologic evidence of BPH.[21,22] This assay may be used if other diagnostics are not available or inconclusive. Canine prostate-specific arginine esterase may also help to screen dogs with preclinical cases of BPH for proactive, preventative treatment options. A commercial laboratory test, using an enzyme-linked immunosorbent-type immunoassay, has been developed that can diagnose BPH using a blood sample (Odelis canine prostate-specific arginine esterase, Virbac, Carros, France). This assay is sensitive (97.1%), specific (92.1%) and shows good repeatability (intraassay coefficient of variation of <3.1%; interassay coefficient of variation of <6.7%).[23] The specific hardware necessary to process the assay is available in Europe and currently undergoing market trials in North America.

BENIGN PROSTATIC HYPERPLASIA TREATMENT

Treatment for BPH focuses on eliminating or decreasing androgen stimulation of the prostate. Orchidectomy is clearly the most effective treatment because it will remove all androgenic stimulation. For nonbreeding males, castration is the treatment of choice and results in marked decrease in size of the prostate (80% by 12 weeks after castration) and dramatic decrease in serum DHT concentrations within days to weeks of surgery.[24,25] For the breeding male, medical options are available. Resolution of BPH is achieved by removing the androgen source of prostatic stimulation. This review considers treatments including 5α-reductase inhibitors, androgen receptor inhibitors, androgen antagonists, aromatase inhibitors and other antiestrogen therapies, and gonadotropin-releasing hormone (GnRH) agonists. Treatments of the past that are no longer in widespread use owing to serious adverse effects, such as estrogens, are not discussed in this review. In men, lower urinary tract symptoms are common sequelae of BPH and an effective treatment is the use of α_1-adrenergic receptor antagonists to relax smooth muscle in the lower urinary tract.[26] Because this issue is not usually a concern in dogs owing to a relative lack of smooth muscle in the canine prostate, this treatment is not used and is not discussed herein.

BENIGN PROSTATIC HYPERPLASIA TREATMENT: ANTIANDROGENS
Finasteride

In North America, the best medical choice for treatment of BPH in dogs is finasteride, an azasteroid that at selectively inhibits the action of 5α-reductase type 2, thus, reducing the conversion of testosterone to DHT,[8] preserving testosterone concentrations while eliminating the production of DHT. The removal of DHT significantly decreases androgenic stimulation to the prostate, which consequently reduces in size owing to apoptosis of prostatic cells.[27] The prostate will reduce by nearly one-half (43%) by 16 weeks of treatment (0.1 mg/kg orally once per day, not to exceed 5 mg per dog per day).[28] A 50% to 70% decrease in prostatic volume has been noted after 16 to 53 weeks of treatment.[29–33] This is enough of a reduction in size and function to cause a resolution of clinical signs in most cases. Treatment can then be tapered to administration every 2 to 3 days, but must be continued for the life of the dog or the prostate will again increase in size and predispose the dog to recurrent clinical signs. Because testosterone itself is not inhibited, its effects on libido and spermatogenesis are preserved.

In humans, side effects include erectile or ejaculatory dysfunction and teratogenic effects in pregnant women, predictably with regard to sexual differentiation in male fetuses. Problems with libido and fertility have not been reported with dogs. In fact, reports indicate normal fertility and libido in dogs on finasteride.[32] Teratogenic effects should not be an issue in dogs because female dogs do not receive finasteride directly. Some veterinary clinicians have reported concerns about male dogs passing the drug onto females through the semen in mating, but passage of the drug in the semen has not been shown to be a concern in humans, the half-life of finasteride is short enough to not be a teratogenic concern even if it were passed in the semen, and humans may have sexual relations during pregnancy, whereas dogs do not. Semen in natural mating in canines is deposited in the cranial vagina and then it is thought that the continual secretion of large volumes of prostatic fluid during ejaculation of the third fraction pushes the sperm-rich fraction through the cervix into the uterus. The use of finasteride greatly decreases the volume of the third fraction, raising the concern that fertility will be decreased in natural matings using male dogs that are receiving finasteride. This concern has led to a variety of anecdotal dosing strategies among clinicians, including discontinuing the use of finasteride a week or two before an anticipated mating, reducing the dosing schedule to once every few days, or only putting the male on finasteride once a year for a few months. One study has tested the fertility of dogs on an active finasteride protocol and found no effect on fertility,[32] so although the concern regarding use of finasteride during natural mating programs makes sense, it may be unwarranted. Certainly, more studies on appropriate dosing regimens for finasteride are needed in the dog. The conventional wisdom at this point would be to continue finasteride treatment (somewhat) continuously until the breeding career of the dog is over, and then consider castration.

Osaterone Acetate

Osaterone acetate (Ypozane, Virbac) is a testosterone analogue with potent antiandrogenic activity attributed to competitive binding to androgen receptors, as well as the overall reduction of androgen receptors, reduction of 5α-reductase, and the inhibition of testosterone transport into prostate cells.[34] In 1 trial, osaterone was administered at a dose of 0.25 mg/kg orally once daily for 7 days to 73 dogs with clinical signs of BPH. By 14 days after the start of the trial, nearly one-half of the dogs had resolution of clinical signs and a 38% average reduction in prostate volume was noted. By 6 months after the start of the trial, 84% of dogs had resolution of clinical signs.[34] Using this same dosing regimen, it was determined that peak serum concentrations were reached by day 7, which may explain the initial rapid effect and then slow tapering of effects in the following weeks.[35] Semen quality and fertility do not seem to be negatively affected by osaterone and may, in some cases, improve.[36] Ypozane is marketed in France and available in some countries in the European Union. It is not licensed in the United States.

BENIGN PROSTATIC HYPERPLASIA TREATMENT: PROGESTINS
Medroxyprogesterone Acetate

Progestins exhibit antiandrogen activity and, therefore, have been used to treat BPH. The antiandrogenic action of progestins is likely due to competitive binding with the androgen receptors and/or suppression of luteinizing hormone secretion via negative feedback.[37] Dogs in 1 study were treated for BPH with medroxyprogesterone acetate and, although 84% showed a decrease in clinical signs, only 53% showed a decrease in prostate volume after 6 weeks of treatment.[38] No effect was noted on semen quality or libido. Concerns regarding the development of diabetes mellitus or mammary nodules have precluded its popular use for BPH treatment.

Delmadinone Acetate

Delmadinone acetate (Tardak, Pfizer Animal Health, Sandwich, Kent, UK) is a progestin with 17 times more potent antiandrogenic activity than progesterone.[34] Treatment of 69 dogs with clinical signs of BPH using a single intramuscular or subcutaneous injection of

3 mg/kg of delmadinone resulted in complete remission of clinical signs by 14 days after the injection in nearly one-half of the dogs and in 83% of the dogs by 6 months after the injection. At 14 days after the injection, a 28% decrease in prostate volume was noted.[34] One of the 69 dogs in the trial developed hypoadrenocorticism, which required treatment to resolve. In another study, delmadinone was administered at a dose of 1.5 mg/kg as a subcutaneous injection at 0, 1, and 4 weeks; adrenocorticotropic hormone and cortisol concentrations were measured during the trial. Adrenocorticotropic hormone stimulation tests were also conducted. There was a significant decrease in basal and 2 hours after adrenocorticotropic hormone stimulation concentrations of cortisol in treated dogs compared with control dogs. The authors concluded that treated dogs may be at risk for developing glucocorticoid insufficiency during treatment if subjected to stressful events.[39] Other side effects were of minimal importance, transient, and affected very few of the dogs; these included increases in appetite, behavior changes, vomiting, diarrhea, asthenia, polyuria, and polydipsia. In a separate study, male beagle dogs given an single injection of 1 mg/kg of delmadinone showed a temporary change in the maturation of epididymal spermatozoa.[33] Tardak is marketed in the UK and currently licensed in Austria, Belgium, Finland, France, Luxemburg, the Netherlands, and the UK. It is not licensed in the United States.

BENIGN PROSTATIC HYPERPLASIA TREATMENT: ANTIESTROGEN THERAPY
Tamoxifen Citrate

Estrogens have been thought to play either a causative or permissive role in the pathogenesis of BPH.[11] Tamoxifen citrate is an antiestrogen drug, marketed under various trade names for breast cancer treatment in women, that has been given at a dose of 2.5 mg per dog once daily for 28 days in male dogs with clinical BPH.[40,41] Prostatic volume decreased by 28% to 50% during the treatment period and volume of the third fraction decreased to a few drops or was absent. Prostate size returned rapidly to or less than pretreatment size after treatment ceased. Testicular size, spermatozoal motility, and normal morphology, libido, and serum testosterone concentration all showed dramatic decreases during treatment, some disappearing altogether, but all gradually returned to pretreatment levels by the end of the monitoring period. Bitches bred to 3 of the male dogs conceived and whelped normal litters. No systemic side effects were noted during the treatment period. Tamoxifen may represent a treatment option. It offers a rapid prostatic response and an apparently reversible contraceptive effect, at least with limited use.

Anastrazole

Anastrazole (Arimidex, AstraZeneca, Cambridge, UK) is a potent, highly selective aromatase inhibitor with no intrinsic hormonal activity that has replaced tamoxifen in many breast cancer treatment protocols for women.[42] Given to dogs at a dose of 0.25 to 1 mg per dog once daily for 28 days, a rapid decrease in prostate volume of 21% was noted with no significant changes in libido, testicular consistency, scrotal diameter, semen volume, count, motility, or morphologic abnormalities.[41] No hematologic or other clinical abnormalities were noted. Anastrazole is available in North America and may present veterinary practitioners with a more rapid alternative to protocols using finasteride.

BENIGN PROSTATIC HYPERPLASIA TREATMENT: GONADOTROPIN-RELEASING HORMONE AGONISTS
Deslorelin Acetate

Deslorelin acetate (Suprelorin, Virbac) and azagly-nafarelin (Gonazon, Intervet, Angers Technopole, France) are potent GnRH agonists that shut down luteinizing hormone release by desensitizing the pituitary gonadotrophs to GnRH and the Leydig cells to luteinizing hormone.[43] GnRH agonists have been used in domestic dogs and in wild carnivores as a reversible contraceptive.[44–48] With no testosterone available, spermatogenesis and libido are suspended after an initial stimulatory period (and therefore no reproduction) and DHT cannot be produced; the prostate gland and testes decrease in volume by up to 60%.[49] These parameters remain suppressed throughout the duration of the treatment, slowly returning to normal ranges usually 2 to 3 months after cessation of the treatment.[44,48,50–53] Male fertility seems to be unaffected after recovery from the treatment.[50,52] Suprelorin must be administered every 6 to 12 months, depending on the formulation used, for as long as suppression is desired. GnRH agonists may be very useful in treating dogs for BPH in situations when nonsurgical, reversible contraception is also a goal during the treatment period. Clients should be aware that reversal times are highly variable, unpredictable, but may be hastened by removal of the implant. GnRH implants are not available commercially for use in dogs in North America at the present time.

PROSTATITIS

Dogs experiencing BPH are predisposed to developing prostatitis. Reports of prostatitis in castrated male dogs are rare and often have a history of recent castration before presentation. Clinical signs of prostatitis will vary largely depending on the chronicity of the infection, with acute cases showing more serious, painful clinical signs and chronic cases often presenting as subclinical. Clinical signs relate to pain, but may manifest as back pain, abdominal pain, a painful, stiff gait, or depression. Semen quality and libido may be diminished. Hematospermia, hematuria, pyospermia, and fever may be present. Because prostatic fluid constantly flows both retrograde into the bladder as well as antegrade out the prepuce, these cases can be misdiagnosed as urinary tract infections. Transrectal digital palpation of the prostate will likely elicit pain in acute cases, but may not in chronic cases. The prostate will feel enlarged in acute cases and may not be bilaterally symmetrical, especially if abscessation is present. Some chronic cases of prostatitis may not have an obvious enlargement because fibrosis may have reduced the size of the prostate. Evaluation of the third fraction of the ejaculate is very helpful, if the dog is not too painful to cooperate with manual collection. Contaminant bacteria (usually Gram-positive cocci) are usually few in number and extracellular. The third fraction of the ejaculate in cases of prostatitis generally is associated with large numbers of Gram-negative rods (although less commonly Gram-positive may be present in large numbers), many of which are inside degenerative neutrophils. Chronic cases of prostatitis also have large numbers of macrophages, with plasma cells and lymphocytes.[19,54] The collection of a sample directly from the prostate via fine needle aspiration has been discouraged because of the concern for seeding the needle track with the infectious agent, but actual evidence of this is lacking.[20] The prostatic fluid will often have a marked number of neutrophils that may show degenerative changes and may have intracellular bacteria. A lack of neutrophils in the third fraction does not entirely rule out prostatitis, because neutrophils may be in a distinct segment of the prostate, not communicating with the secretory ducts. Culture of the third fraction to determine the causative agent should be performed if prostatitis is suspected. Although *Escherichia coli* is the most common pathogen in canine prostatitis, any opportunistic bacteria ascending from the urethra may cause the infection.

Fungal causes are possible, but much less common, and usually part of a systemic fungal infection.[4,55] A complete blood count will often reveal a regenerative leukocytosis, but some dogs may be leukopenic. Ultrasound evaluation of the prostate is valuable and usually shows a heterogenous echogenic appearance to the prostatic parenchyma; distinct hypoechoic regions correspond to abscessation.

Prostatitis Treatment

Because BPH predisposes dogs to prostatic infections, treatment aimed at reduction of the hyperplasia is warranted. For dogs without valuable breeding potential and no signs of systemic infection, castration coupled with antibiotic therapy is the preferred treatment. Otherwise, choose from one of the medical options discussed in this review for BPH treatment. Antibiotic therapy should be based on culture and sensitivity results (or be targeted to *E coli* without culture results) and should consider the unique physiology of the prostate. Owing to the profound inflammation present in acute prostatitis, the blood–prostate barrier is less functional and allows adequate diffusion of drugs that otherwise would not reach therapeutic concentrations in the prostate. Drugs such as broad-spectrum penicillin derivatives or a third-generation cephalosporin may initially be used to good effect. Once the blood–prostate barrier heals after initial improvement, however, diffusion across the barrier is limited to drugs containing specific pharmacokinetic properties and the antibiotic choice must be switched to an antibiotic with those properties. Drug penetration occurs via passive mechanisms of concentration gradients and diffusion. The blood–prostate barrier permits access only to lipophilic drugs and those not highly bound to proteins. In addition, the pH of the prostate is more acidic than the blood (canine prostatic pH ranges from 6.1 to 6.5[56,57]). The phenomenon of ion trapping further determines the concentrations of drugs across the membrane. Each drug will have a charged fraction (ionized) and an uncharged fraction. The uncharged fraction of a lipophilic drug, in a stable system, will equilibrate on both sides of the membrane. The charged portion of the drug, however, will concentrate more on one side or the other, depending on the differing pH on each side. The drug will be most concentrated on the side with the greatest ionization (the greatest charge).[58] Weak bases will, therefore, concentrate in the acidic canine prostatic fluid.

Antibiotic drugs that have proven efficacy in treating prostatic infections are discussed elsewhere in this article. Conventional recommendations have been that treatment for prostatitis should continue for between 4 to 6 weeks in acute cases and 6 to 8 weeks in chronic cases. Those recommendations are currently under review by the International Society for Companion Animal Infectious Diseases, which after review of available veterinary and human medical literature is recommending that antibiotic treatment be 4 weeks for acute cases and 6 weeks for chronic cases or cases with abscessation. Antibiotic treatment for acute cases may be even shorter if accompanied by castration, although objective data on these recommendations are lacking. The dog should be reexamined after the end of the treatment to confirm resolution of the infection.

Trimethoprim

Trimethoprim has the necessary properties to allow diffusion across the blood–prostate barrier and is a weak base with a pK_a of 7.4, therefore concentrating well in the acidic environment of the canine prostate.[59] Trimethoprim has good broad-spectrum activity, but is not effective against anaerobic infections. Pairing with a sulfa drug does not seem to affect prostate penetration.[60] Long-term treatment with trimethoprim, as is required for prostatitis cases, can lead to deleterious side effects, such as keratoconjunctivitis sica, anemia, and folate deficiency.

Fluoroquinolones The fluoroquinolones are amphoteric or zwitterionic in that they are neither purely acidic nor basic, but have qualities of both in clinical settings. They essentially have 2 ionizing groups, one positively charged and one negatively charged. At a pH somewhere in between the 2 groups, there is a minimal amount of charged drug. This is the isoelectric point. At pH values higher or lower than the isoelectric point, the amount of charged drug increases. So, if an amphoteric drug has an isoelectric point close to the pH of plasma, the drug will tend to concentrate in areas where the pH is higher or lower than that of plasma. This is the case with fluoroquinolones and why their concentrations are higher in the prostatic environment.[58] The fluoroquinolones have a good broad spectrum of activity and enrofloxacin is effective against mycoplasma infections. Some studies have indicated that ciprofloxacin may have poor bioavailability owing to decreased prostate penetration,[61–63] but other work suggests that ciprofloxacin can attain therapeutic concentrations in canine prostates.[64] The author is not aware of studies evaluating the efficacy of marbofloxacin in treating prostatitis. Fluoroquinolones do not act efficiently against anaerobic infections.

Macrolides
The macrolides diffuse very well into the prostate, but have poor action against gram-negative bacteria.[65] They should not be used until a sensitivity analysis has been obtained to show that the pathogenic bacteria are gram-positive organisms sensitive to the drug. Examples for veterinary use include erythromycin and tylosin.

Chloramphenicol
Chloramphenicol obtains good concentrations in the prostate and exhibits good activity against many anaerobes. It is highly protein bound, so high doses are required. The toxicity of chloramphenicol in humans is most likely not a concern in adult male dogs. Chloramphenicol, therefore, may be a good choice for an anaerobic prostatic infection.

PROSTATIC ABSCESSATION

Dogs with prostatic abscesses are diagnosed as prostatitis cases with signs of abscessation on ultrasound examination (**Fig. 2**, Video 2). Prostatic abscesses should be treated with the same protocols as dogs with prostatitis, using treatment targeted at BPH (castration or medical) and appropriate antibiotics for the infection. In addition, active drainage of the abscess (if the diameter is >1 cm) is often necessary either via surgical procedures or percutaneous, ultrasound-guided drainage.

Surgical drainage may be accomplished by marsupialization, Penrose drainage, or omentalization. Detailed description of each of these techniques is beyond the scope of this review, but information is available in the literature and in veterinary surgical texts.[66] A summary of each technique is presented herein.

Prostatic Abscessation Treatment

Prostatic omentalization
Omentalization is the current procedure of choice for surgical drainage of prostatic abscesses.[66] The omentum provides an alternate vascular and lymphatic supply and functions well in the presence of infection. As such, it has been used in multiple small animal surgical procedures.[67] The procedure of placing the omentum through the capsule of 20 dogs with prostatic abscessation (intracapsular omentalization) resulted in complete resolution in 19 dogs, with 1 dog showing recurrent abscessation and requiring Penrose drain placement.[68] Minimal to no postoperative complications were reported and most dogs were discharged to their owners 48 hours after surgery.

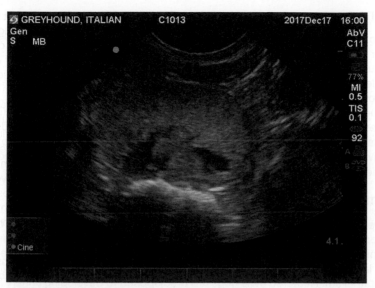

Fig. 2. Cross-sectional view of both lobes of the prostate from an 8-year-old, intact Italian Greyhound showing anechoic pockets of fluid, one in each lobe, consistent with either prostatic cysts or abscesses.

If the abscess is a paraprostatic retention cyst, and not intracapsular, omentalization may still be used to good effect.[69]

Penrose drainage
Penrose drain placement was the treatment of choice before the advent of omentalization techniques. Placement of a Penrose drain within the abscess and leading out through the abdominal wall allows continuous drainage of the abscess. Various techniques are described that differ in the exact placement of the Penrose drains.[70] The duration of time during which the drains are left in place varies with the technique from a few days to a few weeks. Active postoperative monitoring and care are necessary until drainage resolves, the drains are removed, and the wounds close. Complications may include recurrent abscessation, urinary incontinence, subcutaneous edema, anemia, sepsis, shock, hypokalemia, and hypoproteinemia.[71–74]

Marsupialization
Marsupialization is not commonly performed owing to the better postoperative results achieved by omentalization techniques. Marsupialization involves opening the abscess and suturing the edges to the skin to prevent the abscess from closing, allowing continual drainage to the exterior. For treatment of prostatic abscessation, the edges of the opened abscess may be sutured to the external abdominal skin adjacent to the prepuce, or ventral or lateral to the anus.[70] The abscess is thus allowed continual drainage as long as necessary and antibiotic or antiseptic treatments may be placed directly into the abscess. Drainage reportedly continues for 1 to 2 months, but may continue for many months in complicated cases. Active postoperative monitoring and care are necessary until drainage resolves, the drains are removed, and the wounds close. Complications potentially are the same as for Penrose drainage, and may also include fistula formation.[71–73]

PROSTATIC CYSTS

Prostatic cysts may be located within the prostatic parenchyma (retention cysts; see **Fig. 2**) or in a paraprostatic position. Prostatic cysts may not cause any clinical signs or may result in difficulties in urination or defecation. Prostatic cysts may predispose the dog to developing abscessation and, therefore, removal is often recommended, even in the absence of clinical signs. Removal of retention cysts may be done using the techniques described for abscessation, preferably omentalization. Paraprostatic cysts or abscesses do not communicate directly with the prostatic parenchyma and, therefore, local resection is often the treatment of choice.[70] Omentalization may also a good alternative.[69] Concurrent and ongoing treatment for BPH (castration or medical) is recommended.

PROSTATIC NEOPLASIA

Dogs are the only animal, besides man, with a known, significant occurrence of prostatic neoplasia. Adenocarcinomas and transitional cell carcinomas are the most common canine prostatic neoplastic diseases. Evidence suggests that prostatic neoplasia in dogs largely originates from the urothelium or ductular epithelium rather than the acinar epithelium. Neutered male dogs are predisposed to developing urinary bladder transitional cell carcinoma, prostate adenocarcinoma, prostate transitional cell carcinoma, prostate carcinoma, and general prostate tumors.[2] Genetic predispositions exist, making the risk variable for each breed.

Although there are apparent similarities in the disease between dogs and men, important differences also exist. As a result, many screening and treatment modalities used successfully in human medicine fail to be applicable in veterinary medicine. Prostatic neoplasia in men is often diagnosed in the early stages, thanks to heightened awareness and effective diagnostic screening tests (eg, the prostate specific antigen test), and depends on androgens as growth factors. Androgen deprivation therapy is a foundation therapy for men with prostate cancer and they usually respond rapidly and favorably. Most prostatic neoplasia in men is benign or slow growing. In dogs, however, prostatic neoplasia tends to be highly aggressive and metastatic. Canine prostatic neoplasia is not androgen dependent and is more commonly diagnosed in castrated males than intact males.[1–3] Reasons for the increased incidence of prostatic neoplasia in castrated dogs are unknown, but hypotheses include a loss of protective effects of androgens; a shift in the prostatic stroma from actin-positive smooth muscle cells to vimentin-positive mesenchymal cells, which may favor tumor formation; and increased longevity of castrated animals, predisposing them to age-related neoplastic diseases.[6,75] Clinical signs of prostatic neoplasia in dogs resemble those of other prostatic diseases including dysuria, dyschezia, and pain associated with the gait, back, or abdomen. Diagnosis is by history, clinical signs, an irregular painful prostate on transrectal palpation, heterogenous prostatic echogenicity on ultrasound evaluation, neoplastic cells found on cytology, or biopsy results. Cytology from prostatic wash is more likely to yield a diagnosis than an ejaculated sample. Fine needle aspiration can produce a diagnostic sample, but concern has been expressed about seeding the needle track with neoplastic cells. Usually, diagnosis is made at very late stages of the disease and survival times range from days to weeks after diagnosis.[6,76,77] Because of these differences, treatments are palliative and in some cases result in an increased quality of life for only a short time. Many treatment modalities, however, have potential, serious side effects that may result in the death or euthanasia of the dog. This underscores the need to tailor each recommendation to each specific clinical scenario. Clients should be made aware of potential complications, that treatments may not extend the life of the dog, but may alleviate clinical signs.

Prostatic Neoplasia Treatment

Surgery

Prostatic tumors tend to be highly aggressive and metastatic. If, however, there are no signs of metastasis, total prostatectomy may be a suggested therapy. There are some considerations, however, that make total prostatectomy in the dog less likely to produce an acceptable outcome. Even if metastasis has not been documented, there is a high likelihood that it has happened and will manifest itself shortly. Owing to the location of the urethra inside the prostate, urinary incontinence is a common postoperative complication with total prostatectomy. Surgery has also not been shown to increase survival in many cases.[71,72]

Subtotal intracapsular prostatectomy has also been tested, both using traditional surgical instruments and an Nd:YAG laser. In general, survival may be up to 5 times longer than with total prostatectomy and with a lower incidence of urinary incontinence.[78–81] Survival times and postoperative complications are comparable to treatment with piroxicam alone (discussed elsewhere in this article).[77]

Transurethral resection of the prostate has been reported in 3 dogs. Palliation of clinical signs postoperatively was rapid, but survival times remained short and complications included urinary tract infection, seeding of the tumor, and urethral perforation.[82]

Surgical therapy may alleviate clinical signs in some cases, but is associated with an increased risk for complications associated with poor quality of life, and is not associated with increased survival times. The decision to use surgery should be based on individual cases. Postoperative follow-up with systemic therapies to slow the spread of disease will likely aid in a more positive outcome.

Radiation

Radiation therapy has been tried in dogs without extending quality of life and resulting in some cases in severe adverse effects, including chronic colitis, gastrointestinal stricture or perforation, necrotic drainage/ulceration in the skin and subcutaneous tissues, osteopenia, urinary bladder thickening, chronic cystitis, urethral stricture, ileosacral osteosarcoma, pelvic limb edema, and perianal pain.[6,83,84] Survival time was not affected by the adverse effects, but quality of life decreased and owner expense increased. Radiation may play a role in future treatment regimes, but more work must be done to determine the best protocols.

Chemotherapy

The benefits of traditional chemotherapeutic agents have not been well-documented with canine prostatic neoplasia. Work has been done to investigate the chemotherapeutic properties of some nonsteroidal antiinflammatory drugs (NSAIDs). It is thought that cyclooxygenase (COX)-2 inhibition plays a key role through inhibition of angiogenesis, stimulation of apoptosis, and altering immune function.[85] One study evaluating the use of NSAIDs in the treatment of canine prostatic neoplasia noted that a majority of normal and neoplastic prostatic cells expressed COX-1 and that only neoplastic cells expressed COX-2. The study also retrospectively evaluated dogs with prostatic neoplasia that were treated with NSAIDs and those that were not and found that survival time was significantly different between the 2 groups, with 6.9 months in the former group and 0.7 months in the latter.[77] The 2 NSAIDs evaluated were piroxicam and carprofen.

Bisphosphonates

Bisphosphonates are osteoclast inhibitors used in human medicine for treatment of skeletal metastasis of prostatic carcinoma. They have been tested in dogs and seem to have similar benefits of increasing bone density and decreasing pain in some patients.[86] Inhibiting osteoclast activity strengthens bone, which reduces pain and the risk of fracture. It also controls the humoral hypercalcemia of malignancy. Other benefits of bisphosphonates in cancer treatment include inhibition of cancer cell proliferation, induction of apoptosis of cancer cells, angiogenesis inhibition, matrix metalloproteinase inhibition, and cytokine expression alteration.[87]

Samarium-153-ethylenediamine-tetramethylene-phosphonic acid

An injectable radiopharmaceutical, samarium-153-ethylenediamine-tetramethylene-phosphonic acid palliates and may have some curative properties in some restricted cases of canine skeletal metastatic disease (tumors <2 cm in diameter, not invading cortical bone, tumors in the axial skeleton, mineralized tumors, and those with high uptake of technetium (^{99}mTc) medronic acid during scintigraphy).[88] The drug is not currently easily accessible.

Dysuria Therapy

Because dysuria is a common effect of prostatic neoplasia, treatment may be focused on relieving this clinical sign. Tube cystotomy may be used, but owners should be aware of complications, including urinary tract infection and dissemination of the tumor.[89] The presence of the tumor may also cause incontinence to persist. Placement of a metallic urinary stent has been reported, which resulted in immediate restoration of urinary function. The treatment is costly and complications may include loss of the stent, reobstruction, and incontinence. In 1 study, 7 of 12 dogs were scored as having an excellent outcome and mean survival time for all dogs was 20 days.[90]

Prostatic Neoplasia Treatment Summary

No standard protocol for the treatment of prostatic neoplasia in dogs exists, nor is it likely that a standard protocol ever will exist as long as most diagnoses are in the late, terminal stages of the disease, and because individual patient variation and client wishes will always play an important role in deciding the correct treatment regime. At the current time, the best treatment to extend both life expectancy and improve quality of life (for 6 months on average) is the use of COX-2 inhibitors. Some treatments do seem to offer palliative measures to decrease pain and other clinical signs and should be considered as available options on a case-by-case basis, considering owner expectations and concerns, and the current quality of life of the patient.

DISEASE SCREENING

A retrospective survey of intact dogs determined that the most useful time to begin screening intact male dogs for prostatic disease, using ultrasound imaging, was at 40% of that breed's life expectancy.[91] At this time, there was a high probability of detecting prostatic disease before other clinical signs being evident. This measure would allow for early intervention and treatment. No such recommendations have been given for screening neutered males for neoplasia.

SUPPLEMENTARY DATA

Supplementary data related to this article can be found online at https://doi.org/10.1016/j.cvsm.2018.02.012.

REFERENCES

1. Teske E, Naan EC, van Dijk EM, et al. Canine prostate carcinoma: epidemiological evidence of an increased risk in castrated dogs. Mol Cell Endocrinol 2002; 197(1–2):251–5.
2. Bryan JN, Keeler MR, Henry CJ, et al. A population study of neutering status as a risk factor for canine prostate cancer. Prostate 2007;67(11):1174–81.
3. Sorenmo KU, Goldschmidt M, Shofer F, et al. Immunohistochemical characterization of canine prostatic carcinoma and correlation with castration status and castration time. Vet Comp Oncol 2003;1(1):48–56.
4. Johnston SD, Kamolpatana K, Root-Kustritz MV, et al. Prostatic disorders in the dog. Anim Reprod Sci 2000;60-61:405–15.
5. Smith J. Canine prostatic disease: a review of anatomy, pathology, diagnosis, and treatment. Theriogenology 2008;70(3):375–83.
6. LeRoy BE, Northrup N. Prostate cancer in dogs: comparative and clinical aspects. Vet J 2009;180(2):149–62.
7. Russell DW, Wilson JD. Steroid 5[alpha]-reductase: two genes/two enzymes. Annu Rev Biochem 1994;63:25–61.
8. Andriole G, Bruchovsky N, Chung LWK, et al. Dihydrotestosterone and the prostate: the scientific rationale for 5[alpha]-reductase inhibitors in the treatment of benign prostatic hyperplasia. J Urol 2004;172(4, Part 1):1399–403.
9. Wilson JD. The role of 5[alpha]-reductase in steroid hormone physiology. Reprod Fertil Dev 2001;13(8):673–8.
10. Kutzler M, Yeager A. Prostatic diseases. Textbook of veterinary internal medicine. St. Louis: WB Saunders, Elsevier; 2005. p. 1809–19.
11. Habenicht UF, Schwarz K, Schweikert HU, et al. Development of a model for the induction of estrogen-related prostatic hyperplasia in the dog and its response to the aromatase inhibitor 4-hydroxy-4-androstene-3,17-dione: preliminary results. Prostate 1986;8(2):181–94.
12. Rhodes L, Ding VDH, Kemp RK, et al. Estradiol causes a dose-dependent stimulation of prostate growth in castrated beagle dogs. Prostate 2000;44(1):8–18.
13. Berry SJ, Strandberg JD, Saunders WJ, et al. Development of canine benign prostatic hyperplasia with age. Prostate 1986;9:363–73.
14. Krawiec DR, Heflin D. Study of prostatic disease in dogs: 177 cases (1981-1986). J Am Vet Med Assoc 1992;200(8):1119–22.
15. Krakowski L, Wachockaa A, Brodzkia P, et al. Sperm quality and selected biochemical parameters of seminal fluid in dogs with benign prostatic hyperplasia. Anim Reprod Sci 2015;160:120–5.
16. Ruel Y, Barthez PY, Mailles A, et al. Ultrasonographic evaluation of the prostate in healthy intact dogs. Vet Radiol Ultrasound 1998;39(3):212–6.
17. Atalan G, Holt PE, Barr FJ, et al. Ultrasonographic estimation of prostatic size in canine cadavers. Res Vet Sci 1999;67:7–15.
18. Powe JR, Canfield PJ, Martin PA. Evaluation of the cytologic diagnosis of canine prostatic disorders. Vet Clin Pathol 2004;33:150–4.
19. Kraft M, Brown M, LeRoy E. Cytology of the canine prostate. Ir Vet J 2008;61: 320–4.
20. Kustritz MVR. Collection of tissue and culture samples from the canine reproductive tract. Theriogenology 2006;66(3):567–74.
21. Bell FW, Klausner JS, Hayden DW, et al. Evaluation of serum and seminal plasma markers in the diagnosis of canine prostatic disorders. J Vet Intern Med 1995;9. https://doi.org/10.1111/j.1939-1676.1995.tb03288.x.

22. Pinheiro D, Machado J, Viegas C, et al. Evaluation of biomarker canine-prostate specific arginine esterase (CPSE) for the diagnosis of benign prostatic hyperplasia. BMC Vet Res 2017;13(1):76.
23. Levy, Mimouni P, Fontbonne A, et al. Performance evaluation of the new blood test Odelis CPSE in the diagnosis of benign prostatic hyperplasia (BPH) in dogs. 6th EVSSAR meeting. Wroclaw, Poland, June 5–6, 2009.
24. Huggins C, Clark P. Quantitative studies on prostatic secretion: the effect of castration and estrogen injections on the normal and hyperplastic prostate gland of the dog. J Exp Med 1940;72:747–62.
25. Society for Theriogenology. The role of dihydrotestosterone in prostate physiology: comparisons among rats, dogs, and primates. Annual meeting of the Society for Theriogenology. Kansas City (MO), August 15–17, 1996.
26. Rossi M, Roumeguere T. Silodosin in the treatment of benign prostatic hyperplasia. Drug Des Devel Ther 2010;4:291–7.
27. Sirinarumitr K, Sirinarumitr T, Johnston SD, et al. Finasteride-induced prostatic involution by apoptosis in dogs with benign prostatic hypertrophy. Am J Vet Res 2002;63(4):495–8.
28. Sirinarumitr K, Johnston SD, Kustritz MVR, et al. Effects of finasteride on size of the prostate gland and semen quality in dogs with benign prostatic hypertrophy. J Am Vet Med Assoc 2001;218(8):1275–80.
29. Cohen SM, Werrmann JG, Rasmusson GH, et al. Comparison of the effects of new specific azasteroid inhibitors of steroid 5α-reductase on canine hyperplastic prostate: suppression of prostatic DHT correlated with prostate regression. Prostate 1995;26(2):55–71.
30. Laroque PA, Prahalada S, Gordon LR, et al. Effects of chronic oral administration of a selective 5α-reductase inhibitor, finasteride, on the dog prostate. Prostate 1994;24(2):93–100.
31. Laroque PA, Prahalada S, Molon-Noblot S, et al. Quantitative evaluation of glandular and stromal compartments in hyperplastic dog prostates: effect of 5-alpha reductase inhibitors. Prostate 1995;27(3):121–8.
32. Iguer-Ouada M, Verstegen JP. Effect of finasteride (Proscar MSD) on seminal composition, prostate function and fertility in male dogs. J Reprod Fertil Suppl 1997;51:139–49.
33. Lange K, Cordes EK, Hoppen HO, et al. Determination of concentrations of sex steroids in blood plasma and semen of male dogs treated with delmadinone acetate or finasteride. J Reprod Fertil Suppl 2001;57:83–91.
34. Albouy M, Sanquer A, Maynard L, et al. Efficacies of osaterone and delmadinone in the treatment of benign prostatic hyperplasia in dogs. Vet Rec 2008;163(6):179–83.
35. Allix V, Sillon M, Mezzasalma T, et al. Pharmacokinetics of osaterone acetate after repeated oral administration at 0.25 mg/kg/day for 7 days. Proceedings of the 31st World Small Animal Veterinary Congress. Prague, Czech Republic, October 11–14, 2006.
36. Fontaine E, Mir F, Vannier F, et al. Fertility after osaterone acetate treatment in breeding dogs suffering from prostatic diseases. Reprod Domest Anim Suppl 2010;45(3):60.
37. Romagnoli S, Concannon PW. Clinical use of progestins in bitches and queens: a review. In: Concannon PW, England G, Verstegen J, et al, editors. Recent advances in small animal reproduction. Ithaca (NY): International Veterinary Information Service; 2003.
38. Bamberg-Thalen B, Linde-Forsberg C. Treatment of canine benign prostatic hyperplasia with medroxyprogesterone acetate. J Am Anim Hosp Assoc 1993;29:221–6.

39. Court EA, Watson ADJ, Church DB, et al. Effects of delmadinone acetate on pituitary-adrenal function, glucose tolerance and growth hormone in male dogs. Aust Vet J 1998;76(8):555–60.

40. Corrada Y, Arias D, Rodrìguez R, et al. Effect of tamoxifen citrate on reproductive parameters of male dogs. Theriogenology 2004;61(7–8):1327–41.

41. Gonzalez G, Guendulain C, Maffrand C, et al. Comparison of the effect of the aromatase inhibitor, anastrazole, to the antioestrogen, tamoxifen citrate, on canine prostate and semen. Reprod Domest Anim 2009;44:316–9.

42. Plourde PV, Dyroff M, Dukes M. Arimidex®: a potent and selective fourth-generation aromatase inhibitor. Breast Cancer Res Treat 1994;30(1):103–11.

43. Junaidi A, Williamson PE, Martin GB, et al. Pituitary and testicular endocrine responses to exogenous gonadoptrophin-releasing hormone (GnRH) and luteinising hormone in male dogs treated with GnRH agonist implants. Reprod Fertil Dev 2007;19(8):891–8.

44. Trigg TE, Wright PJ, Armour AF, et al. Use of a GnRH analogue implant to produce reversible long-term suppression of reproductive function in male and female domestic dogs. J Reprod Fertil Suppl 2001;57:255–61.

45. Bertschinger HJ, Asa CS, Calle PP, et al. Control of reproduction and sex related behaviour in exotic wild carnivores with the GnRH analogue deslorelin: preliminary observations. J Reprod Fertil Suppl 2001;57:275–83.

46. Bertschinger HJ, Trigg TE, Jochle W, et al. Induction of contraception in some African wild carnivores by downregulation of LH and FSH secretion using the GnRH analogue deslorelin. Reprod Suppl 2002;60:41–52.

47. Jewgenow K, Dehnhard M, Hildebrandt TB, et al. Contraception for population control in exotic carnivores. Theriogenology 2006;66(6–7):1525–9.

48. Trigg TE, Doyle AG, Walsh JD, et al. A review of advances in the use of the GnRH agonist deslorelin in control of reproduction. Theriogenology 2006;66(6–7):1507–12.

49. Palm J, Reichler IM. The use of deslorelin acetate (Suprelorin) in companion animal medicine. Schweiz Arch Tierheilkd 2012;154(1):7–12.

50. Lacoste D, Dube D, Trudel C, et al. Normal gonadal functions and fertility after 23 months of treatment of prepubertal male and female dogs with the GnRH agonist [D-Trp6, des-Gly-NH2(10)]GnRH ehtylamide. J Androl 1989;10(6):456–65.

51. Cavitte JC, Lahiou N, Mialot JP, et al. Reversible effects of long-term treatment with D-Trp6-LH-RH-microcapsules on pituitary-gonadal axis, spermatogenesis and prostate morphology in adolescent and adult dogs. Andrologia 1988;20(3):249–63.

52. Goericke-Pesch S, Spang A, Schulz M, et al. Recrudescence of spermatogenesis in the dog following downregulation using a slow release GnRH agonist implant. Reprod Domest Anim 2009;44:302–8.

53. Junaidi A, Williamson PE, Cummins JM, et al. Use of a new drug delivery formulation of the gonadatrophin-releasing hormone analogue Deslorelin for reversible long-term contraception in male dogs. Reprod Fertil Dev 2003;15(6):317–22.

54. Dorfmann M, Bartsani J. Diseases of the canine prostate gland. Compend Contin Educ Vet 1995;17:791–810.

55. Reed LT, Balog KA, Boes KM, et al. Pathology in practice. J Am Vet Med Assoc 2010;236(4):411–3.

56. Fair WR, Cordonnier JJ. The pH of prostatic fluid: a reappraisal and therapeutic implications. J Urol 1978;120(6):695–8.

57. Meares EM. Prostatitis. A review. Urol Clin North Am 1975;2:3–27.

58. Wagenlehner FME, Weidner W, Sörgel F, et al. The role of antibiotics in chronic bacterial prostatitis. Int J Antimicrob Agents 2005;26(1):1–7.
59. Madsen PO, Whalen PR. Interaction between antimicrobial agents and prostatic tissue extract and fluid. Infection Suppl 1978;6(1):75–7.
60. Fowler JE Jr. Antimicrobial therapy for bacterial and nonbacterial prostatitis. Urology 2002;60(6):24–6.
61. Png J, Tan E, Foo K, et al. A comparative study of the distribution of ofloxacin and ciprofloxacin in prostatic tissues after simultaneous oral ingestion. Br J Urol 1997; 79(5):781–4.
62. Bergeron M. The pharmacokinetics and tissue penetration of the fluoroquinolones. Clin Invest Med 1989;12(1):20–7.
63. Naber K, Sorgel F, Kinzig M, et al. Penetration of ciprofloxacin into prostatic fluid, ejaculate and seminal fluid in volunteers after an oral dose of 750 mg. J Urol 1993;150(5 Pt 2):1718–21.
64. Albarellos GA, Montoya L, Waxman S, et al. Ciprofloxacin and norfloxacin pharmacokinetics and prostatic fluid penetration in dogs after multiple oral dosing. Vet J 2006;172(2):334–9.
65. Stamey TA, Meares EM, Winningham G. Chronic bacterial prostatitis and the diffusion of drugs into the prostatic fluid. J Urol 1970;103:187–94.
66. Freitag T, Jerram RM, Walker AM, et al. Surgical management of common canine prostatic conditions. Compend Contin Educ Vet 2007;29(11):656–8, 660, 662–3.
67. Hosgood G. The omentum–the forgotten organ: physiology and potential surgical applications in the dog and cat. Compend Contin Educ Vet 1990;12:45–51.
68. White RA, Williams JM. Intracapsular prostatic omentalization: a new technique for management of prostatic abscesses in dogs. Vet Surg 1995;24(5):390–5.
69. Bray JP, White RAS, Williams JM. Partial resection and omentalization: a new technique for management of prostatic retention cysts in dogs. Vet Surg 1997; 26(3):202–9.
70. Basinger RR. Surgical management of prostatic diseases. Compend Contin Educ Vet 1987;29:993–9.
71. Basinger RR, Rawlings CA, Barsanti JA. Urodynamic alterations associated with clinical prostatic diseases and prostatic surgery in 23 dogs. J Am Anim Hosp Assoc 1989;25:385–92.
72. Hardie EM, Barsanti JA, Rawlings CA. Complications of prostatic surgery. J Am Anim Hosp Assoc 1984;20:50–6.
73. Matthiesen DT, Marretta SM. Complications associated with the surgical treatment of prostatic abscessation. Probl Vet Med 1989;1:63–7.
74. Mullen HS, Matthiesen DT, Scavelli TD. Results of surgery and postoperative complications in 92 dogs treated for prostatic abscessation by a multiple Penrose drain technique. J Am Anim Hosp Assoc 1990;26:369–79.
75. Shidaifat F, Daradka M, Al-Omari R. Effect of androgen ablation on prostatic cell differentiation in dogs. Endocr Res 2004;30(3):327–34.
76. Cornell KK, Bostwick DG, Cooley DM, et al. Clinical and pathologic aspects of spontaneous canine prostate carcinoma: a retrospective analysis of 76 cases. Prostate 2000;45(2):173–83.
77. Sorenmo KU, Goldschmidt MH, Shofer FS, et al. Evaluation of cyclooxygenase-1 and cyclooxygenase-2 expression and the effect of cyclooxygenase inhibitors in canine prostatic carcinoma. Vet Comp Oncol 2004;2(1):13–23.
78. Goldsmid SE, Bellenger CR. Urinary incontinence after prostatectomy in dogs. Vet Surg 1991;20(4):253–6.

79. Hardie EM, Stone EA, Spaulding KA, et al. Subtotal canine prostatectomy with the neodymium: yttrium-aluminum-garnet laser. Vet Surg 1990;19(5):348–55.
80. L'Eplattenier HF, Van Nimwegen SA, Van Sluijs FJ, et al. partial prostatectomy using Nd:YAG laser for management of canine prostate carcinoma. Vet Surg 2006; 35(4):406–11.
81. Vlasin M, Rauser P, Fichtel T, et al. Subtotal intracapsular prostatectomy as a useful treatment for advanced-stage prostatic malignancies. J Small Anim Pract 2006;47(9):512–6.
82. Liptak JM, Brutscher SP, Monnet E, et al. Transurethral resection in the management of urethral and prostatic neoplasia in 6 dogs. Vet Surg 2004;33(5):505–16.
83. Anderson CR, McNiel EA, Gillette EL, et al. Late complications of pelvic irradiation in 16 dogs. Vet Radiol Ultrasound 2002;43(2):187–92.
84. Arthur JJ, Kleiter MM, Thrall DE, et al. Characterization of normal tissue complications in 51 dogs undergoing definitive pelvic region irradiation. Vet Radiol Ultrasound 2008;49(1):85–9.
85. Hayes A. Cancer, cyclo-oxygenase and nonsteroidal anti-inflammatory drugs – can we combine all three? Vet Comp Oncol 2007;5(1):1–13.
86. Fan TM, de Lorimier L-P, Charney SC, et al. Evaluation of intravenous pamidronate administration in 33 cancer-bearing dogs with primary or secondary bone involvement. J Vet Intern Med 2005;19(1):74–80.
87. Milner RJ, Farese J, Henry CJ, et al. Bisphosphonates and cancer. J Vet Intern Med 2004;18(5):597–604.
88. Lattimer JC, Corwin LA Jr, Stapleton J, et al. Clinical and clinicopathologic response of canine bone tumor patients to treatment with samarium- 153-EDTMP. J Nucl Med 1990;31(8):1316–25.
89. Williams JM, White RAS. Tube cystostomy in the dog and cat. J Small Anim Pract 1991;32(12):598–602.
90. Weisse C, Berent A, Todd K, et al. Evaluation of palliative stenting for management of malignant urethral obstructions in dogs. J Am Vet Med Assoc 2006; 229(2):226–34.
91. Mantziaras G, Alonge S, Faustini M, et al. Assessment of the age for a preventive ultrasonographic examination of the prostate in the dog. Theriogenology 2017; 100:114–9.

Population Control in Small Animals

Margaret V. Root Kustritz, DVM, PhD, MMedEd

KEYWORDS

- Ovariohysterectomy • Castration • Immunocontraception • Overpopulation

KEY POINTS

- Optimal age for ovariohysterectomy (OHE) or castration has not been defined in the scientific literature.
- Bitches and queens are significantly less likely to develop mammary neoplasia, which has a high incidence and potentially high morbidity and mortality, if spayed when young.
- Tom cats exhibit undesirable behaviors that preclude them being good pets and should be castrated young unless they are intended for breeding.
- There is no compelling reason to castrate male dogs when young unless it is needed to control reproductive behaviors or prevent indiscriminate breeding.
- Alternatives to surgical sterilization that may be available in the future include intratesticular injection and immunization against GnRH.

INTRODUCTION
Pet Overpopulation

Attitudes about pet ownership and ready availability of dogs and cats for purchase or adoption, and presence of feral populations of dogs and cats in the United States are associated with overpopulation of these species. It is estimated that about 8% of the owned populations of dogs and cats in the United States is euthanized annually at humane organizations.[1] Sexually intact animals adopted from humane organizations may be returned or may reproduce, both of which would repopulate those shelters. For this reason, many humane organizations now perform ovariohysterectomy (OHE)/ovariectomy or castration on all dogs and cats before they are adopted.

Disclosure Statement: The author has nothing to disclose.
This article contains information excerpted with permission from Root Kustritz MV, Slater MR, Weedon GR, Bushby PA. Determining optimal age for gonadectomy in the dog: a critical review of the literature to guide decision making. Clin Ther 2017;9:167–211; and Root Kustritz MV. Current and proposed research in canine and feline non-surgical sterilization. Clin Ther 2012;4:225–31.
Department of Veterinary Clinical Sciences, University of Minnesota College of Veterinary Medicine, 1365 Gortner Avenue, St Paul, MN 55108, USA
E-mail address: rootk001@umn.edu

Veterinarians also stress OHE and castration to cat and dog owners for population control and to improve animal health. Gonadectomy is the most common elective surgery performed on dogs in the United States, with reported prevalence of 67% in female dogs and 61% in male dogs, and 81% in female cats and 83% in male cats.[2] Surgical sterilization is expensive and not readily available to help control owned and free-roaming populations in developing countries, where such populations negatively impact animal and human health. For these reasons, there is growing research in nonsurgical alternatives.

Sterilization Versus Contraception

Contraception is reversible control of reproduction and usually is the goal in human medicine. Drugs are available that have been demonstrated to safely suppress estrus in females and spermatogenesis in males of canid and felid species for varying periods of time. These drugs include progestogens, such as megestrol acetate, medroxyprogesterone acetate, and proligestone; androgens, such as testosterone esters and mibolerone; gonadotropin-releasing hormone (GnRH) agonists, such as deslorelin, nafarelin, and buserelin; GnRH antagonists, such as acyline; and prolactin.[3] There are no approved contraceptive drugs for dogs and cats available in North America at this time.

Sterilization is permanent cessation of reproduction and usually is the goal in small animal veterinary medicine. Associated with that complete cessation of fertility is decrease in reproductive physiology and behaviors that society has deemed unacceptable in pets, including exudation of serosanguinous vulvar discharge associated with heat in bitches, yowling and lordosis in queens, mounting in stud dogs, and urine spraying in tom cats. Current research is geared toward identification of a sterilant product or procedure that is 100% effective at decreasing fertility for the reproductive life of the animal, that is completely safe to that animal and to other species that may encounter distributed compounds, and that is administered as a single application in the animal's life.

SURGICAL METHODS OF POPULATION CONTROL

Surgical methods for sterilization in bitches and queens are OHE, ovariectomy, hysterectomy (also known as ovary-sparing spay), and tubal ligation. Tubal ligation is not described. Ovariectomy is commonly practiced throughout the world, although OHE remains the standard of practice in the United States for reasons that are not clear. One could hypothesize that ovariectomy would be preferred to OHE because is it less technically complicated, duration of surgery should be shorter, and morbidity and pain should be less.[4] Studies done to date have not consistently borne this out with several showing no difference between the two techniques in surgery time, length of incision, and pain score on recovery.[5,6] Short-term complications, such as bleeding at the pedicles, are equally likely between the two procedures, because it is usually the ovarian pedicles, not the broad ligament or uterine stump, from which significant postoperative hemorrhage occurs.[4] Long-term complications are pathologies of the uterus. Pyometra is only likely to occur after ovariectomy or after OHE (uterine stump pyometra) if ovarian tissue is left behind. There is no literature documenting incidence of ovarian remnant syndrome after ovariectomy compared with OHE. Finally, uterine neoplasia could occur after ovariectomy but incidence of uterine neoplasia in dogs is low, at 0.03%.[4] No studies to date have demonstrated differences in long-term medical concerns, such as obesity and urethral sphincter mechanism incompetence, when comparing dogs having undergone ovariectomy to OHE.[4]

Hysterectomy, popularly called ovary-sparing spay, is less well researched. Use of this procedure is supported by some based on limited research suggesting that estrogen and nonestrogenic secretory factors from the ovaries positively impact lifespan and may impact other aspects of health in dogs.[7] Dogs that have undergone hysterectomy continue to cycle but should not have the serosanguinous vulvar discharge of heat, which arises in the uterus. In the few studies in the literature describing side effects of hysterectomy, short-term concerns were possible abnormalities in length of estrous cycling, and apparent increase in signs of false pregnancy in a cohort of dogs hysterectomized during diestrus.[8,9] Long-term complications reported in one study were ovarian cysts and fibrosis, inflammation of the uterine stump, and mammary neoplasia.[10] Risk of the long-term complication of inflammation and potential pyometra of the uterine stump is greatly decreased by ligation at the cervix, leaving behind no endometrial tissue.

In male dogs, castration is the most common surgical sterilization technique. Vasectomy is described and seems to be associated long term with degeneration of the seminiferous tubules and with possible formation of spermatoceles or sperm granulomas in some dogs.[11,12] There is nothing to suggest that vasectomy diminishes secretion of testosterone, so vasectomized dogs would still be predisposed to testosterone-dependent disease.

Most published research about pros and cons of sterilization surgery in female dogs and cats describes OHE and in male dogs and cats describes castration, so that is the focus of this article. This article also focuses more on medical concerns than on behavioral concerns. It is difficult to draw conclusions of any kind from currently published behavioral studies evaluating effect of gonadectomy on behavior because those studies vary greatly in methods and reporting of data.

Ovariohysterectomy/Castration in Cats

The primary benefit of OHE in queens is decreased incidence of mammary neoplasia. Mammary neoplasia is common in cats, with a reported incidence of 2.5% and reported malignancy rate of greater than 90%.[13,14] Cats spayed before their first estrus are significantly protected from developing mammary neoplasia with age, with intact queens reported to have seven times the risk of developing mammary tumors compared with spayed queens.[15] The primary detriment to spaying in queens is development of obesity, which is caused by decline in metabolic rate and can therefore be countered with appropriate diet.[16] Because of the high incidence and high morbidity and mortality of mammary neoplasia in queens left intact, spaying of all queens not intended for breeding is recommended as early in life as possible.

The primary benefits of castration of tom cats are behavioral. Intact tom cats demonstrate aggressive reproductive behaviors and mark their territory with foul-smelling urine sprayed on vertical surfaces. These behaviors are readily reduced by castration.[17,18] The only reported detriment to castration in tom cats is decreased metabolic rate and subsequent obesity, as described for queens. For these reasons, castration of all tom cats not intended for breeding is recommended as early in life as possible.

Ovariohysterectomy/Castration in Dogs

Concerns have been expressed by veterinarians, dog breeders, and pet owners or guardians about the need to better understand effects of gonadectomy on individual animal health. To best meet needs of dog owners, veterinarians must maintain an awareness of studies published and, most critically, the value they bring to the question of suitable age for gonadectomy in dogs. The question about impact of gonadectomy on health is one of causation: does gonadectomy at certain ages cause or prevent specific health issues? Answering this type of question requires a large body of high-quality data of varying types ranging from laboratory studies to clinical trials and observational studies of populations. No single study can prove causation. Many studies to date on this topic have been performed on small or unique populations of dogs and data from those studies may or may not readily be extrapolated to dogs seen by veterinarians in private practice. Researchers, article reviewers, and readers of publications must be aware of possible biases in measurement and must pay attention to whether or not findings that are statistically significant have any practical implications in veterinary practice. Peer-reviewed publications should include an in-depth assessment of the study limitations and generalizability; studies that do not provide this should be assessed with extra caution. Veterinarians should be careful to read articles in their entirely whenever possible rather than to rely on brief summaries that do not permit the reader to make their own decisions regarding value of the data as presented to their clinical practice.

The primary reported benefits of OHE in bitches are decreased incidence of mammary neoplasia and pyometra. Reported incidence of mammary cancer in bitches is 3.4%, with malignancy rate of about 50%.[19–24] Detriments reported include other cancers, including transitional cell carcinoma, lymphosarcoma, osteosarcoma, hemangiosarcoma, and mast cell tumors; orthopedic disorders including hip dysplasia and cranial cruciate ligament injury; obesity; and urethral sphincter mechanism incompetence.[25] Reports of these benefits and detriments vary in number of studies and quality of those studies (**Table 1**). It has been well demonstrated that OHE early in life provides the greatest protection against development of mammary neoplasia with age.[26] OHE at any age is protective against pyometra. Because of the high incidence and morbidity of mammary cancer, it generally is recommended that bitches be spayed before their first estrus. Research regarding effect of age of gonadectomy on all of these disorders is ongoing.

The primary reported benefits of castration in male dogs are decreased incidence of testicular neoplasia and testosterone-dependent disease including benign prostatic hypertrophy. Castration at any age is protective against testicular neoplasia and benign prostatic hypertrophy and these generally are benign diseases that are cured by castration at the time of diagnosis. Detriments are similar to those reported for bitches (see **Table 1**). There are no compelling medical reasons evident at this time to castrate male dogs early in life. Testosterone-dependent behaviors, such as mounting, roaming, and urine-marking, have been demonstrated to be decreased but not necessarily abolished by about 50% to 70% with castration and may be a reason for castration for some dog owners, as may inability or unwillingness to prevent that male dog from mating indiscriminately.[27,28]

Dog owners and breeders are aware of the body of literature describing possible detriments of OHE and castration. Veterinarians need to develop a means of communicating this large amount of contradictory data. One way to help clients think through the information is to provide them with an idea of the varying impacts of the disorders the veterinarian believes to be associated with gonadectomy. In one example of this method, veterinarians generated a morbidity score for various disorders that was multiplied by incidence of those disorders to create an impact score (**Table 2**).[29] Positive impact scores were associated with better health after gonadectomy and negative impact scores with worse health after gonadectomy. For female dogs, benefits of OHE outweighed detriments and prepubertal spay was recommended; for male dogs, benefits of castration did not outweigh detriments until the animal was likely to develop age-related, benign diseases of the reproductive tract, or about

Table 1
Reports in the veterinary literature evaluating association between gonadectomy and various disorders in dogs

Disorder	Increased, Decreased, or No Change with Gonadectomy (Number of Studies)	Extent of Change	Characteristics of Published Studies
Mammary neoplasia	Decreased (5) No change (2)	OR, 0.01 if spayed at <1 y of age; one-third less likely if neutered, one-half as likely if neutered, 2 times as likely if intact	Cause and effect not identified. Effect of age at time of gonadectomy identified. One study breed-specific. Two studies with small sample size.[†]
Prostatic neoplasia	Increased (4) No change (1)	OR, 2.4–4.3	Cause and effect not identified. Effect of age at time of gonadectomy not identified.
Transitional cell carcinoma	Increased (2)	OR, 2.0–4.4	Cause and effect not identified. Effect of age at time of gonadectomy not identified. One study from unique population.
Osteosarcoma	Increased (2) No change (1)	OR, 1.6–2.0 RR, 3.8	Cause and effect not identified. Effect of age at time of gonadectomy not identified. Variation by gender. Two studies breed-specific.
Hemangiosarcoma	Increased (5) No change (2)	OR, 1.6–9.0 RR, 5.3–6.1	Cause and effect not identified. Effect of age at time of gonadectomy not identified. Variation by gender. Four studies breed-specific. Four studies from unique populations.
Lymphoma	Increased (5) No change (3)	OR, 1.1–4.3	Cause and effect not identified. Effect of age at time of gonadectomy not identified. Variation by gender. Four studies breed-specific. Three studies from unique populations.
Cutaneous mast cell tumor	Increased (6) No change (5)	OR, 0.1–4.1	Cause and effect not identified. Effect of age at time of gonadectomy not identified. Variation by gender. Four studies breed-specific. Four studies from unique populations.

(continued on next page)

	Table 1 (*continued*)		
Disorder	**Increased, Decreased, or No Change with Gonadectomy (Number of Studies)**	**Extent of Change**	**Characteristics of Published Studies**
Obesity	Increased (3)	OR, 1.6; gonadectomized dogs twice as likely compared with intact dogs	Cause and effect not identified in dogs. Effect of age at time of gonadectomy not identified. One study from a unique population.
Cranial cruciate ligament injury	Increased (11) Decreased (1) No change (2)	OR, 0.5–3.0; two studies showed increased incidence with age (gonadectomy at 6 mo or 1 y)	Cause and effect not identified. Variation by gender. Three studies breed-specific. Seven studies from unique populations.
Patellar luxation	Increased (2) No change (1)	OR, 1.3–3.1	Cause and effect not identified. Effect of age at time of gonadectomy not identified.
Hip dysplasia	Increased (5) Decreased (1) No change (4)	1.5 times more likely HR, 1.7 OR, 0.9–1.2	Cause and effect not identified. One study showed effect of age at time of gonadectomy identified. Variation by gender. Four studies breed-specific. Three studies from unique populations.
Urinary incontinence	Increased (6)	HR, 0.9–1.2 OR, 4.9 RR, 7.8	Cause and effect not identified. Effect of age at time of gonadectomy identified. Two studies breed-specific. One study from unique population.
Lifespan	Increased (2) Decreased (1)	Castrated males live 13.8%–18.0% longer; spayed females live 23.0%–26.3% longer	Cause and effect not identified. Effect of age at time of gonadectomy not identified. One study breed-specific and from unique population.

Abbreviations: HR, hazard ratio; OR, odds ratio; RR, relative risk.

2.5 years of age. Use of this kind of tool also gives veterinarians an opportunity to talk with clients about other topics in preventive medicine. For example, this provided a real way to demonstrate to clients the concerns associated with obesity, which had a high impact score in females and males.

Another technique is to provide clients with some idea of positives and negatives for their specific animal. This requires specific knowledge of predispositions caused by age, breed, and other factors for all of the disorders described. An example previously

| Table 2 | | |
| Impact[a] on health of male and female dogs after gonadectomy | | |
Disorder	Female Dog	Male Dog
Mammary neoplasia	+24	—
Pyometra	+100	—
Surgical complications	−20	−16
Osteosarcoma	−2	−2
Hemangiosarcoma	−2	−2
Transitional cell carcinoma	−7	−7
Prostate neoplasia	—	−3
Testicular neoplasia	—	+5
Urethral sphincter mechanism incompetence	−66	—
Benign prostatic hypertrophy	—	+368
Rupture of the cranial cruciate ligament	−11	−11
Obesity	−14	−13

Positive impact score, benefit from gonadectomy; negative impact score, detriment from gonadectomy.

[a] Impact score Is derived from incidence and severity of disease.

described is the following[30]: You are a veterinarian speaking to the owner of an 8-week-old female Labrador Retriever that is not intended for breeding. This dog would benefit greatly from spaying before her first estrus as a means of preventing mammary gland tumors, which are extremely common relative to other diseases of concern and cause substantial morbidity. Because of her breed, reported detriments of spaying include an increased predisposition to cranial cruciate ligament injury, hemangiosarcoma, and obesity. However, there is a low incidence of hemangiosarcoma, and obesity is readily controlled with diet and exercise, which leaves cranial cruciate ligament injury as the most important possible detriment. Because the incidence of cranial cruciate ligament rupture is lower than that of mammary gland neoplasia, you choose to recommend spaying and educate the owner about maintenance of optimal body condition and other management techniques that minimize potential for cranial cruciate ligament injury. The best age at which to perform the spay must include considerations of when the dog's first estrus is likely to occur and how young one can spay a dog before greatly increasing risk of urethral sphincter mechanism incompetence. The likely recommendation for this bitch would be OHE at about 5 to 6 months of age. The scenario might be different if this dog came from a line with a history of cranial cruciate ligament injury, or if the owner had had a previous dog with that injury and was seriously concerned about the morbidity of the condition and cost of repair. Then the conversation would have to revolve around lack of knowledge of how timing of gonadectomy affects incidence of orthopedic disease, and how there is still some benefit in decreasing incidence of mammary neoplasia if we spay after the dog goes through puberty, albeit a decreasing benefit. This owner may elect to wait until the dog has gone through estrus once and spay at 12 to 18 months of age.

NONSURGICAL METHODS OF POPULATION CONTROL
Intratesticular Injection

Another direct way to induce sterility is to destroy germ cells without removing the gonads. Sterilizing agents have been described that are injected directly into the testes, epididymes, or vas deferens.[3] The first such products approved, including Neutersol and Zeuterin, were no longer commercially available at the time of this writing. Zinc arginine is injected directly into the testes of puppies, with dose based on testicular size. The manufacturer of Zeuterin recommended puppies be sedated before intratesticular injection was performed and cautioned against extratesticular movement of the compound, which is associated with severe inflammation of scrotal tissue. An inflammatory and fibrous reaction within the testis impairs continuing spermatogenesis but does not completely inhibit testosterone production.[31] Long-term effect on behavior and development of androgen-dependent disease is not clear. Intratesticular injection is safe if administered properly and requires only one application. The drug is expensive and the need for sedation limits its use, especially for free-roaming populations that may require management without veterinary oversight.

Immunocontraception

Immunocontraception relies on humoral and cell-mediated immune responses against specific proteins or tissues involved in reproduction. Humoral immunity is mediated by antibody production by B cells exposed to extracellular antigens. Cell-mediated immunity is mediated by cytotoxic T cells, killer T cells, and macrophages, which often are activated by intracellular antigens including virus-infected cells. Antibodies may bind to regions of interest, blocking receptors and subsequent hormone responses, such as stimulation of release of GnRH, or directly blocking reproductive events, such as fertilization. Immunosterilization requires cell-mediated destruction of reproductive proteins or tissues. Primary concerns with immunocontraception are lack of antigenicity of many reproduction-specific proteins or tissues, desire not to block function of those proteins in nontarget tissues, and inflammatory response associated with the immune reaction that may damage surrounding tissue.

Because many of the proposed targets are recognized as "self" and therefore do not elicit an immune response, investigators have tried several things to enhance immune response. These include conjugation to other large proteins and packaging of antigen to create a repeat of antigens every 50 to 100 Å, as is a common presentation on bacteria and viruses that stimulate a strong immune response. Many reproductive targets are immunologically privileged because they are sequestered from the immune response early in embryologic development. Although these may be antigenic when administered systemically, the tissues may still be protected from the immune response. For example, spermatozoa are protected from the immune system by the blood-testis barrier and neurons producing GnRH are protected by the blood-brain barrier.

Potential immunogens include GnRH, luteinizing hormone, follicle-stimulating hormone (FSH); receptors for those hormones; zona pellucida (ZP); and specific proteins associated with germ cells or reproductive organs. GnRH is a small peptide hormone and is highly conserved, raising concerns about inadvertent immunization of nontarget species in any compound distributed as an oral bait or otherwise introduced into the environment. Increased antigenicity requires conjugation of GnRH with a larger protein; those that have been used include tetanus toxoid and keyhole limpet hemocyanin. There have been many studies completed evaluating use of homologous or heterologous ZP proteins for immunocontraception. One example of a specific protein that could be used as an immunocontraceptive agent is a protein called "maternal antigen that embryos require," which is expressed solely by oocytes.

Research in immunocontraception has mostly involved ZP or GnRH-based vaccines. Vaccines using porcine ZP in dogs cause erratic estrous cycling and do not consistently prevent pregnancy long-term. Vaccines using recombinant canine ZP proteins conjugated to diphtheria toxin in dogs caused a rise in titers and subsequent inhibition of ovarian follicular development but did not prevent estrous cycling and pregnancy in all cases. Most ZP vaccine studies in dogs were associated with at least short-term infertility in more than 75% of cases but were associated with prolonged proestrus bleeding and estrous behavior and with ovarian cystic disease.[32–34] In cats, vaccines developed using ZP proteins from dogs, cats, mink, and ferrets all were demonstrated to induce a significant, measurable antibody response but did not protect against pregnancy because the antibodies did not bind to the queen's own ZP in vitro.[35,36] It may be that variation in sperm binding sites on the ZP vary enough between species to minimize the effect of antibodies raised against ZP proteins.

Another reported problem with immunocontraceptive ZP vaccines evaluated to date is the adjuvant used. In one study in cats, using Freund's complete adjuvant, 7 of 10 cats developed granulomatous reactions at the injection site and in distant tissues including lymph nodes and brain. One of the 10 cats died of a vaccine-associated sarcoma at the injection site, and 3 of 10 suffered from hypercalcemia and compromised renal function.[37] Granulomatous reactions also have been reported at the injection site in dogs. A commercial ZP vaccine with Freund's adjuvant (SpayVac, Wildlife Inc., North Saanich BC, Canada) was available from 2002 to 2005 through a Canadian company. As of this writing, no ZP vaccine is commercially available for use in companion animal species.

GnRH-based immunocontraceptive vaccines may be a more viable alternative. A recent study in cats using multiple tandem repeats of GnRH conjugated to proteins from *Pasteurella* sp showed high titers against GnRH, lack of follicular development, and no estrous cycling or pregnancy for up to 20 months after vaccination.[38] GnRH conjugated to hemocyanin from the keyhole limpet and adjuvanted with a commercial preparation using *Mycobacterium avium* (AdjuVac, USDA APHIS National Wildlife Research Center, Fort Collins, CO) has been demonstrated to decrease testosterone and sperm count in male dogs and cats; work in bitches and queens is ongoing.[39] A commercial GnRH vaccine using AdjuVac (GonaCon, USDA APHIS National Wildlife Research Center, Fort Collins, CO) is reported to be undergoing registration for use in hoofstock by the US Department of Agriculture. There are no reports of a commercial vaccine for companion animals as of this writing.

FUTURE POSSIBILITIES
Targeted Cytotoxins

Targeted toxins work by binding to specific cells associated with reproductive function and destroying those cells only.[39] This is analogous to chemotherapy. For this to work, a purified toxin must be attached to some sort of transport molecule for delivery to a specific target and that transport molecule must bind to the cell of interest and not to nontarget cells. One example that has been published is conjugation of pokeweed antiviral protein to GnRH. As GnRH binds to gonadotrophs in the pituitary and is taken up, the toxin is introduced as well and function of those cells inhibited, decreasing release of FSH and luteinizing hormone. Another example is linking of a cytotoxic fragment of exotoxin A from *Pseudomonas aeruginosa* to a ligand that binds the G-protein-coupled receptor for FSH that is expressed specifically in testicular Sertoli cells and ovarian granulosa cells. With binding, cells that express receptors for FSH are selectively destroyed. Problems lie in specificity of targeting to the cells of interest and ensuring nonreproductive tissues are not accidentally destroyed. For example, FSH receptors are not uncommonly expressed in tissues of the urinary tract in females of some species.

Gene Silencing

Gene silencing most commonly is accomplished with a class of double-stranded RNA molecules. These molecules, when introduced into a cell containing genes with homologous DNA, block transcription and effectively abolish expression of that gene.[40] Specific types of RNA used in this way, small interfering RNAs and small temporal RNAs, are themselves regulated by the enzyme Dicer. As a group, these are referred to as interfering RNAs (iRNAs). Introduction of iRNAs to cells of interest decreases gene transcription for a variable amount of time. Specificity of the iRNA is vital, to ensure mRNA of a desirable gene is not blocked unintentionally. Similarly, targeting of the iRNA to specific tissues is vital to ensure that production of the protein of interest is abolished as completely as possible but that transcription is not blocked in nontarget tissues requiring that gene product. Because gene silencing does not permanently shut down cell function, the challenge is to create long-term infertility from a transient silencing event. Examples of how this might be achieved include by silencing inhibitory factors that control apoptosis (controlled cell death) or otherwise altering secretion of gene products required for maintenance of the germ cell population. Another question that has not yet been answered is what percentage of active cells must be silenced to effect a change in reproduction. For example, if a system could be created that silences 50% of kisspeptin secretion, would that alter GnRH secretion or is there a much lower threshold needed, such that a much higher percentage of cells must be silenced to effect change?

SUMMARY

The Red Queen Hypothesis in evolutionary biology states that continuing adaptation is needed in order for a species to maintain its relative fitness among the systems with which it is coevolving. Reproduction is a biologic imperative for animals, and is a complex system with built-in safeguards and fail-safes that have not yet been identified. For example, kisspeptin is produced primarily in the arcuate nucleus and anteroventral periventricular area of the hypothalamus but kisspeptin neurons also are scattered elsewhere in the brain.[41] There is evidence of stem cells permitting follicular renewal in mammalian species.[42] Surgical sterilization may be too broad in its attempts to completely prevent fertility and reproductive behaviors by removing tissues without recognizing nonreproductive functions of those tissues or impact of their removal on other systems through endocrine or other pathways. Current research continues to deepen the understanding of animal reproduction to lead toward the stated goal of complete control of animal reproduction.

REFERENCES

1. New JC, Welch WJ, Hutchison JM, et al. Birth and death rate estimates of cats and dogs in US households and related factors. J Appl Anim Welf Sci 2004;7: 229–41.
2. Trevejo R, Yang M, Lund EM. Epidemiology of surgical castration of dogs and cats in the United States. J Am Vet Med Assoc 2011;238:898–904.
3. Kutzler M, Wood A. Non-surgical methods of contraception and sterilization. Theriogenology 2006;66:514–25.
4. vanGoethem B, Schaefers-Okkens A, Kirpensteijn J. Making a rational choice between ovariectomy and ovariohysterectomy in the dog: a discussion of the benefits of either technique. Vet Surg 2006;35:136–43.

5. Harris KP, Adams VJ, Fordyce P, et al. Comparison of surgical duration of canine ovariectomy and ovariohysterectomy in a veterinary teaching hospital. J Small Anim Pract 2013;54:579–83.

6. Peeters ME, Kirpensteijn J. Comparison of surgical variables and short-term postoperative complications in healthy dogs undergoing ovariohysterectomy or ovariectomy. J Am Vet Med Assoc 2011;238:189–94.

7. Waters DJ, Kengeri SS, Clever B, et al. Exploring mechanisms of sex differences in longevity: lifetime ovary exposure and exceptional longevity in dogs. Aging Cell 2009;8:752–5.

8. Hoveler R, Evers P, Hoffmann B. Investigations on endocrine responses in the bitch following hysterectomy. Eur J Endocrinol 1987;(Suppl 116.3):S110–1.

9. Hoffmann B, Hoveler R, Hasan SH, et al. Ovarian and pituitary function in dogs after hysterectomy. J Reprod Fertil 1992;96:837–45.

10. Kaszak I, Kanafa S, Ruszczak A, et al. Different mammary tumors, ovarian cysts, uterocervical stump inflammation in hysterectomized bitch. Anim Sci Pap Rep 2016;4:399–403.

11. Perez-Marin CC, Lopez R, Dominguez JM, et al. Clinical and pathological findings in testis, epididymis, deferens duct and prostate following vasectomy in a dog. Reprod Domest Anim 2006;41:169–74.

12. Zhang Y, Wang X, Chen Z, et al. Long-term reproductive consequences of no-scalpel vasectomy in Beagles. J Huazhong Univ Sci Technolog Med Sci 2012; 32:899–905.

13. Verstegen J, Onclin K. Mammary tumors in the queen. Proceedings, Society for Theriogenology. Columbus (OH), September 16-20, 2003. p. 239–45.

14. Hayes HM, Milne KL, Mandel CP. Epidemiological features of feline mammary carcinoma. Vet Rec 1981;108:476–9.

15. Dorn CR, Taylor DON, Schneider R, et al. Survey of animal neoplasms in Alameda and Contra Costa counties, California. II. Cancer morbidity in dogs and cats from Alameda county. J Natl Cancer Inst 1968;40:307–18.

16. Root MV, Johnston SD, Olson PN. Effect of prepuberal and postpuberal gonadectomy on heat production measured by indirect calorimetry in male and female domestic cats. Am J Vet Res 1996;57:371–4.

17. Hart BL, Barrett RE. Effects of castration on fighting, roaming, and urine spraying in adult male cats. J Am Vet Med Assoc 1973;163:290–2.

18. Hart BL, Cooper L. Factors relating to urine spraying and fighting in prepubertally gonadectomized cats. J Am Vet Med Assoc 1984;184:1255–8.

19. Dorn CR, Taylor DON, Frye FL, et al. Survey of animal neoplasms in Alameda and Contra Costa counties, California. I. Methodology and description of cases. J Natl Cancer Inst 1968;40:295–305.

20. Moe L. Population-based incidence of mammary tumors in some dog breeds. J Reprod Fertil Suppl 2001;57:439–43.

21. Richards HG, McNeil PE, Thompson H, et al. An epidemiological analysis of a canine-biopsies database compiled by a diagnostic histopathology service. Prev Vet Med 2001;51:125–36.

22. Cotchin E. Neoplasms in small animals. Vet Rec 1951;63:67–72.

23. Brodey RS, Goldschmidt MH, Roszel JR. Canine mammary gland neoplasms. J Am Anim Hosp Assoc 1983;19:61–90.

24. Moulton JE, Taylor DON, Dorn CR, et al. Canine mammary tumors. Pathol Vet 1970;7:289–320.

25. Root Kustritz MV, Slater MR, Weedon GR, et al. Determining optimal age for gonadectomy in the dog: a critical review of the literature to guide decision making. Clin Ther 2017;9:167–211.

26. Schneider R, Dorn CR, Taylor DON. Factors influencing canine mammary cancer development and postsurgical survival. J Natl Cancer Inst 1969;43:1249–61.

27. Hopkins SG, Schubert TA, Hart BL. Castration of adult male dogs: effects on roaming, aggression, urine marking, and mounting. J Am Vet Med Assoc 1976; 168:1108–10.

28. Nielsen JC, Eckstein RA, Hart BL. Effects of castration on problem behaviors in male dogs with reference to age and duration of behavior. J Am Vet Med Assoc 1997;211:180–2.

29. Root Kustritz MV. Use of an impact score to guide client decision-making about timing of spay-castration of dogs and cats. Clin Ther 2012;4:481–5.

30. Root Kustritz MV. Determining the optimal age for gonadectomy of dogs and cats. J Am Vet Med Assoc 2007;231:1665–75.

31. Root Kustritz MV, Brazzell J, Swanson J, et al. Histopathologic changes in testes three days after administration of zinc gluconate neutralized with arginine as an intratesticular injection for contraception. Clin Ther 2014;6:473–9.

32. Purswell BJ, Kolster KA. Immunocontraception in companion animals. Theriogenology 2006;66:510–3.

33. Barber MR, Fayrer-Hosken RA. Evaluation of somatic and reproductive immunotoxic effects of the porcine zona pellucida vaccination. J Exp Zool 2000;286: 641–6.

34. Barber MR, Lee SM, Steffens WL, et al. Immunolocalization of zona pellucida antigens in the ovarian follicle of dogs, cats, horses and elephants. Theriogenology 2001;55:1705–17.

35. Levy JK, Mansour M, Crawford PC, et al. Survey of zona pellucida antigens for immunocontraception of cats. Theriogenology 2005;63:1334–41.

36. Jewgenow K, Rohleder M, Wegner I. Differences between antigenic determinants of pig and cat zona pellucida proteins. J Reprod Fertil 2000;119:15–23.

37. Munson L, Harrenstein LA, Acton AE, et al. Immunologic responses and adverse reactions to Freunds-adjuvanted porcine zona pellucida immunocontraceptives in domestic cats. Vaccine 2005;23:5646–54.

38. Robbins SC, Jelinski MD, Stotish RL. Assessment of the immunologic and biological efficacy of two different doses of a recombinant GnRH vaccine in domestic male and female cats (Felis catus). J Reprod Immunol 2005;64:107–19.

39. Root Kustritz MV. Current and proposed research in canine and feline nonsurgical sterilization. Clin Ther 2012;4:225–31.

40. McManus MT, Sharp PA. Gene silencing in mammals by small interfering RNAs. Nat Rev Genet 2002;3:737–47.

41. Roa J, Navarro VM, Tena-Sempere M. Kisspeptins in reproductive biology: consensus knowledge and recent developments. Biol Reprod 2011;85:650–60.

42. Johnson J, Canning J, Kaneko T, et al. Germline stem cells and follicular renewal in the postnatal mammalian ovary. Nature 2004;428:145–50.

Contraception in Dogs and Cats

Cheryl S. Asa, BS, MA, PhD*

KEYWORDS

- Contraception • Fertility control • Canine • Feline

KEY POINTS

- Contraception in dogs and cats allows temporary, nonsurgical management of reproduction.
- Steroid hormone–based methods can have serious side effects, but use of the minimum effective dose can avoid these problems.
- Gonadotropin-releasing hormone (GnRH) agonists offer the most promise for dog and cat contraception, but the implant product used in Europe and Australia is not approved in the United States.
- GnRH or other vaccines might also be appropriate, but they have not been adequately tested in dogs and cats.
- Considerably more research is necessary to identify better contraceptive options for these species.

Permanent sterilization of young dogs and cats is much more common in North America than reversible contraception for managing reproduction. There is increasing interest, however, in reversible contraception, particularly when temporary or nonsurgical approaches to fertility control are preferred. Unfortunately, the choices are limited. Due to the high cost of bringing pharmaceutical products to market, the simplest option is frequently extralabel use in dogs and cats of drugs tested and approved for human application. The most commonly used human contraceptives are methods based on steroid hormones, for example, the combination birth control pill containing synthetic estrogen and progestin, long-acting implants, or injections containing only a progestin. Some of these products have been tested in dogs and cats, with results varying by product and dose. The most important outcome of those trials has been the recognition of profound species differences, especially in the

The author has nothing to disclose.
AZA Reproductive Management Center, Saint Louis Zoo, 1 Government Drive, St Louis, MO 63110, USA
* 244 Mitchell Brook Road, Norwich, VT 05055.
E-mail address: asa@stlzoo.org

occurrence of side effects, many of which can be life threatening. This review summarizes those outcomes as well as the other contraceptive options available for potential use in dogs and cats.

CONTRACEPTIVE METHODS USING STEROID HORMONES
Estrogen

Synthetic estrogens are especially effective at preventing the luteinizing hormone (LH) surge associated with ovulation, which makes them a good candidate for contraception. They also have been associated, however, with serious side effects, although those vary by species.

Estrogen contraception in dogs
Synthetic estrogens, especially diethylstilbestrol, were formerly used for mismating in dogs. They are no longer recommended, however, due to concerns about both efficacy and safety.[1,2] In particular, estrogen can cause potentially fatal suppression of bone marrow and aplastic anemia in dogs.[3] A more recent study[4] showed, however, that a single treatment with estradiol benzoate could be both effective and safe for early pregnancy termination in dogs.

Estrogen contraception in cats
There is no similar history of estrogen treatment of fertility control in cats, but concerns for safety seem to have precluded their use, despite the lower sensitivity of cats compared with dogs to estrogen-induced aplastic anemia.[3]

Progestins

Synthetic progestins, in particular, megestrol acetate (MA), medroxyprogesterone acetate (MPA), and proligestone (PROL), have been used for decades to control fertility in cats and dogs. Progestins have a negative feedback effect on the hypothalamus and pituitary, such that continuous high concentrations suppress production of follicle-stimulating hormone (FSH) and LH, which in turn prevents stimulation of follicle growth and ovulation. Sufficient estrogen production, however, may continue to stimulate some follicle growth and estradiol production,[5] so that estrous behavior may still occur. Other contraceptive effects include impeding the movement of sperm and eggs to the site of fertilization and interfering with implantation.[6,7]

Synthetic formulations differ in how strongly they bind to receptors for other steroid hormones, such as androgens and glucocorticoids,[8–10] which determines potential side effects.[11,12] For example, binding to androgen receptors can cause masculinization,[13] and binding to glucocorticoid receptors can disrupt glucose activity and suppress immune function.[14]

Increased appetite and weight gain are common with progestin treatment,[15] with hair loss and discoloration also reported.[16] More serious side effects, evident especially at higher doses in carnivores, such as dogs and cats, include uterine and mammary gland proliferation and tumor development, growth hormone (GH) stimulation, suppression of the immune system, and altered glucose metabolism, which can be associated with diabetes mellitus.

Progestin-based contraceptives are marketed in various forms, such as pills, slow-release depot injections, and implants. Not all products are available in all countries, however, and they may be marketed under different brand names in different regions of the world. Actions of the 3 progestins most commonly used in dogs and cats, including side effects, are summarized.

Megestrol acetate

Approved in the United States and Canada for contraception in dogs but not cats, MA is currently only available through compounding pharmacies in pill form since the brand Ovaban formerly produced by Intervet (Merck Animal Health, Madison, NJ)/Schering-Plough became unavailable. MA was also previously available in the United States as the compounded product FeralStat (WestLab Pharmacy, Gainesville, FL), specifically for preventing reproduction in feral cat colonies. MA as Megace (Bristol-Myers Squibb), marketed for humans in the United States, is sometimes used off-label for other species. MA is currently available in Europe as Ovarid (Virbac Animal Health).

MA has both antiandrogenic and antiestrogenic effects but is a cortisol agonist, which has made it useful for treating some dermatologic conditions in cats,[14] but caution is needed to prevent more profound immune suppression.

Medroxyprogesterone acetate

MPA is most commonly used in dogs and cats in its injectable formulation (Depo-Provera; Pfizer, New York, NY). Of the synthetic progestins currently available, MPA is the most androgenic[17] and immunosuppressive.[18]

Proligestone

Another injectable progestin, PROL is not available in the United States, Canada, or Mexico but is approved in Europe for contraception in dogs and cats as Delvosteron (MSD Animal Health New Zealand). The contraceptive action of PROL is primarily antigonadotrophic, that is, blocking ovulation via LH suppression, but it is less progestogenic than other synthetic progestins. Thus, the progesterone-caused overstimulation of mammary and uterine tissue is not observed,[19] but PROL can affect adrenal function, which may disrupt glucose homeostasis and cause immunosuppression.[20] That adrenal effect, however, was found to be less severe than that caused by MA.[21]

Progestin contraception in dogs

Progestin-based contraceptives, which have been used in female dogs and cats for many decades, are in general effective, but most products and dosing regimens have been associated with potentially serious side effects.

Uterine pathology The association between progestin treatment and uterine pathology, especially cystic endometrial hyperplasia, has been well documented.[22,23] This effect on endometrial growth is exacerbated if the uterus has been sensitized by estrogen, either endogenous (as during proestrus) or exogenous administration.[24] Thus, if progestin contraception of dogs is considered, treatment should not be initiated when estradiol is elevated, as during proestrus. Protocols based on lower doses initiated during deep anestrus, however, when endogenous estradiol is minimal, can be safe.[16,25] Alternatively, treatment with PROL is less likely to result in uterine abnormalities due primarily to its low binding affinity to progesterone receptors.[19]

Mammary tumors Progestin-based contraceptives, with the possible exception of PROL,[26] also can stimulate mammary tumor growth in dogs.[23] Progestins may affect mammary tissue via stimulation of GH and possibly insulinlike growth factor 1 in dog mammary glands.[27] High doses, but not low doses, are more likely to cause mammary tumors, including carcinomas.[28]

Diabetes mellitus The GH release stimulated by progestins also may contribute to development of diabetes mellitus.[23,29] Although PROL may carry lower risk to uterine and mammary tissue, its high affinity for the glucocorticoid receptor and its effect on GH and the adrenal gland may influence glucocorticoid dynamics.[30]

Acromegaly High doses of MPA have resulted in acromegaly, a condition due to chronically high GH concentrations that cause abnormal growth of head, paws, and internal organs as well as skin thickening and folding.[31]

Immunosuppression A further complication of progestin effects on the adrenal gland is suppression of the immune response. Because this effect can extend beyond the treatment period,[20] a lower response to infection can be prolonged. MPA and MA are reported to have equal potency in adrenal suppression.[32]

Other effects Progestins have not been found to alter prolactin secretion, but minor effects on thyroid-stimulating hormone have been reported.[5] The more androgenic progestins, but not MA, can masculinize developing fetuses.[33]

Use in male dogs Progestins have been administered to reduce behaviors that might be supported by testosterone[34] as well as for contraception.[35] Because behavior can be challenging to quantify, evidence linking suppression of testosterone to reduction in aggressive behavior is weak. Use of progestins to reduce undesirable male-type behavior can be more effective if initiated before puberty, that is, before learned behavior patterns are established.[34]

Progestins have been more successful at suppressing sexual behaviors but not for sufficient suppression of spermatogenesis to ensure contraceptive efficacy. A high dose of MPA did reduce sperm motility and numbers,[35] but whether the dose required to sustain infertility could be safe is questionable.

Potentially safe treatment protocols Although progestins can have numerous side effects, those were primarily found with higher doses. That, plus the observation that those progestin effects were exacerbated when treatment began during proestrus or estrus, prompted development of safer protocols. Initiating treatment during deep anestrus and using a lower dose calculated by body weight can avoid serious side effects.[25] Because of its association with a lower incidence of side effects, PROL might also be considered.

Progestin contraception in cats

Progestins are effective in suppressing reproduction in cats. Although a range of side effects similar to those detected in dogs have been reported, the likelihood of uterine pathology seems lower in cats. Listlessness, docility, and general changes in temperament, have been reported for cats treated with MA.[36]

Mammary tumors As with dogs, MPA and MA have been associated with mammary tumors in cats,[37] although no link to GH has been shown, even though both MA and PROL can stimulate GH release in cats as well as dogs.[38]

Immunosuppression Among progestins, MA, in particular, can affect activity of the adrenal gland, which can result in suppression of immune response.[14] In comparing MA and PROL, however, significant adrenal suppression was seen only in cats treated with MA, suggesting that PROL may be a safer alternative.[21]

Diabetes mellitus MA has been reported to cause symptoms of diabetes mellitus.[39] Similar to effects on the adrenal gland, MA but not PROL caused significant changes in insulin concentrations.[21] MA effects on the adrenal and on insulin levels were reported to regress when treatment was discontinued.[36]

Effects on future fertility Although kittens in first litters after MPA treatment were small, weak, or even stillborn, subsequent litters were normal, demonstrating eventual complete reversal of the contraceptive effect.[40]

Use in male cats Rather than for contraception, progestins, such as MPA and MA, have been used in male cats primarily to reduce objectionable behaviors, such as urine marking. Although not as extensively studied as in female cats, mammary hypertrophy and adenocarcinomas also have been associated with exogenous progestins in male cats.[41]

Potentially safe treatment protocols As with dogs, using the lowest effective dosage can achieve contraception while avoiding serious side effects.[42] The recommended dose of FeralStat (MA compounded with lactose powder for palatability), promoted for limiting reproduction in feral cat colonies in the United States, is within the range considered safe, although there are no published reports on FeralStat efficacy of that low dose.

Androgens

In females, androgen treatment can interfere with fertility by negative feedback on LH, blocking its ovulatory surge. Androgens have also been used for contraception in males, although somewhat less successfully. The synthetic androgen mibolerone, approved for use as a contraceptive agent In the United States for dogs, and sometimes used in cats,[43] may no longer be on the market. In Europe, dogs and cats are also sometimes treated with other androgens that are approved for human or veterinary use in those countries.

Androgen contraception in dogs

In male dogs, androgen administration can achieve contraception by interfering with spermatogenesis subsequent to suppression of LH. It can also directly stimulate libido and prostatic growth.[43]

Mibolerone, as an oral preparation given daily, is the androgen most frequently used for fertility control in female dogs, reportedly for periods up to 5 years.[2] The most common side effect is clitoral hypertrophy; others include vaginal discharge, vaginitis, and male-type behavior, such as increased mounting and aggression. Androgens are contraindicated for pregnant female cats, because masculinization of female fetuses can occur, and before puberty, because they can hasten epiphyseal closure.

Androgen contraception in cats

Although not approved for use in cats, mibolerone and other androgens can be effective in preventing reproduction,[44] but they are contraindicated due to potentially fatal liver toxicity.[45]

CONTRACEPTIVE METHODS USING PROTEIN HORMONES: GONADOTROPIN-RELEASING HORMONE AGONISTS

Hypothalamic gonadotropin-releasing hormone (GnRH) stimulates the endocrine cascade necessary for reproduction in both male and female mammals. When administered continuously, however, GnRH causes down-regulation of the pituitary gonadotrophs (LH and FSH), so that gonadal hormones are no longer produced.[46] The similar action in both male and female mammals makes it a potentially effective and reversible contraceptive for either gender. There are currently 2 commercially available GnRH agonists: an injectable formulation of leuprolide acetate (Lupron Depot; AbbVie, North Chicago, IL) marketed for human use, and deslorelin acetate in slow-release implant form (Suprelorin, Virbac Animal Health Australia, Milperra, NSW) approved for use in dogs in Australia, New Zealand, and the European Union. A related product, Suprelorin-F (Virbac Animal Health Australia), is indexed, not approved, by the Food and Drug Administration, that is, provisionally available, in the United States only for treatment of adrenal gland disease in domestic ferrets; its use off-label is prohibited, so it cannot be used in dogs or cats. Although not licensed for cats, Suprelorin is widely used clinically, where available, for both cats and dogs.

A disadvantage of using GnRH agonists for contraception is the initial stimulation phase, or flare, which may stimulate estrus and ovulation. Females can be separated from males for 3 weeks to 4 weeks after implant insertion, or a progestin, such as MA, can be given daily during the week before and week after implantation to prevent the flare.[47] A subsequent study with greyhounds, however, found this regimen not effective.[48] For males, additional time must be allowed after the stimulation phase for passage of sperm already in the tract.[49] A further disadvantage is the large individual variability in duration of efficacy. Suprelorin is available in 2 formulations with minimum efficacies of 6 months and 12 months, but suppression commonly extends beyond those times.[50,51]

No side effects of GnRH agonists have been reported beyond those generally seen after surgical castration or ovariohysterectomy, for example, weight gain. The primary endocrine difference with GnRH agonist treatment is that the agonist suppresses LH and FSH, whereas after gonadectomy these hormones are elevated due to the absence of gonadal hormone negative feedback.

Gonadotropin-Releasing Hormone Agonist Contraception in Dogs

Suprelorin was developed and is approved only for male dogs, where its efficacy has been well established.[46] It also has been widely used off-label, however, for female dogs in Europe since it became commercially available there.[52] Treatment can be initiated during any cycle stage, although if started during the luteal phase (metestrus) it can exacerbate subclinical endometrial hyperplasia.[52] Stimulation of fertile estrus is common, and deslorelin in a fast-release implant (Ovuplant, Virbac Animal Health Australia) is sometimes used to induce estrus and ovulation in dogs.

Gonadotropin-Releasing Hormone Agonist Contraception in Cats

Suprelorin is also regularly used off-label as a reversible contraceptive in both male and female cats in Europe.[51,53] Initiation of Suprelorin treatment of female cats during proestrus or estrus can stimulate ovulation, which can be fertile.[51] Although pregnancy can go to term with the implant in place, disruption of maternal behavior and lactation resulting in death of the kittens is possible.[54] Reversibility has been documented both in female cats, with normal litters and maternal care,[54] and in male cats.[55]

CONTRACEPTIVE VACCINES
Porcine Zona Pellucida Vaccines

A vaccine that prevents sperm penetration of the zona pellucida, which surrounds the oocyte, has been used successfully to prevent fertilization in many wild ungulates, especially free-ranging horses in the United States.[56] Another porcine zona pellucida (pZP)-based product (SpayVac, North Saanich, BC, Canada; SpayVac-for-Wildlife, Canada) was only available in the United States in the early 2000s. pZP has not been a consistently successful contraceptive when applied to dogs or cats.[57] The primary problem seems to have been identifying an adjuvant that renders the vaccine effective without generating unacceptable side effects, such as injection site reactions.[58]

Gonadotropin-Releasing Hormone Vaccines

As with pZP, vaccines against GnRH have been more successful contraceptive agents in ungulates than in other species. There are currently several such products available in the United States and around the world, marketed under various names (eg, Equity, Improvac, and Improvest; Zoetis Animal Health, Parsippany, NJ). A GnRH vaccine specifically for dogs (Canine Gonadotropin Releasing Factor Immunotherapeutic; Pfizer) was only available in the United States for a short time.

BARRIER CONTRACEPTION DEVICES IN DOGS

Two intrauterine devices (IUDs) have been designed especially for dogs. One uses a copper-coated, flexible, Y-shaped design that allows an arm of the Y to be placed in each uterine horn (Biotumer, Buenos Aires, Argentina). It was shown effective for at least 2 years, and no side effects were detected, although 1 of 9 female dogs showed persistent estrus while the device was in place.[59] This product seems, however, no longer available.

The other IUD designed for dogs, Dogspiral (www.dogspiral.vet), consists of a stainless steel spiral coated with copper, silver, or gold. There are no published reports of its use, but information is available at the Dogspiral Web site, in addition to an analysis by the Alliance for Contraception in Cats and Dogs (www.acc-d.org).

The general concern about the use of IUDs in dogs is the potential for a foreign body reaction resulting in uterine pathology,[60] because the basic mode of action of IUDs is to provoke a local inflammatory response.

SUMMARY

Unfortunately, there are few choices for temporary, reversible fertility control in dogs and cats, particularly in North America. Most research focuses on controlling stray dog and cat populations, but the aim is permanent sterilization. Shorter-term methods, however, are also being pursued that might find application for pets.

REFERENCES

1. Bowen RA, Olson PN, Behrendt MD. Efficacy and toxicity of estrogens commonly used to terminate canine pregnancy. J Am Vet Med Assoc 1985;186:783–8.
2. Concannon PW, Meyers-Wallen VN. Current and proposed methods for contraception and termination of pregnancy in dogs and cats. J Am Vet Med Assoc 1991;198:1214–25.
3. Weiss DJ, Bonagura JD. Aplastic anemia. In: Kirk RW, editor. Current veterinary therapy XI: small animal practice. 1992. p. 479–84.
4. Tsutsui T, Mizutani W, Hori T, et al. Estradiol benzoate for preventing pregnancy in mismated dogs. Theriogenology 2006;66:1568–72.
5. Beijerink NJ, Bhatti SF, Okkens AC, et al. Adenohypophyseal function in bitches treated with medroxyprogesterone acetate. Domest Anim Endocrinol 2007;32:63–78.
6. Brache V, Faundes A, Johansson E. Anovulation, inadequate luteal phase and poor sperm penetration in cervical mucus during prolonged use of Norplant implants. Contraception 1985;31:261–73.
7. Attardi B. Progesterone modulation of the luteinizing hormone surge: regulation of hypothalamic and pituitary progestin receptors. Endocrinology 1984;115:2113–22.
8. Duncan GL, Lyster SC, Hendrix JW, et al. Biologic effects of melengestrol acetate. Fertil Steril 1964;15:419–32.

9. Fekete G, Szeberényi S. Data on the mechanism of adrenal suppression by medroxyprogesterone acetate. Steroids 1965;6:159–66, missing p. 163.

10. Kloosterboer HJ, Vonk-Noordegraaf CA, Turpijn EW. Selectivity in progesterone and androgen receptor binding of progestagens used in oral contraceptives. Contraception 1988;38:325–32.

11. Sloan JM, Oliver IM. Progestogen-induced diabetes in the dog. Diabetes 1975; 24:337–44.

12. Selman PJ, Mol JA, Rutteman GR, et al. Effects of progestin administration on the hypothalamic-pituitary-adrenal axis and glucose homeostasis in dogs. J Reprod Fertil Suppl 1997;51:345–54.

13. Wilkins L. Masculinization of female fetus due to use of orally given progestins. JAMA 1960;172:1028–32.

14. Middleton DJ, Watson A, Howe C, et al. Suppression of cortisol responses to exogenous adrenocorticotrophic hormone, and the occurrence of side effects attributable to glucocorticoid excess, in cats during therapy with megestrol acetate and prednisolone. Can J Vet Res 1987;51:60–5.

15. Romatowski J. Use of megestrol acetate in cats. J Am Vet Med Assoc 1989;194: 700–2.

16. Evans JM, Sutton DJ. The use of hormones, especially progestagens, to control oestrus in bitches. J Reprod Fertil Suppl 1989;39:163–73.

17. Labrie C, Cusan L, Plante M, et al. Analysis of the androgenic activity of synthetic "progestins" currently used for the treatment of prostate cancer. J Steroid Biochem 1987;28:379–84.

18. Hapgood JP, Koubovec D, Louw A, et al. Not all progestins are the same: implications for usage. Trends Pharmacol Sci 2004;25:554–7.

19. Van Os JL, Oldenkamp EP. Oestrus control in bitches with proligestone, a new progestational steroid. J Small Anim Pract 1978;19:521–9.

20. Selman PJ, Mol JA, Rutteman GR, et al. Progestin treatment in the dog. II. Effects on the hypothalamic-pituitary-adrenocortical axis. Eur J Endocrinol 1994;131: 422–30.

21. Church DB, Watson ADJ, Emslie DR, et al. Effects of proligestone and megestrol on plasma adrenocorticotrophic hormone, insulin and insulin-like growth factor-1 concentrations in cats. Res Vet Sci 1994;56:175–8.

22. Brodey RS, Fidler IJ. Clinical and pathologic findings in bitches treated with progestational compounds. J Am Vet Med Assoc 1966;149:1406–15.

23. Nelson LW, Kelly WA. Progestogen-related gross and microscopic changes in female beagles. Vet Pathol 1976;13:143–56.

24. Noakes DE, Dhaliwal GK, England GC. Cystic endometrial hyperplasia/pyometra in dogs: a review of the causes and pathogenesis. J Reprod Fertil Suppl 2001;57: 395.

25. Jöchle W. Pet population control in Europe. J Am Vet Med Assoc 1991;198: 1225–30.

26. van Os JL, van Laar PH, Oldenkamp EP, et al. Oestrus control and the incidence of mammary nodules in bitches, a clinical study with two progestogens. Vet Q 1981;3:46–56.

27. Selman PJ, Mol JA, Rutteman GR, et al. Progestin-induced growth hormone excess in the dog originates in the mammary gland. Endocrinology 1994;134:287–92.

28. Misdorp W. Progestagens and mammary tumors in dogs and cats. Acta Endocrinologica 1991;125(Suppl 1):27–31.

29. Selman PJ, Mol JA, Rutteman GR, et al. Progestin treatment in the dog. I. Effects on growth hormone, insulin-like growth factor I and glucose homeostasis. Eur J Endocrinol 1994;131:413–21.
30. Selman PJ, Wolfswinkel J, Mol JA. Binding specificity of medroxyprogesterone acetate and proligestone for the progesterone and glucocorticoid receptor in the dog. Steroids 1996;61:133–7.
31. Concannon P, Altszuler N, Hampshire J, et al. Growth hormone, prolactin, and cortisol in dogs developing mammary nodules and an acromegaly-like appearance during treatment with medroxyprogesterone acetate. Endocrinology 1980; 106:1173–7.
32. Briggs MH, Briggs M. Glucocorticoid properties of progestogens. Steroids 1973; 22:555–9.
33. Grumbach MM, Ducharme JR, Moloshok RE. On the fetal masculinizing action of certain oral progestins. J Clin Endocrinol Metab 1959;19:1369–80.
34. Knol BW, Egberink-Alink ST. Treatment of problem behaviour in dogs and cats by castration and progestagen administration: a review. Vet Q 1989;11:102–7.
35. England GCW. Effect of progestogens and androgens upon spermatogenesis and steroidogenesis in dogs. J Reprod Fertil Suppl 1997;51:123–38.
36. Houdeshell JW, Hennessey PW. Megestrol acetate for control of estrus in the cat. Vet Med Small Anim Clin 1977;72:1013–7.
37. Hernandez FJ, Fernandez BB, Chertack M, et al. Feline mammary carcinoma and progestogens. Feline Pract 1975;5:45–8.
38. Mol JA, van Garderen E, Rutteman GR, et al. New insights in the molecular mechanism of progestin-induced proliferation of mammary epithelium: induction of the local biosynthesis of growth hormone (GH) in the mammary glands of dogs, cats and humans. J Steroid Biochem Mol Biol 1996;57:67–71.
39. Middleton DJ. Megestrol acetate and the cat. Veterinary Annual 1986;26:341–7.
40. Harris TW, Wolchuk N. The suppression of estrus in the dog and cat with long-term administration of synthetic progestational steroids. Am J Vet Res 1963;24: 1003–6.
41. Hayden D, Johnston S, Kiang D, et al. Feline mammary hypertrophy/fibroadenoma complex: clinical and hormonal aspects. Am J Vet Res 1981;42:1699–703.
42. Romagnoli S. Progestins to control feline reproduction: Historical abuse of high doses and potentially safe use of low doses. J Feline Med Surg 2015;17:743–52.
43. Romagnoli S. Non-surgical contraception in dogs and cats. World Small Animal Veterinary Association World Congress 2009. p. 7.
44. Burke TJ, Reynolds HA, Sokolowski JH. A 180-day tolerance-efficacy study with mibolerone for suppression of estrus in the cat. Am J Vet Res 1977;38:469–76.
45. Shille VM, Sojka NJ. Feline reproduction. In: Ettinger SJ, Feldman EC, editors. Textbook of veterinary internal medicine. 4th edition. Philadelphia: W. B. Saunders and Co; 1995. p. 1690–8.
46. Trigg TE, Wright PJ, Armour AF, et al. Use of a GnRH analogue implant to produce reversible long-term suppression of reproductive function in male and female domestic dogs. J Reprod Fertil Suppl 2001;57:255–61.
47. Wright PJ, Verstegen JP, Onclin K, et al. Suppression of the oestrous responses of bitches to the GnRH analogue deslorelin by progestin. J Reprod Fertil Suppl 2001;57:263–8.
48. Sung M, Armour AF, Wright PJ. The influence of exogenous progestin on the occurrence of proestrous or estrous signs, plasma concentrations of luteinizing hormone and estradiol in deslorelin (GnRH agonist) treated anestrous bitches. Theriogenology 2006;66:1513–7.

49. Junaidi A, Williamson P, Martin G, et al. Pituitary and testicular endocrine responses to exogenous gonadotrophin-releasing hormone (GnRH) and luteinising hormone in male dogs treated with GnRH agonist implants. Reprod Fertil Dev 2007;19:891–8.
50. Trigg TE, Doyle AG, Walsh JD, et al. A review of advances in the use of the GnRH agonist deslorelin in control of reproduction. Theriogenology 2006;66:1507–12.
51. Goericke-Pesch S. Reproduction control in cats: new developments in non-surgical methods. J Feline Med Surg 2010;12:539–46.
52. Romagnoli S, Stelletta C, Milani C, et al. Clinical use of deslorelin for the control of reproduction in the bitch. Reprod Domest Anim 2009;44:36–9.
53. Fontaine C. Long-term contraception in a small implant: a review of Suprelorin (deslorelin) studies in cats. J Feline Med Surg 2015;17:766–71.
54. Goericke-Pesch S, Georgiev P, Atanasov A, et al. Treatment of queens in estrus and after estrus with a GnRH-agonist implant containing 4.7 mg deslorelin; hormonal response, duration of efficacy, and reversibility. Theriogenology 2013;79: 640–6.
55. Goericke-Pesch S, Georgiev P, Antonov A, et al. Reversibility of germinative and endocrine testicular function after long-term contraception with a GnRH-agonist implant in the tom—a follow-up study. Theriogenology 2014;81:941–6.
56. Kirkpatrick JF, Turner JW Jr, Liu IKM, et al. Applications of pig zona pellucida immunocontraception to wildlife fertility control. J Reprod Fertil Suppl 1996;50: 183–9.
57. Kutzler M, Wood A. Non-surgical methods of contraception and sterilization. Theriogenology 2006;66:514–25.
58. Munks M. Progress in development of immunocontraceptive vaccines for permanent non-surgical sterilization of cats and dogs. Reprod Domest Anim 2012;47: 223–7.
59. Volpe P, Izzo B, Russo M, et al. Intrauterine device for contraception in dogs. Vet Rec 2001;149:77–9.
60. Nomura K. Induction of canine deciduoma in some reproductive stages with the different conditions of corpora lutea. J Vet Med Sci 1997;59:185–90.

Moving?

Make sure your subscription moves with you!

To notify us of your new address, find your **Clinics Account Number** (located on your mailing label above your name), and contact customer service at:

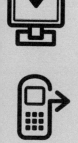

Email: journalscustomerservice-usa@elsevier.com

800-654-2452 (subscribers in the U.S. & Canada)
314-447-8871 (subscribers outside of the U.S. & Canada)

Fax number: 314-447-8029

Elsevier Health Sciences Division
Subscription Customer Service
3251 Riverport Lane
Maryland Heights, MO 63043

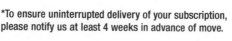

*To ensure uninterrupted delivery of your subscription, please notify us at least 4 weeks in advance of move.